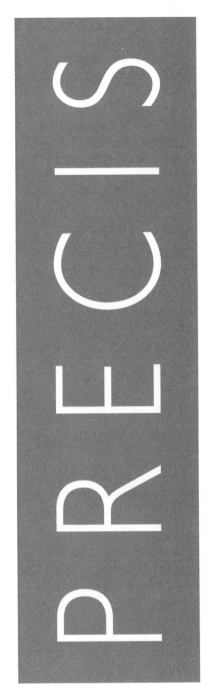

an update in obstetrics and gynecology

Oncology

Third Edition

Precis: An Update in Obstetrics and Gynecology represents the knowledge and experience of experts in the field and does not necessarily reflect policy of the American College of Obstetricians and Gynecologists (ACOG). This publication describes methods and techniques of clinical practice that are accepted and used by recognized authorities. The recommendations do not dictate an exclusive course of treatment or of practice. Variations taking into account the needs of the individual patient, resources, and limitations unique to the institution or type of practice may be appropriate.

Medicine is an ever-changing field. As new research and clinical experience emerge, changes in treatment and drug therapy are required. Every effort has been made to ensure that the drug dosage schedules contained herein are accurate and in accordance with standards accepted at the time of publication. Readers are advised, however, to check the product information literature of each drug they plan to administer to be certain that there have been no changes in the dosage recommended or in the contraindications for administration. This recommendation is of particular importance for new or infrequently used drugs.

Lists of Web sites provided throughout this volume were prepared by ACOG Resource Center librarians from other sources and are provided for information only. Referral to these Web sites does not imply ACOG endorsement. The lists are not meant to be comprehensive; the exclusion of a Web site does not reflect the quality of that site. Please note that Web sites and URLs are subject to change without warning. Web sites were verified on June 15, 2007.

Library of Congress Cataloging-in-Publication Data

Precis: an update in obstetrics and gynecology. Oncology. -- 3rd ed.
p. ; cm.
   Includes bibliographical references and index.
   ISBN 978-1-932328-45-5 (alk. paper)
   1. Generative organs, Female--Cancer. 2. Breast--Cancer. 3. Cancer in women. I. American College of Obstetricians and Gynecologists. II. Title: Precis. Oncology. III. Title: Oncology.
   [DNLM: 1. Genital Neoplasms, Female. WP 145 P9228 2008]
RC280.G5P74 2008
616.99'465--dc22

                              2007044580

The American College of Obstetricians and Gynecologists
409 12th Street, SW
PO Box 96920
Washington, DC 20090-6920

12345/21098

Contents

Contributors

EDITORIAL COMMITTEE

Jonathan Berek, MD, Chair

Ross Berkowitz, MD

Robert Bristow, MD

Joanna M. Cain, MD

Daniel Clarke-Pearson, MD

Barbara Goff, MD

Stephen C. Rubin, MD

Peter E. Schwartz, MD

ADVISORY COMMITTEE

Donald R. Coustan, MD

Kenneth L. Noller, MD

Roger P. Smith, MD

AUTHORS

Ronald D. Alvarez, MD

Kim A. Boggess, MD

John F. Boggess, MD

Jesus Gonzalez Bosquet, MD

Dennis S. Chi, MD

William A. Cliby, MD

Don S. Dizon, MD

Tracy Gaudet, MD

Mary Louise Gemignani, MD

Noah D. Kauff, MD

Robert D. Legare, MD

John R. Lurain, MD

David H. Moore, MD

R. Wendel Naumann, MD

T. Michael Numnum, MD

Richard T. Penson, MD

Peter G. Rose, MD

Mark Spitzer, MD

Joan L. Walker, MD

Shelley W. Wroth, MD

STAFF

Sterling B. Williams, MD, MS
Vice President of Education

Rebecca D. Rinehart
Director of Publications

Nikoleta Dineen
Editor

Preface

Education is a lifelong process. In no field is this process more important than in medicine. As scientific advances unfold, new techniques and technologies emerge, knowledge expands, and the art and science of medicine undergo dynamic change. Progress in medicine is ongoing, and so too must be the continuing medical education of those who practice it.

Precis: An Update in Obstetrics and Gynecology is intended to meet the continuing education needs of obstetricians and gynecologists. It is a broad, yet concise, overview of information relevant to the specialty. As in earlier editions, the emphasis is on innovations in clinical practice, presented within the context of traditional approaches that retain their applicability to patient care.

Precis is an educational resource for preparation for the cognitive assessment of clinical knowledge, regardless of the form of the assessment—formal or informal, structured or independent. It is one of the recognized vehicles useful in preparing for certification and accreditation processes, and it is designed to complement those evaluations while serving as a general review of the field.

Each year, one volume of this five-volume set is revised. This process provides continual updates that are critical to the practice of obstetrics and gynecology and echoes the dynamic nature of the field. The focus is on new and emerging techniques, presented from a balanced perspective of clinical value and cost-effectiveness in practice. Hence, discussion of traditional medical practice is limited. The information has been organized to unify coverage of topics into a single volume so that each volume can stand on its own merit.

This third edition of *Precis: Oncology* reflects current thinking on optimal practice. The information is intended to be a useful tool to assist practicing obstetrician–gynecologists in maintaining current knowledge in a rapidly changing field and to prepare them better for the role of primary care practitioner for women.

Some information from the previous edition continues to be of value and, thus, has been retained and woven into the new structure. The efforts of authors contributing to previous editions, as well as the work of those authors providing new material, must be recognized with gratitude. Collectively, they represent the expertise of the specialty. With such a breadth of representation, differences of opinion are inevitable and have been respected.

Other *Precis* volumes are *Primary and Preventive Care*, Third Edition; *Obstetrics*, Third Edition; *Gynecology*, Third Edition, and *Reproductive Endocrinology*, Third Edition. Each is an educational tool for review, reference, and evaluation. Precis establishes a broad scientific basis for the delivery of quality health care for women. Rather than being a statement of American College of Obstetricians and Gynecologists (ACOG) policy, Precis serves as an intellectual approach to education. An effort has been made, however, to achieve consistency within *Precis* and with other ACOG recommendations. Variations in patient care, based on individual needs and resources, are encouraged as an integral part of the practice of medicine.

—THE EDITORS

Introduction

Over the past few years we have witnessed an extraordinary increase in our basic knowledge of the biology and pathophysiology of cancer and have been able to apply it to improved patient care. The new edition of *Precis: Oncology* strives to reflect this progress by providing updated information on the role of genetics in cancer, preventive strategies, therapeutic modalities, supportive care, and psychosocial issues.

This new edition of *Precis: Oncology* offers practicing obstetrician–gynecologists insight into the latest techniques for preventing, detecting, and managing cancer. The information has been updated completely to provide an overview of each topic with emphasis on new advances.

An entire chapter is devoted to screening and prevention strategies for all types of gynecologic and nongynecologic cancer. Likewise, the genetic basis of cancer has been described in detail to aid physicians in diagnosis and counseling patients at risk. The chapter on breast cancer covers all forms of imaging and techniques for screening and diagnosis. Information on preinvasive cervical neoplasia has been expanded to highlight important new guidelines for screening and management, with detailed explanations of specific changes.

New trends in more immediate and less invasive treatment modalities, including the role of immunosuppression, have been covered. Besides having expertise in diagnostic and therapeutic techniques, physicians need to appreciate the role of palliative care and psychosocial issues. Accordingly, special topics, such as cancer in pregnancy, quality-of-life considerations, and integrative medicine, have been included in this volume to present a balanced approach to patient care.

Aside from providing focused, current, and clinically relevant content, much attention is devoted to the visual presentation of the concepts. The new volume features tables, boxes, and figures to highlight clinical considerations, including information on staging that appears strategically within the respective chapters. Each chapter is accompanied by a list of national organizations that provide additional resources.

Finally, information in *Precis: Oncology*, Third Edition, has been revised to conform to the latest recommendations of the American College of Obstetricians and Gynecologists (ACOG) while also acknowledging controversies. As the discipline of gynecologic oncology evolves, clinicians are encouraged to keep abreast of new developments in the field. The authors, editors, and ACOG staff hope this volume will become a helpful resource in your practice and your continuing medical education. We dedicate this *Precis* to our patients, their families, and their loved ones.

—Jonathan S. Berek, MD
Editor

Cancer Prevention and Screening in Women

Joan L. Walker, MD

Cancer screening and prevention recommendations are important in all well-woman visits. These recommendations are particularly important for women with a history of cancer because their risk of a second cancer is higher. The American Cancer Society (ACS) has noted that cancer mortality could be decreased by one half if Americans followed the recommended screening guidelines that are available. Recommendations have been formulated for all relevant cancer screenings by the American College of Obstetricians and Gynecologists (ACOG) and other groups and should be monitored for updates (Table 1).

RISK ASSESSMENT

Family history is a key component of risk assessment, and the quality of the history and the recognition of potential genetic risks are important in the screening patterns recommended to patients. It also is important to update that information in subsequent visits to determine whether a new diagnosis of cancer in the family may have occurred. "Genetics and Gynecologic Cancer," "Cancer of the Breast," and "Cancer of the Ovary, Peritoneum, and Fallopian Tube" outline appropriate procedures for reviewing specific points in the family history. Precise risk estimates and counseling are critical in making informed decisions regarding genetic testing and interventions based on individual risk.

MODIFIABLE RISKS OF CANCER

Risks of cancer can be modified with screening and treatment of patients with preinvasive lesions, prophylactic surgery for individuals at high risk, or behavioral and lifestyle changes. Few chemoprevention strategies have the appropriate risk/benefit ratio to recommend their routine implementation. Tamoxifen and raloxifene use in a woman at high risk for breast cancer is an example of an important chemopreventive advance.

The American Cancer Society estimates that two thirds of cancer cases in the United States are associated with behavioral risk factors that may be modified by smoking cessation, dietary choices, exercise, and weight control. Of the preventable cancer cases, one third of the 500,000 cancer deaths are attributable to exposure to cigarettes or other tobacco products. The combination of tobacco products and excess consumption of alcoholic beverages is associated not only with lung cancer but also with specific malignancies of the head, neck, and upper gastrointestinal system. It also is associated with the promotion of gynecologic malignancies such as vulvar and cervical can-

cers. The ACOG Committee Opinion No. 316 (October 2005), "Smoking Cessation During Pregnancy," outlines the risks to the fetus and ways to motivate women to stop smoking when they become pregnant, and these tools are helpful in the lifelong effort to stop smoking. Pharmacotherapy for assistance in smoking cessation and prevention of relapse includes nicotine replacement, varenicline, and antidepressants. Pregnant women should not use these agents. However, they may use nicotine, when all other attempts to stop smoking have failed and benefits outweigh risks.

TABLE 1. Suggested Routine Cancer Screening Guidelines

Topic	Guideline
General health counseling and cancer evaluation	All women should have a general health evaluation annually or as appropriate that should include relevant cancer screening for personal risk and counseling for risk reduction.
Breast cancer	Mammography should be performed every 1–2 years beginning at age 40 years and yearly beginning at age 50 years. All women should have an annual clinical breast examination as part of the physical examination. Despite a lack of definitive data for or against breast self-examination, this procedure has the potential to detect palpable breast cancer and can be recommended. Digital mammography or MRI should be used for specific risk categories.
Cervical cancer	Cervical cytologic evaluation should be performed annually beginning 3 years after initiation of sexual intercourse but no later than age 21 years. Cervical cytologic screening can be performed every 2–3 years after three consecutive negative test results if the patient is 30 years or older with no high-risk history. Annual cervical cytologic evaluation also is an option for women aged 30 years and older. The use of a combination of cervical cytologic evaluation and HPV DNA screening is appropriate for women aged 30 years and older. If this combination is used, women who receive negative results on both tests should be rescreened no more frequently than every 3 years. In women older than 70 years with low risk and negative Pap test history, cessation of testing can be considered.
Colorectal cancer screening for women at average risk starting at age 50 years*	Preferred method: • Colonoscopy every 10 years Other appropriate methods: • Fecal occult blood testing or fecal immunochemical testing[†] every year • Flexible sigmoidoscopy every 5 years • Fecal occult blood testing or fecal immunochemical testing[†] every year plus flexible sigmoidoscopy every 5 years • Double contrast barium enema every 5 years
Endometrial cancer	Screening asymptomatic women for endometrial cancer and its precursors is not recommended at this time.
Lung cancer	Available screening techniques are not cost-effective for normal-risk individuals; CT screening recommendations may be changing for high-risk individuals with significant carcinogen (for example, nicotine) exposure.
Ovarian and fallopian tube cancer	There are no effective techniques for the routine screening of asymptomatic, low-risk women for ovarian cancer. Screening and prevention measures for high-risk women are outlined in "Cancer of the Ovary, Peritoneum, and Fallopian Tube."
Skin cancer	Evaluate and counsel regarding exposure to ultraviolet rays.

Abbreviations: MRI indicates magnetic resonance imaging; HPV, human papillomavirus; CT, computed tomography.

*The American College of Gastroenterology recommends that African Americans begin screening with colonoscopy at age 45 years because of increased incidence and earlier age of onset of colorectal cancer. (Agrawal S, Bhupinderjit A, Bhutani MS, Boardman L, Nguyen C, Romero Y, et al; Committee of Minority Affairs and Cultural Diversity, American College of Gastroenterology. Colorectal cancer in African Americans [published erratum appears in Am J Gastroenterol 2005;100:1432]. Am J Gastroenterol 2005;100:515–23; discussion 514.)

[†]Both fecal occult blood testing and fecal immunochemical testing require two or three samples of stool collected by the patient at home and returned for analysis. A single stool sample obtained by digital rectal examination for fecal occult blood testing or fecal immunochemical testing is not adequate for the detection of colorectal cancer.

Data from Routine cancer screening. ACOG Committee Opinion No. 356. American College of Obstetricians and Gynecologists. Obstet Gynecol 2006;108:1611–3 and Colonoscopy and colorectal cancer screening and prevention. ACOG Committee Opinion No. 384. American College of Obstetricians and Gynecologists. Obstet Gynecol 2007;110:1199–202.

An important cancer risk-reduction strategy for women is counseling and behavioral modification to promote exercise, healthy nutrition, and maintenance of an ideal body weight. The strongest scientific rationale for the association of obesity and cancer is found in postmeno-pausal breast cancer and endometrial cancer, but obesity is associated with an increase in death rates for colon, esophageal, and kidney cancer as well. The relative risk of death for all cancer types for a body mass index (BMI; expressed as weight in kilograms divided by height in meters squared) of 25–29.9 is 1.08; for a BMI of 30–34.9, 1.23; for a BMI of 35–39.9, 1.32; and for a BMI of 40 or higher, 1.62. The relative risk of breast cancer death increases to 1.63 (1.44–1.85) for a BMI of 30–34.9, and it is even higher for endometrial cancer (relative risk, 2.53; 2.02–3.18) (1). The following is relevant to obesity, but independently associated with prevention: Greater consumption of vegetables and fruit is associated with a decreased risk of lung, esophageal, stomach, and colorectal cancers. Alcohol consumption is associated with cancer of mouth, pharynx, larynx, esophagus, and liver. Consuming more than one alcoholic drink per day also is associated with an increased risk of breast cancer.

Calcium intake may be an important dietary strategy for prevention of adenomas of the colon and, possibly colon cancer. Getting an optimal amount of intentional physical activity, as well as adding foods that decrease cancer risk, will assist in overall prevention of increased cancer risk due to obesity. A minimum of 30 minutes of moderate to vigorous activity per day on most days of the week is believed to reduce the risk of chronic disease. Women committed to 60 minutes of vigorous activity daily on most days of the week are less likely to become obese.

SKIN CANCER

Approximately 1 million cases of basal cell and squamous cell carcinoma of the skin are diagnosed annually in the United States. Approximately 27,530 women are expected to receive the diagnosis of melanoma in 2008, and nearly 3,020 are expected to die of this cancer (2). Early identification of melanoma may reduce mortality, and finding less aggressive skin cancer earlier may make surgical treatment easier and less disfiguring. Nonmelanomatous skin cancer risk factors include personal history of skin cancer, actinic keratosis, race (white), high lifetime number of severe sunburns, and family history of skin cancer. Risk factors for melanoma include a high number of moles larger than 2 mm and the presence of atypical moles. Risk also is increased in patients who have red or light-colored hair, actinic lentigines, heavy sun exposure, growth of a mole, and skin that burns easily (3).

The mainstay of primary prevention remains the avoidance of sun exposure where possible and the use of hats, clothing, and sunscreen to reduce ultraviolet exposure and sunburn. Early detection with self-examination of the skin and the reporting of any changes are important for every woman. Routine screening for skin cancer is recommended by the ACS every 3 years for individuals aged 20–40 years and then annually. This recommendation is not supported by the U.S. Preventive Services Task Force, which recommends visual inspection of the skin of patients who are seen by their primary care physicians for other visits only, not routine screening. Individuals at higher risk may benefit from skin mapping and yearly or more frequent evaluation of all skin surfaces for changes or new lesions.

LUNG CANCER

Lung cancer is primarily a disease of smokers or individuals exposed to appreciable secondhand smoke, so primary prevention is the cessation of smoking or prevention of smoking, as well as avoidance of other pulmonary carcinogens (see "Modifiable Risks of Cancer"). Other risk factors include occupational exposure to other carcinogens such as asbestos, beryllium, uranium, and radon. Attention has been directed to whether women have a greater susceptibility to tobacco carcinogens and to the potential cause of the observed gender-based risk difference.

Screening for lung cancer in women with high risk based on nicotine exposure has not been recommended because of the poor outcome demonstrated in trials conducted in the 1970s. The International Early Lung Cancer Action Program recently published results that challenge these traditional screening guidelines. These data make a strong case for screening high-risk individuals because of an observed improved survival rate for patients who received their diagnosis of stage I cancer with computed tomography (CT) (92% 10-year survival). This study is controversial, however, because of the lack of a control group, the potential for inclusion of less aggressive lesions, and concerns about how mortality is measured. In addition, the hypothetical risks of CT radiation exposure have been cited against this study's conclusions. At present the National Lung Screening Trial is continuing, and its control group design may eliminate the potential bias cited for the data from the International Early Lung Cancer Action Program. The data from this trial, however, raise questions about whether CT should be used in screening protocols for high-risk individuals and may change the screening recommendations over time to include CT screening.

BREAST CANCER

Breast cancer is the most common cancer in women, with an estimated 182,460 cases and 40,480 deaths predicted in 2008 (2). Survival rates, however, are excellent in most women with early-stage breast cancer that is found during regularly timed, routine screening mammographic examinations.

Breast cancer risk is influenced by early childbearing, breast-feeding, maintaining a healthy weight, and physical activity of 45–60 minutes per day on 5 or more days per week, along with a healthy diet and limited intake of alcoholic beverages (4). The role of estrogen and progesterone in the proliferation of breast cancer remains elusive, although recent results of the Women's Health Initiative suggest that postmenopausal estrogen therapy alone may not increase the risk of breast cancer but rather may decrease it. The way in which using various progestins affects the risk of breast cancer is not known, although medroxyprogesterone may increase the risk, according to the results of this trial. Risk reduction with weight control using diet and exercise is optimal. The use of raloxifene therapy for risk reduction for women with average risk is controversial but may be an option for women with osteoporosis who derive a secondary benefit of decreasing breast cancer risk.

Breast cancer screening remains the mainstay for early detection. Mammography should be performed every 1–2 years beginning at 40 years, and then yearly beginning at 50 years. Women at increased risk may consider beginning mammography at an earlier age, undergoing additional testing (for example, magnetic resonance imaging of the breast), or having more frequent examinations.

The benefits of digital mammography compared with film mammography have been tested, and overall, the diagnostic accuracy was similar. However, for women younger than 50 years with the diagnosis of heterogeneously dense or extremely dense breasts based on mammographic examination, there was an advantage to digital approaches. Digital mammography also has the advantage of reducing the radiation dose by 15–40%, depending on breast thickness. Computer-aided detection systems add to the sensitivity of both approaches. Achieving accurate results with mammography is considered more important than the method by which the results are achieved, particularly in postmenopausal women.

COLORECTAL CANCER

Colorectal cancer risk is associated with premenopausal obesity, alcohol consumption, smoking at an early age, diet (calorie excess and folate and methionine deficiency), and genetic predisposition. Risk is inversely related to the consumption of low-fat dairy products, fish, poultry, vegetables, fruit, and fiber. Aspirin and other nonsteroidal antiinflammatory drugs have an approximate 30–50% rate of risk reduction. Risk reduction has been advocated in the form of calorie restriction; exercise; folate, methionine, and calcium supplementation; use of aspirin or other nonsteroidal antiinflammatory drugs; and screening. The hypothesis of insulin resistance and hyperinsulinemia as the mechanism of excess colon cancer risk secondary to obesity has been suggested but is unproven. There is a 50% risk reduction in individuals with the highest level of physical activity. The Women's Health Initiative confirmed earlier reports that estrogen therapy in menopausal women reduces the risk of colorectal cancer by 30–40%. It had been speculated that the cause of the associated benefit was that hormone users may have been healthier, but that idea has been put to rest by this randomized, controlled trial with adequate power to demonstrate the benefit.

The American College of Obstetricians and Gynecologists has issued guidelines for colorectal cancer screening based on modified ACS guidelines. According to ACOG, screening for colorectal cancer, using one of the methods listed in Table 1, is indicated for all women 50 years or older who are at average risk. For women at increased risk, screening and surveillance guidelines also have been published (Table 2).

CERVICAL CANCER

The 2008 publication of the ACS estimates of cancer incidence warns of an increased number of cervical cancer cases in the United States, with the 2006 estimated incidence of 9,710 cases increased to 11,070 in 2008 (2). Cervical cancer is one of the few types of cancer for which primary prevention is possible. In 2006, the U.S. Food and Drug Administration approved the human papillomavirus (HPV) vaccine for use in females aged 9–26 years. The Centers for Disease Control and Prevention recommends that this vaccine be routinely given to all females aged 11–12 years. The vaccine is effective against HPV genotypes 6, 11, 16, and 18. It is expected to reduce the incidence of cervical cancer by as much as 70% in approximately 20 years if all girls who have not been exposed to HPV are vaccinated. The remaining HPV high-risk types, however, will continue to cause abnormal Pap test results and will be responsible for a lingering risk of cancer, especially if Pap testing and cervical cancer screening guidelines are ignored in unvaccinated or partially protected vaccinated individuals.

Guidelines have been changed to delay the beginning of screening until 3 years after the onset of vaginal intercourse, or at age 21 years. Abnormal Pap test results in young women with initial exposure to HPV frequently resolve without intervention and with little risk of development of cancer in that window; this fact resulted in the change in the recommendation for initiating screening. Annual screening with the Pap test is recommended from age 21 years to 30 years. Women then may consider the combined HPV testing with Pap testing to improve the sensitivity of the screening result. A negative high-risk HPV test result, in combination with a normal Pap test cytologic finding, may allow women to decrease their screening interval to every 3 years because of the improved sensitivity (or lower false-negative rate). The American College of Obstetricians and Gynecologists recommends consideration of cessation of screening at age 70 years if a woman has had three normal screening test results during the past 10 years (5). Women with prior cervical, vaginal, vulvar, or anal cancer or recent changes should continue screening on a more frequent basis as dictated by their individual circumstances.

High incidence rates of cervical cancer usually are caused by nonadherence to screening recommendations. Prevention with vaccination, therefore, may help decrease the incidence rates of cervical cancer appreciably.

OVARIAN CANCER AND FALLOPIAN TUBE CANCER

Risks for ovarian cancer include a family history of ovarian cancer and related types of cancer, length of ovarian function (for example, early menarche, late menopause, cessation of function with pregnancy, and use of oral con-

TABLE 2. American Cancer Society Guidelines for Colorectal Cancer Screening and Surveillance for Women at Increased Risk or High Risk

Risk Category	Age to Begin	Recommendation	Comment
Increased Risk			
Women with a single, small (less than 1 cm) adenoma	At 3–6 years after the initial polypectomy	Colonoscopy*	If the examination result is normal, the patient thereafter can be screened as per average-risk guidelines.
Women with a large adenoma (1 cm or greater), multiple adenomas, or adenomas with high-grade dysplasia or villous change	Within 3 years after the initial polypectomy	Colonoscopy*	If normal, repeat examination in 3 years; if normal then, the patient can thereafter be screened as per average-risk guidelines.
Personal history of curative-intent resection of colorectal cancer	Within 1 year after cancer resection	Colonoscopy*	If normal, repeat examination in 3 years; if normal then, repeat examination every 5 years.
Either colorectal cancer or adenomatous polyps in any first-degree relative before age 60 years, or in two or more first-degree relatives at any age (if not a hereditary syndrome)	Age 40 years, or 10 years before the youngest case in the immediate family	Colonoscopy*	Every 5–10 years. Colorectal cancer in relatives more distant than first degree does not increase risk substantially above the average-risk group.
High Risk			
History of familial adenomatous polyposis	Puberty	Early surveillance with endoscopy, and counseling to consider genetic testing	If the genetic test result is positive, colectomy is indicated. These patients are best referred to a center with experience in the management of familial adenomatous polyposis.
Family history of hereditary nonpolyposis colon cancer	Age 21 years	Colonoscopy and counseling to consider genetic testing	If the genetic test result is positive or if the patient has not had genetic testing, screen every 1–2 years until age 40 years, then annually. These patients are best referred to a center with experience in the management of hereditary nonpolyposis colon cancer.
Inflammatory bowel disease, chronic ulcerative colitis, or Crohn disease	Cancer risk begins to be significant 8 years after the onset of pancolitis, or 12–15 years after the onset of left-sided colitis	Colonoscopy with biopsies for dysplasia	Every 1–2 years. These patients are best referred to a center with experience in the surveillance and management of inflammatory bowel disease.

*If colonoscopy is unavailable, not feasible, or not desired by the patient, double-contrast barium enema alone or the combination of flexible sigmoidoscopy and double-contrast barium enema are acceptable alternatives. Adding flexible sigmoidoscopy to double-contrast barium enema may provide a more comprehensive diagnostic evaluation than double-contrast barium enema alone in finding considerable lesions. A supplementary double-contrast barium enema may be needed if a colonoscopic examination fails to reach the cecum, and a supplementary colonoscopy may be needed if a double-contrast barium enema identifies a possible lesion or does not visualize the entire colorectum adequately.

Smith R, von Eschenbach A, Wender R, Levin B, Byers T, Rothenberger D, et al. American Cancer Society guidelines for the early detection of cancer: update of early detection guidelines for prostate, colorectal, and endometrial cancers. CA Cancer J Clin 2001;51:38–75.

traceptives). Women may decrease their risk of this cancer if they have had full-term pregnancies, have breast-fed, have used birth control pills (risk reduction as high as 50%), and have undergone tubal ligation (with reports of variable risk reduction rates). Ovarian cancer prevention is most effective with prophylactic bilateral salpingo-oophorectomy in appropriate candidates after completion of childbearing (6). The specific strategies for managing women with a family history of breast or ovarian malignancies or other relevant genetic syndromes are well outlined in "Genetics and Gynecologic Cancer," "Cancer of the Breast," and "Cancer of the Ovary, Peritoneum, and Fallopian Tube." Although rare, fallopian tube cancer is associated with similar risk factors, particularly an inherited predisposition, and it must be considered in risk reduction strategies.

Screening for ovarian cancer cannot be recommended for the general population (6). Measurement of CA 125 levels and transvaginal ultrasonography have increased the rates of unnecessary surgery and failed to improve detection rates of early-stage disease. The Prostate, Lung, Colon, and Ovary Cancer Screening Trial arrived at the nationwide conclusion that unnecessary surgery was performed based on abnormal ultrasound findings and elevated CA 125 level measurements. This conclusion resulted in a reevaluation of the use of ultrasonography and CA 125 decision points for diagnostic intervention. This study recommended that the cutoff for normal CA 125 level be changed to less than 65 units/mL. The size of the ovarian mass also was important in the study in differentiating cancer from benign processes. Women with lesions of at least 7 cm had a 26% risk of cancer, whereas women with smaller lesions had a 1.5% cancer risk. The low incidence and lack of a preinvasive stage suggest that any mass screening of women at average risk would not be effective, although continuing research is pursuing new serum tests for women with suggestive symptoms or higher risk to assess whether earlier diagnosis is possible.

ENDOMETRIAL CANCER

Nearly 40,000 women receive the diagnosis of endometrial cancer every year. Traditional risk factors for endometrial cancer are early menarche (relative risk [RR], 1.5–2), late menopause (RR, 2–3), nulliparity (RR, 3), anovulation (polycystic ovary syndrome; RR greater than 5), obesity RR 2–5), tamoxifen use (RR, 3–7), diabetes (RR 3), and age (RR, 2–3). The use of tamoxifen has been demonstrated to increase the risk of endometrial cancer to 2–3 cases per 1,000 women per year. The use of raloxifene has a rate of 1.25 endometrial cancer cases per 1,000 women per year (7). There is concern that women at increased risk of breast cancer (BRCA carriers) may be at higher risk of endometrial cancer than the general population. Family history of endometrial cancer at an age younger than 50 years increases a woman's risk 10-fold. Family history of colon cancer is associated with endometrial cancer and also hereditary nonpolyposis colorectal cancer due to DNA mismatch repair enzyme abnormalities or Lynch syndrome. Women with these mismatch repair gene defects are eligible for screening and prophylactic hysterectomy with bilateral salpingo-oophorectomy. Endo-

metrial cancer is the most common cancer in women with these disorders. Reduced risk of endometrial cancer is seen with oral contraceptive use (RR, 0.3–0.5).

Preventive measures for reducing the risk of endometrial cancer include weight control in the form of a healthy diet and daily exercise. Anovulation, including that in perimenopause, can be treated with oral contraceptives, a progestin-containing intrauterine device, or the use of continuous progestin to decrease the risk of continuous estrogen stimulation.

There is no screening strategy for endometrial cancer. The use of endometrial biopsies for evaluation of the endometrium in women at high risk due to tamoxifen use failed to show an ability to prevent endometrial cancer. Pap testing detects less than 50% of endometrial cancer cases, and usually only in the face of existing symptoms, such as bleeding. At present, the success of treatment of patients with endometrial adenocarcinoma is dependent on early diagnosis, not screening.

CANCER OF THE VULVA AND VAGINA

The risk factors of vaginal cancer and vulvar cancer are similar to the risk factors of cervical cancer. Exposure to some skin carcinogens, such as direct and prolonged exposure to coal tars, has been shown to increase local vulvar cancer patterns (for example, in coal-mining regions). There is an increase in the incidence of vulvar intraepithelial neoplasia, particularly in younger women, based on the data from Surveillance, Epidemiology, and End Results. Older women have cancer that may develop independent of HPV infection and can be associated with vulvar lichen sclerosis. It is expected that the HPV vaccination program will reduce the incidence of the HPV-related lesions in all of the lower genital tract, including vulvar intraepithelial neoplasia, vaginal intraepithelial neoplasia, vulvar cancer, and vaginal cancer.

The physical examination is the only screening appropriate for vulvar cancer. Vulvar self-examination should be encouraged, especially in women treated for cervical neoplasia. Women with symptoms of vulvar irritation need to be examined for inflammatory conditions or premalignant lesions. Biopsy of the vulva and vagina is needed for confirmation of the diagnosis. Removal of precancerous lesions of the vulva or vagina is expected to prevent future cases of invasive cancer.

References

1. Calle EE, Rodriguez C, Walker-Thurmond K, Thun MJ. Overweight, obesity, and mortality from cancer in a prospectively studied cohort of U.S. adults. N Engl J Med 2003; 348:1625–38.

2. American Cancer Society. Cancer facts and figures 2008. Atlanta (GA): ACS; 2008. Available at: http://www.cancer.

org/downloads/STT/2008CAFFfinalsecured.pdf. Retrieved February 20, 2008.

3. Lanni SM, Nunley JR. Dermatoses. Clin Update Womens Health Care 2007;VI:1–137.

4. Kushi LH, Byers T, Doyle C, Bandera EV, McCullough M, McTiernan A, et al. American Cancer Society Guidelines on Nutrition and Physical Activity for cancer prevention: reducing the risk of cancer with healthy food choices and physical activity. American Cancer Society 2006 Nutrition and Physical Activity Guidelines Advisory Committee [published erratum appears in CA Cancer J Clin 2007;57:66]. CA Cancer J Clin 2006;56:254–81; quiz 313–4.

5. Cervical cytology screening. ACOG Practice Bulletin No. 45. American College of Obstetricians and Gynecologists. Obstet Gynecol 2003;102:417–27.

6. Elective and risk-reducing salpingo-oophorectomy. ACOG Practice Bulletin No. 89. American College of Obstetricians and Gynecologists. Obstet Gynecol 2008;111:231–41.

7. Vogel VG, Costantino JP, Wickerham DL, Cronin WM, Cecchini RS, Atkins JN, et al. Effects of tamoxifen vs raloxifene on the risk of developing invasive breast cancer and other disease outcomes: the NSABP Study of tamoxifen and raloxifene (STAR) P-2 Trial. National Surgical Adjuvant Breast and Bowel Project (NSABP) [published errata appear in JAMA 2006;296:2926, JAMA 2007; 298:973]. JAMA 2006;295:2727–41.

Genetics and Gynecologic Cancer

Robert D. Legare, MD

Advances in human genetics and molecular biology have led to greater insight into the hereditary and somatic mutations associated with cancer development. The malignant phenotype ultimately arises from the serial acquisition of mutations within specific genes, and incremental understanding of this process is beginning to revolutionize how we perform risk assessment, prevention, and treatment for patients with cancer. As we advance to an era of personalized medicine, new predictive, prognostic, and therapeutic tools will be available to the obstetrician–gynecologist that will have practical implications for the day-to-day primary care of patients.

HEREDITARY BREAST AND OVARIAN CANCER

Approximately 5–10% of cases of breast and ovarian cancer are associated with hereditary risk. Breast and ovarian cancer syndrome, the prototypic hereditary cancer syndrome, is largely accounted for by deleterious *BRCA1* and *BRCA2* gene mutations, discovered in 1994 and 1995, respectively. Both *BRCA1*, located on chromosome 17, and *BRCA2*, located on chromosome 13, are tumor suppressor genes important in the repair of damaged DNA and cell cycle kinetics.

The inheritance of a single recessive mutation is responsible for this autosomal dominant cancer syndrome and is explained by Knudson's "two-hit" hypothesis (Fig. 1). In normal cells, two separate somatic mutations

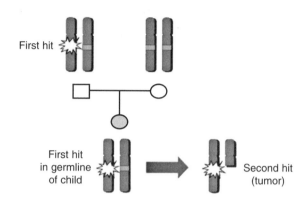

FIG. 1. The Two-Hit Hypothesis. American Society of Clinical Oncology. Cancer genetics and cancer predisposition testing. 2nd edition. Alexandria (VA): ASCO; 2004. Reprinted with permission from the American Society of Clinical Oncology.

(two hits) are required to inactivate a tumor suppressor gene. Each mutation is a low-probability event, so it is relatively rare for one cell to have both of its alleles inactivated. In hereditary cancer syndromes, every cell inherits a germline mutation in one of the alleles (ie, the first hit). In these cases, a second hit in at least one cell in the target organ is statistically much more likely and can be sufficient for the malignant phenotype. It is important to remember that hereditary risk can arise through the paternal, as well as maternal, lineage. Germline mutations in either gene, therefore, increase the likelihood that cancer will develop during the lifetime of the individual. Approximately 16% of mutations in families with site-specific hereditary breast cancer are not found by standard *BRCA1* and *BRCA2* DNA sequencing or large *BRCA1* genomic rearrangement analysis and are believed to be caused by either an undiscovered gene or mutations within *BRCA1* and *BRCA2* that are missed by current testing methods. Most cases of hereditary breast or ovarian cancer and site-specific ovarian cancer are associated with *BRCA1* or *BRCA2* mutations.

More than 1,863 different mutations have been reported throughout the 22 coding exons of *BRCA1* and 1,380 different mutations throughout the 26 coding exons of *BRCA2*, including frameshift, missense, and nonsense mutations. Most mutations are unique and limited to a given family; however, some mutations have a higher frequency in certain populations because of the founder effect. For example, the *BRCA1 185delAG*, *BRCA1 5382insC*, and *BRCA2 6714delT* mutations are found in 1.05%, 0.11%, and 1.36% of the Ashkenazi Jewish population, respectively. Together, these three founder mutations may occur in 1 in 40 Ashkenazi Jews (1). Founder mutations in other populations, such as the *BRCA1 C4446T* and *BRCA2 8765delAG* mutations in French Canadians and the *BRCA2 999de15* mutation in the Icelandic population, have been characterized.

Cancer Risk Assessment Based on Molecular Alterations

The lifetime risk of breast cancer up to age 70 years associated with a *BRCA1* mutation is estimated to be between 50% and 85%, with a significant risk of early-onset breast cancer. This contrasts with the approximate 12.5% lifetime risk in the general population. Moreover, second primary breast cancer may occur in 40–60% of women over 10 years, higher than the 0.7–1.0% risk per year in the setting of sporadic breast cancer. Carriers of *BRCA2* mutations have a slightly lower lifetime risk of developing breast cancer compared with carriers of *BRCA1* mutation, and early-onset breast cancer is less common.

The lifetime risk of epithelial ovarian cancer ranges from approximately 16% to 44% for *BRCA1* mutation carriers and from 10% to 20% for *BRCA2* mutation carriers (2). This contrasts with an estimated 1.7% lifetime risk in the general population. Additionally, reports have suggested the average age of individuals with ovarian cancer to be younger in *BRCA1* carriers compared with *BRCA2* carriers (54 years and 62 years, respectively).

In males, *BRCA2* mutations carry approximately a 6% risk of breast cancer by the time an individual is aged 70 years and a threefold to fourfold increased relative risk of prostate cancer by age 80 years. Although low, the risk of pancreatic cancer in men and women carrying a *BRCA2* mutation was estimated to be approximately 2–3% by age 80 years. There is some evidence of additional cancer risks influenced by an absent *BRCA* protein, such as fallopian tube cancer, primary peritoneal cancer, and melanoma. Papillary serous carcinoma of the endometrium may be associated with *BRCA1* mutations in Ashkenazi Jews (3). However, further studies need to be conducted to substantiate these findings.

Prognostic Use of Molecular Information

Breast cancer associated with *BRCA1* mutations has distinguishing phenotypic characteristics. Of cases of breast cancer associated with *BRCA1* mutations, 80–90% are negative for immunohistochemical expression of the estrogen receptor, progesterone receptor, and HER-2 receptor (ER–PR–HER-2–; triple negative) and are typically high-grade ductal carcinomas that are aneuploid with increased S-phase fraction, pushing borders, and lymphocytic infiltration. Most also are found to be basaloid on DNA microarray analysis and immunohistochemistry testing (CK5/6 positive, EGFR +) (4). Such primary tumor characteristics have been associated with more aggressive clinical behavior and worse prognosis in the general population of women with breast cancer. The *BRCA2* tumors typically are positive for expression of estrogen receptor and progesterone receptor with HER-2 receptor expression similar to that of sporadic breast tumors.

There have been conflicting data on the prognosis of breast cancer in *BRCA* mutation carriers. It is likely that survival is similar to, or worse than, that in sporadic breast cancer. Based on histopathology, it is surprising that survival of *BRCA1* patients is not significantly more unfavorable. One possible contributing factor to this discrepancy may lie in the apparent increase in medullary carcinoma, a prognostically favorable subtype, which appears more commonly in *BRCA1* mutation carriers. In addition, ductal carcinoma in situ, considered a precursor lesion to invasive breast cancer, is part of the *BRCA* phenotype and, whereas not incorporated into current pretest probability modeling, may influence mutation risk assessment.

Phenotypic characteristics of breast cancer, when considered in combination with age at diagnosis and family history, may increase the probability that the disease is associated with a germline mutation. A recent retrospective analysis of triple-negative breast cancer found that 11.3% of patients had a *BRCA1* mutation. In women younger than 50 years, the *BRCA1* mutation prevalence was 16%; in women younger than 50 years with a strong family history (defined as more than one first- or second-degree relative with breast or ovarian cancer or one with breast and ovarian cancer), the mutation prevalence was 29%. In women aged 50 years or older with a strong family history, the mutation prevalence was 27%, although there were no *BRCA1* mutations noted in this age group in the absence of a strong family history (5).

Ovarian cancer in the setting of a germline *BRCA* mutation usually has high-grade serous histology and typically is not associated with mucinous histology or borderline tumors. Compared with its somatic counterparts, ovarian cancer arising in the *BRCA* setting appears to have a better prognosis, possibly because of greater sensitivity to platinum agents (6).

Fallopian tube cancer and primary peritoneal cancer also are part of the *BRCA* syndrome. In 16–43% of women with primary fallopian tube cancers, *BRCA* mutations have been identified (7). In women with primary peritoneal cancer, *BRCA* mutations are found in approximately 10% of cases (8).

Other Hereditary Breast Syndromes and Ovarian Cancer Syndromes

Whereas *BRCA1* and *BRCA2* mutations contribute to most cases of hereditary breast and ovarian cancer, less common hereditary cancer syndromes can be identified by associated clinical characteristics and confirmed with molecular testing (Table 3). Germline *p53* mutations are associated with Li–Fraumeni syndrome. This syndrome is characterized by bone and soft tissue sarcomas, leukemia, brain tumors, and adrenocortical carcinomas, as well as breast carcinoma, which is the most common malignancy in adults. Li–Fraumeni syndrome is associated with a 50% risk of carcinoma by age 35 years and a 70–90% lifetime risk of cancer development. Germline mutations in the *PTEN* gene are associated with Cowden syndrome, which is characterized by multiple hamartomas, including papillomas and trichilemmomas, thyroid disease, uterine leiomyomata, macrocephaly, mental retardation, and breast cancer.

Both benign and malignant breast tumors occur in Muir–Torre syndrome, a syndrome associated with hereditary nonpolyposis colorectal cancer (HNPCC), which will be discussed later. Peutz–Jeghers syndrome, associated with germline mutations in the *STK11* gene and characterized by benign gastrointestinal polyps and abnormal pigmentation, is associated with an increased risk of breast cancer, including early-onset and bilateral disease.

Peutz–Jeghers syndrome also is associated with ovarian sex cord tumors with annular tubules and adenoma malignum (minimal deviation adenocarcinoma) of the cervix. Unlike the aforementioned disorders, which are inherited in an autosomal dominant fashion, ataxia–telangiectasia is inherited in an autosomal recessive fashion and is associated with cerebellar ataxia, oculocutaneous telangiectasia, radiation hypersensitivity, leukemia or lymphoma, and breast cancer in mutation carriers.

Identifying Patients at Risk and Referral for Genetic Counseling

Identifying patients at a risk high enough to be considered appropriate for genetic counseling and testing is fundamental to practitioners in a primary care setting (9). Family history remains the cornerstone of hereditary risk assessment. Factors that have been associated with the presence of a *BRCA* mutation include breast cancer diagnosed before age 50 years, bilateral breast cancer, ovarian cancer, Ashkenazi Jewish ancestry, multiple affected gen-

TABLE 3. Hereditary Cancer Syndromes Associated With Gynecologic Malignancy

Hereditary Cancer Syndrome	Clinical Features	Identified Gene(s)	Inheritance Pattern
Breast and ovarian cancer syndrome	Breast (including in males), ovarian, pancreatic, and prostate cancer; melanoma	*BRCA1* and *BRCA2*	Autosomal dominant
Hereditary nonpolyposis colorectal cancer syndrome	Colorectal, endometrial, ovarian, gastric, hepatobiliary, small bowel, and brain cancer	*MLH1, MSH2, MSH6, PMS1,* and *PMS2*	Autosomal dominant
Li–Fraumeni syndrome	Soft tissue sarcomas; leukemia; breast, brain, adrenocortical, pancreatic, lung, and possibly prostate cancer; melanoma; and gonadal germ cell tumors	*p53*	Autosomal dominant
Cowden syndrome	Thyroid cancer, breast cancer, mucocutaneous lesions, and colonic neoplasms	*PTEN*	Autosomal dominant
Peutz–Jeghers syndrome	Abnormal melanin deposits, gastrointestinal tract polyposis and cancer, sex cord tumors with annular tubules, breast cancer, and adenoma malignum of the cervix	*STK11*	Autosomal dominant
Ataxia–telangiectasia	Cerebellar ataxia, oculocutaneous telangiectasia, radiation hypersensitivity, leukemia, lymphoma, many other tumors, and breast cancer in carriers	*ATM*	Autosomal recessive
Nevoid basal cell carcinoma (Gorlin) syndrome	Ovarian fibromas and fibrosarcomas	*PTCH*	Autosomal dominant

erations, and the presence of breast cancer and ovarian cancer in the same individual (Box 1). The presence of ovarian cancer in a family with breast cancer strongly increases the pretest probability of an inherited *BRCA* mutation. As previously noted, triple-negative breast tumors in premenopausal women or postmenopausal women with a strong family history of breast cancer increase the probability of an associated germline *BRCA* mutation. Limitations to family history that can affect hereditary risk assessment include family size, small numbers of females within a pedigree, and adopted status. These limitations should not preclude referral for genetic counseling.

Women thought to be at high risk of breast and ovarian cancer syndrome who elect to further investigate that possibility should be referred, whenever possible, for formal cancer risk assessment. Ideally, this assessment would include a multidisciplinary team of specialists composed of genetic counselors as well as physicians and surgeons specifically trained and focused on clinical cancer genetics. This team also should include psychologists, psychiatrists, and social workers.

Several statistically based models have been developed specifically to estimate the risk of *BRCA1* and *BRCA2* carrier status based on personal and family medical history. These models have been developed to aid in determining whether an individual's probability of harboring a germline mutation is sufficient to merit consideration of genetic testing. The first is a software model called *BRCA*PRO. The calculation is based on observations in referral populations in which the majority of women tested were affected with breast or ovarian cancer. *BRCA*PRO

adjusts risk according to the Bayesian theorem, but it may overestimate or underestimate carrier risk depending on the family characteristics present.

A second model is an empiric model derived by Myriad Genetics Laboratories. These data were obtained from a series of 238 women with a positive family history who developed breast cancer before age 50 years or who developed ovarian cancer at any age. The development of ovarian cancer within such families significantly increased the chance of finding a *BRCA1* or *BRCA2* mutation. The Myriad model was later applied to 10,000 tested individuals by observational data. These risk estimates are calculated directly from the clinician's completed test request form, which usually contains history obtained only from the patient's verbal report without documentation of pathology. Because of each model's limitations, it is recommended that hereditary cancer risk assessment be performed by experienced clinicians to ensure that the most accurate assessment is calculated. Several other models may be used to determine pretest probability.

In reviewing recommendations for women who are *BRCA* mutation carriers, it is important to remember that risk assessment can reassure the women who have overestimated their hereditary risk based on cancer within the family by determining a calculated low risk of harboring a germline *BRCA* mutation. Likewise, women from a known *BRCA*-positive family who test negative (true negative) for a mutation revert their cancer risk back to that of the general population risk and receive the recommendation to follow general population cancer screening guidelines. Finally, women who test negative for a *BRCA* mutation in a family with a history of breast or ovarian cancer but without a known mutation have received a relatively uninformative test result that may not influence screening or preventive recommendations.

Screening and Follow-up of High-Risk Patients

In individuals found to be positive for hereditary breast and ovarian cancer susceptibility syndrome, management includes discussion regarding cancer screening and surveillance, prophylactic surgery, and cancer prevention. Often research protocols are available, and patients should be advised strongly to enroll, when possible.

Recommendations for cancer screening of individuals with a *BRCA1* or *BRCA2* cancer-predisposing mutation have been made by a task force convened by the Cancer Genetics Studies Consortium, the American College of Obstetricians and Gynecologists, and the National Comprehensive Cancer Network. Given the evolving but limited prospective data sets regarding benefit of specific interventions, patients must be counseled regarding the limited knowledge about strategies to reduce risk in combination with individual preference regarding follow-up decisions.

BOX 1

Features Associated With *BRCA* Mutations

- Early-onset breast cancer
- Ovarian cancer in a family with a history of breast cancer
- Breast and ovarian cancer in the same woman
- Bilateral breast cancer
- Multiple cases of breast or ovarian cancer occurring over several generations
- Ashkenazi ancestry with breast or ovarian cancer
- Male breast cancer
- Triple-negative breast cancer in a woman younger than 50 years, or in a woman older than 50 years with a family history of breast or ovarian cancer
- Ductal carcinoma in situ at a young age with family history
- Fallopian tube or primary peritoneal cancer

The following screening regimen is based on data from families with cancer-predisposing *BRCA1* or *BRCA2* mutations and addresses the elevated breast cancer risk beginning in a woman's late 20s or early 30s. It is recommended that individuals predisposed to an inherited breast cancer risk consider monthly breast self-examination beginning at age 18 years, clinical breast examination 2–4 times annually beginning at age 25 years, annual mammography beginning at age 25 years, and annual breast magnetic resonance imaging (MRI) beginning at age 25 years. Annual MRI screening often is interdigitated between annual mammographic screenings of breasts every 6 months. This strategy is thought to further decrease the development of interval breast cancer in this high-risk population.

Although the sensitivity of MRI appears to be superior to that of mammography and breast ultrasonography for the detection of invasive cancer in high-risk women, the specificity is debated and appears to be directly related to the clinical experience of the radiologist. Several studies have supported the use of MRI in women having an increased breast cancer risk. The detection of small foci of breast disease in women carrying a *BRCA* germline mutation (undetectable with mammography) has supported the integration of screening MRI in germline carriers (10).

Men with *BRCA* mutations, particularly *BRCA2* mutations, also may be at increased risk for breast cancer, and evaluation of any breast mass or change is advisable. However, there are insufficient data to recommend a formal surveillance program.

The ovarian cancer screening measures that are now available have limited sensitivity and specificity and have not been shown to reduce ovarian cancer mortality. Nevertheless, the Cancer Genetics Studies Consortium task force and the National Comprehensive Cancer Network recommend the following examinations for women carrying a deleterious *BRCA1* or *BRCA2* gene mutation: annual or semiannual pelvic examination beginning at age 25–35 years, annual or semiannual transvaginal ultrasonography with color Doppler beginning at age 25–35 years (preferably on day 1–10 of the cycle for premenopausal women), and annual or semiannual serum CA 125 measurement beginning at age 25–35 years. Serum screening can be associated with a high false-positive rate, especially in premenopausal women, and often is not offered by physicians even to germline mutation carriers. Promising data provide the first prospective evidence demonstrating that the previous surveillance strategy used in women carrying a *BRCA* germline mutation may result in the diagnosis of early-stage ovarian tumors (11). Transvaginal ultrasonography has limitations in detecting early-stage disease, and it is not clear that screening improves survival rates. For this reason, risk-reducing surgery generally is recommended for women who do not wish to have children in the future.

Prophylactic Surgery

Prophylactic mastectomy removes breast tissue, but minimal residual breast tissue remaining postoperatively still may be at risk for cancer development. In a study of 6,039 women found to carry *BRCA* gene mutation or to have a family history of breast cancer or both who underwent prophylactic mastectomy, there was an estimated 90–94% reduction rate in breast cancer risk and an 81–94% reduction rate in breast cancer-related deaths. Additional prospective data regarding 251 individuals carrying a *BRCA* germline mutation demonstrated the detection of two cases of occult intraductal breast cancer within the 29 individuals choosing risk-reducing mastectomy. Although only a small percentage of women from high-risk families choose to undergo prophylactic bilateral mastectomy, those who do generally feel content with their decision. In a follow-up study of high-risk women who pursued preventive surgery, approximately 74% reported a reduced emotional concern regarding breast cancer development and seemed to naturally sustain other psychologic and social functioning (12).

Bilateral prophylactic salpingo-oophorectomy reduces the risk of ovarian cancer by 95% in mutation carriers, and recent prospective data suggest this intervention improves overall survival and cancer-specific survival in this high-risk population (13, 14). The risk of primary peritoneal carcinomatosis does not appear to be affected by salpingo-oophorectomy. A study conducted by the National Cancer Institute found that women from families at high risk of ovarian cancer had an equal rate of primary peritoneal cancer after oophorectomy compared with the rate of primary peritoneal cancer in women who did not have the procedure. The absolute risk is fairly low, approximately 3%, after bilateral salpingo-oophorectomy. When performing the surgery, it is important to remove as much of the fallopian tube as possible. Of cases of occult cancer at the time of risk-reducing surgery, 30–50% will be in the fallopian tube (15). Further studies are necessary to investigate whether the uterus should be removed to ensure complete removal of the fallopian tubes and to determine the role of omental biopsy (Box 2).

Prophylactic oophorectomy reduces the risk of breast cancer by approximately 50% in carriers of a *BRCA* germline mutation (16). Additionally, in 21 of 36 women carrying a *BRCA* germline mutation who received the diagnosis of breast cancer and underwent bilateral salpingo-oophorectomy either before or within 6 months of their cancer diagnosis, only 1 of 15 women (4.8%) had a relapse, compared with the 7 of 15 women (47%) who retained their ovaries. An update combining data from two large prospective cohorts that included 871 mutation carriers evaluating risk-reducing salpingo-oophorectomy suggests similar benefit in *BRCA1* and *BRCA2* mutation carriers in regard to risk reduction of ovarian cancer (17). However, *BRCA2* mutation carriers derived a statistically significant reduction in breast cancer risk with a hazard ratio of 0.28 (*P*=.036), whereas *BRCA1* mutation carriers derived a small but not statistically significant benefit from risk-reducing salpingo-oophorectomy. Risk-reducing salpingo-oophorectomy reduced the risk of estrogen receptor–positive breast cancer, more common in *BRCA2* mutation carriers, but not estrogen receptor–negative breast cancer (hazard ratio, 0.22; *P*=.06 versus hazard ratio, 1.27; *P*=.58). Because of study results, it is now advocated that after comprehensive counseling, *BRCA*-heterozygous women consider risk-reducing prophylactic salpingo-oophorectomy to reduce the risk of ovarian cancer and breast cancer.

As preventive oophorectomy is becoming more common after the identification of an inheritable mutation, specific recommendations are emerging related to this surgical procedure and the pathologic examination of the tissue removed. Research facilities are especially well equipped to study prophylactic oophorectomy and have the resources to help integrate clinically relevant data into practice. When a prophylactic bilateral salpingo-oophorectomy is performed, it is imperative to remove the ovaries and fallopian tubes completely. In addition, peritoneal washings should be submitted and the peritoneal surfaces carefully examined. The surgeon should be prepared to perform a staging procedure when unanticipated findings are encountered. Pathologists should perform serial sectioning on submitted specimens, including the ovaries and fallopian tubes, to define more accurately the presence of occult malignancy, which is reported to be present in at least 2.5% of women undergoing risk-reducing salpingo-oophorectomy (18). It is recommended that the entire ovarian epithelium be evaluated and the fallopian tube be sectioned every 2–3 mm (Box 3 and Fig. 2).

After comprehensive cancer genetic counseling, most women are pleased with their decision to pursue surgical intervention for ovarian cancer prevention. Although approximately 93% of high-risk women who underwent prophylactic oophorectomy expressed no regret about their decision, 50% preferred more information about the risk and benefits of hormone therapy (HT) before making decisions about surgery (19). In a study of the use of HT after bilateral salpingo-oophorectomy in premenopausal *BRCA* gene mutation carriers, results consistent with previous publications were found: short-term HT use is reasonable for women experiencing a compromise in quality of life (20). Most clinicians recommend discontinuing use before or at the time of expected menopause. Women in this situation must assume at least a theoretical increase in breast cancer risk.

Chemoprevention

The National Surgical Adjuvant Breast and Bowel Project P-1 prevention trial assessed the use of tamoxifen (a selec-

BOX 2

Pros and Cons of Concurrent Hysterectomy

Pros
- Hormonal therapy with unopposed estrogen can be administered.
- There is an increased risk of endometrial cancer in women taking tamoxifen.
- Women of Ashkenazi descent with *187delAG* and *5385 ins C* site mutations are at increased risk for uterine papillary serous carcinoma.

Cons
- There is increased risk for complications and morbidity.
- A day surgery procedure is converted to an inpatient admission.

BOX 3

Essential Points of Risk-Reducing Surgery

- Obtain preoperative ultrasonography and CA 125 measurement results.
- Discuss the possibility of detecting occult malignancy with patients, and be prepared for resection and staging of cancer.
- Transect ovarian vessels 2 cm proximal to the ovary to avoid leaving remnants.
- Remove as much fallopian tube as possible.
- If adhesions are present, perform dissection carefully to ensure complete removal of the ovaries and fallopian tube.
- Obtain washings.
- Inspect peritoneal surfaces carefully for the presence of early primary peritoneal cancer.
- Discuss the pros and cons of removing the uterus at the time of risk-reducing surgery.
- Make pathologists aware that surgery is being done for risk reduction. The entire ovarian epithelium should be evaluated, and fallopian tubes should be sectioned serially and evaluated every 2–3 mm.
- If possible, encourage patients to have their surgery at centers specializing in research of hereditary cancer so that they may participate in research trials.

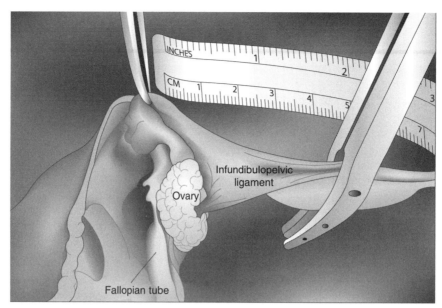

■ **FIG. 2.** Risk-reducing salpingo-oophorectomy. Care is taken to remove as much of the fallopian tube as possible and to excise the ovary completely with a 2-cm margin on the infundibulopelvic ligament. Illustration: John Yanson. Karlan BY, Berchuck A, Mutch D. The role of genetic testing for cancer susceptibility in gynecologic practice. Obstet Gynecol 2007;110:155–67.

tive estrogen receptor modulator) in women identified by the Gail model to have an increased breast cancer risk estimated at 1.66% at 5 years. This study reported a 49% reduction in breast cancer with the use of tamoxifen for 5 years. It was concluded that tamoxifen risk reduction was most beneficial in women with an elevated risk of breast cancer who were younger than 50 years because premenopausal women did not seem to be at increased risk of deep vein thrombosis or uterine cancer compared with their postmenopausal counterparts. However, tamoxifen reduced the incidence of breast cancer that was estrogen receptor positive, but not estrogen receptor negative.

Because breast cancer occurring in women with *BRCA1* mutations is more likely to be estrogen receptor negative, it is difficult to estimate the benefit of tamoxifen prophylaxis without specifically testing the effect in women with *BRCA1* or *BRCA2* cancer-predisposing mutations. To assess the effect of tamoxifen in *BRCA* carriers, complete *BRCA* sequencing analysis was performed on 288 of the 315 women who developed invasive breast carcinoma within the National Surgical Adjuvant Breast and Bowel Project P-1 tamoxifen trial. However, only 19 women (6.6%) were found to be heterozygous for *BRCA* mutations. Because of the small number of cases and wide confidence intervals, conclusions could not be drawn from these data. However, data from the Breast Cancer Clinical Study Group suggest a 50% and 60% decrease in contralateral breast cancer in *BRCA1* and *BRCA2* mutation carriers with the use of tamoxifen (21). This protective effect was not seen in women who had undergone oophorectomy. Nevertheless, because there are significant adverse consequences of tamoxifen treatment, including a

higher rate of endometrial cancer and thromboembolic episodes such as pulmonary embolism, each patient should be counseled appropriately, enabling her to make the best personal decision. The Study of Tamoxifen and Raloxifene trial, which demonstrated the benefit of raloxifene therapy for reduction in rates of invasive breast cancer in high-risk women, has not yielded any data on *BRCA* mutation carriers. Finally, based on the phenotype of *BRCA1* malignancy, other nonhormonal agents are being studied as possible risk-reducing agents.

One case–control study has found a substantial decreased risk of ovarian cancer in women with *BRCA* mutations who took oral contraceptives, with an odds ratio of 0.56 for *BRCA1* mutation carriers and an odds ratio of 0.39 for *BRCA2* mutation carriers (22). Women need to be counseled regarding the possible increased risk of breast cancer with this intervention.

Treatment Strategies Based on Molecular Alterations

It is hoped that molecular insights into cancer predisposition syndromes will lead to novel and effective targeted therapies to manage these disorders successfully. The mutations *BRCA1* and *BRCA2* play a critical role in the repair of double-strand DNA breaks by homologous recombination, also called the Fanconi anemia/*BRCA* repair pathway, so cells deficient in *BRCA* proteins may possess significant sensitivity to cisplatin, possibly because of the inability to repair platinum-DNA adducts. It may be through the same deficiency in a specific DNA repair pathway that *BRCA*-deficient cells have profound sensitivity to the inhibition of poly(adenosine diphosphate–ribose) polymerase activity (23). Indeed poly (adenosine diphosphate–ribose) polymerase inhibitors are now being studied in the treatment of patients with *BRCA*-associated breast and ovarian cancer.

HEREDITARY NONPOLYPOSIS COLORECTAL CANCER SYNDROME

Initially called *Lynch syndrome*, this disorder was later termed *hereditary nonpolyposis colorectal cancer (HNPCC)* and is believed to be responsible for an estimated 3–5% of colorectal cancer (24). Because endometrial cancer is not generally recognized as an inherited tumor type, HNPCC is reviewed with emphasis on the related extracolonic gynecologic malignancies.

The colorectal cancer seen in families with a history of HNPCC occurs at an average age of 44 years, develops primarily in the right side of the colon (proximal to the splenic flexure), and progresses more rapidly. Individuals with an HNPCC gene mutation have a lifetime risk of colorectal cancer of approximately 80%. In addition to colorectal cancer, patients and family members are more susceptible to a wide variety of extracolonic malignancies. Women heterozygous for an HNPCC mutation also have a 60% risk of endometrial cancer and a 12% risk of ovarian cancer by age 70 years. The mean age at diagnosis is 48 years for endometrial cancer and 42 years for ovarian cancer (25). Other risk factors that have been well documented include transitional cell carcinoma of the ureter and renal pelvis and adenocarcinomas of the stomach, small bowel, biliary system, pancreas, and brain (Fig. 3).

Families meeting the established Amsterdam criteria are most likely to hold an inherited HNPCC gene mutation as the primary cause of the associated cancer in the family. The Amsterdam criteria (Table 4) require the presence of at least three family members with colorectal cancer, extending over at least two generations, with at least one person receiving the diagnosis before age 50 years and one affected person being a first-degree relative of the other two. As many as 70% of families meeting these criteria link to one of the known HNPCC genes. Nevertheless, because families not meeting these criteria have been found to harbor an HNPCC mutation, less restrictive guidelines, called the Amsterdam II criteria (Table 4), were established and include the characteristic clinicopathologic features of HNPCC. Lastly, the Bethesda criteria (Box 4) are primarily focused on a specific patient rather then the entire family and are the least strict of the three sets of guidelines (26).

Hereditary nonpolyposis colorectal cancer is an autosomal dominant condition that is caused by one of several DNA mismatch repair gene mutations. These genes normally function to correct DNA errors during cellular replication. The identified mismatch repair genes that mutate in HNPCC include *hMLH1*, *hMSH2*, *hPMS1*, *hPMS2*, and *hMSH6*. The replication error repair phenotype associated with HNPCC can be associated with microsatellite instability (MSI). Because these five genes do not account for the entire HNPCC syndrome, there still remain undiscovered genes, as well as possible mutations within the known inherited genes, missed with current testing methods. Nevertheless, *hMLH1* and *hMSH2* are thought to account for an estimated 70% of families with a history of HNPCC, and all five genes are now available

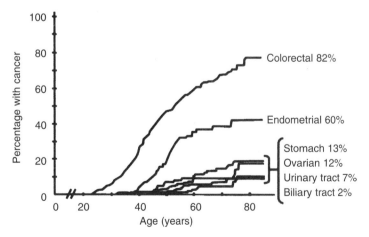

■ FIG. 3. Cancer risks in hereditary nonpolyposis colorectal cancer. Aarnio M, Sankila R, Pukkala E, Salovaara R, Aaltonen LA, de la Chapelle A, et al. Cancer risk in mutation carriers of DNA-mismatch-repair genes. Int J Cancer 1999;81:214–8. Copyright © 1999 Wiley-Liss, Inc. Reprinted with permission of Wiley-Liss, inc., a subsidiary of John Wiley & Sons, Inc.

TABLE 4. Amsterdam and Amsterdam II Criteria for the Clinical Diagnosis of Hereditary Nonpolyposis Colorectal Cancer

Amsterdam Criteria	Amsterdam II Criteria
Three or more family members, one of whom is a first-degree relative* of the other two, with a confirmed diagnosis of colorectal cancer	Three or more family members, one of whom is a first-degree relative* of the other two, with HNPCC-related cancer
Two successive affected generations	Two successive affected generations
One or more occurrences of colon cancer diagnosed before age 50 years	One or more occurrences of HNPCC-related cancer diag-before age 50 years
Exclusion of familial adenomatous polyposis	Exclusion of familial adenomatous polyposis

Abbreviation: HNPCC indicates hereditary nonpolyposis colorectal cancer.
*Parent, child, or sibling.

for clinical testing. Full gene sequencing was thought to be the best method for searching for a family mutation; however, Southern blot analysis has become commercially available and is believed to identify up to 32% of HNPCC mutations (specifically large rearrangements of *MLH1* and *MSH2*) not detectable by sequencing technology.

BOX 4

Bethesda Guidelines for Hereditary Nonpolyposis Colorectal Cancer (2004)

- Colorectal cancer diagnosis established in an individual younger than 50 years
- Presence of synchronous, metachronous colorectal, or other hereditary nonpolyposis colorectal cancer associated tumors, regardless of age
- Colorectal cancer with the microsatellite instability histology* diagnosis established in an individual younger than 60 years
- Colorectal cancer diagnosis established in one or more first-degree relatives with a hereditary nonpolyposis colorectal cancer–related tumor, with one cancer diagnosis established in an individual younger than 50 years
- Colorectal cancer diagnosis established in two or more first- or second-degree relatives of any age

*Presence of tumor-infiltrating lymphocytes, Crohn-like lymphocytic reaction, mucinous or signet-ring differentiation, or medullary growth pattern.
Umar A, Boland CR, Terdiman JP, Syngal S, de la Chapelle A, Ruschoff J, et al. Revised Bethesda Guidelines for hereditary nonpolyposis colorectal cancer (Lynch syndrome) and microsatellite instability. J Natl Cancer Inst 2004;96:261–8.

In accordance with published studies, the American Gastroenterological Association recommends the consideration of MSI testing when a person meets any of the first three Bethesda criteria (Box 4). Microsatellite instability testing is an evaluation of repeating DNA sequences in the colorectal tumor. Colorectal cancer testing positive for MSI indicates an increased probability of an HNPCC gene mutation. Approximately 80% of HNPCC colon cancer will be MSI positive, compared with only 10–15% of noninherited tumors. Therefore, because the sensitivity of MSI in HNPCC-related tumors is not 100%, HNPCC mutation analysis should still be pursued in compelling families with a history of colorectal or endometrial cancer found to be MSI negative. However, because immunohistochemistry studies of the HNPCC gene products with MSI analysis have been reported to enhance the mutation detection rate, it is a reasonable strategy to better specify the defective HNPCC gene before performing direct DNA analysis.

Screening and Follow-up of High-Risk Patients

Recommendations for colorectal cancer screening in HNPCC have been published by several authors on the basis of expert and consensus opinion. It is recommended that individuals with germline mutations start colonoscopy at age 25 years or 5 years before the youngest age at which a family member received the diagnosis of colorectal cancer—whichever comes first—and to continue this practice annually. It has been reported that colorectal screening decreases morbidity and mortality from colorectal cancer in the children of patients with HNPCC (27).

Based on the expert opinion, annual screening for endometrial cancer is recommended beginning at age 25–35 years. There is no consensus on the optimal method of screening, but choices include annual pelvic examination, endometrial aspiration, and transvaginal ultrasonography. The effectiveness of these tools remains uncertain.

Some experts have recommended screening for ovarian and genitourinary cancer when these tumors have been observed in the family, although insufficient data exist to recommend a specific regimen. Proposed methods of screening for ovarian cancer include transvaginal ultrasonography and serum CA 125 measurement as well as urine analysis for genitourinary tumors.

Chemoprevention

No chemopreventive strategies clearly have been proved to be effective in the specific setting of HNPCC. However, research focusing on cyclooxygenase-2 inhibitors, aspirin, and other nonsteroidal antiinflammatory drugs is ongoing.

Prophylactic Surgery

For patients with HNPCC who have previously received the diagnosis and been treated for colon cancer, prophylactic colectomy is a reasonable option to consider because of the high risk of metachronous colon malignancies. This surgical prophylaxis also is reasonable in carriers who received a diagnosis of adenomas at a young age or in those who are unable to undergo routine colonoscopy.

There is insufficient evidence to recommend for or against prophylactic hysterectomy and oophorectomy to reduce risk, and women who are carriers of HNPCC germline mutations should be counseled appropriately. Recently, a retrospective study identified 61 HNPCC mutation carriers who underwent prophylactic hysterectomy and 47 germline carriers who underwent prophylactic bilateral salpingo-oophorectomy (25). This cohort was then compared with 210 mutation carriers who did not undergo prophylactic hysterectomy and 223 who did not undergo prophylactic salpingo-oophorectomy. In the control group, 69 cases (33%) of endometrial cancer developed with an average of 7.4 years of follow-up, and 12 cases (5%) of ovarian cancer developed with an average of 10.6 years of follow-up. In contrast, no patients in the prophylactic group developed cancer after being monitored for an average of 13.3 years and 11.2 years, respectively. There were no cases of primary peritoneal cancer after risk-reducing surgery. While we await prospective data, prophylactic total abdominal hysterectomy with bilateral salpingo-oophorectomy at the time of colorectal surgery for individuals with HNPCC should be considered. Hereditary nonpolyposis colorectal cancer carriers should be counseled regarding the benefits and risks of prophylactic total abdominal hysterectomy with bilateral salpingo-oophorectomy after childbearing.

SOMATIC MUTATIONS AND GYNECOLOGIC CANCERS

Somatic mutations are at the core of the multistep process of tumorigenesis. Through better understanding of this process, coupled with the advancement of targeted therapies focused on specific mutations, more effective treatments are being developed. In breast cancer, the use of the monoclonal antibody trastuzumab in the management of invasive tumors that overexpress HER-2 has led to a 50% decrease in cancer recurrence in the adjuvant setting and has improved survival in stage IV disease. Avastin, a monoclonal antibody that targets the vascular endothelial growth factor receptor, has improved disease-free survival in stage IV breast cancer (28) and is being studied in early and recurrent ovarian cancer.

Gene expression profiles are being developed and used to help guide decisions related to treatment. For example, Oncotype DX is approved by the U.S. Food and Drug Administration to assess the risk of recurrence and the benefit from chemotherapy in patients with estrogen receptor–positive, node-negative breast cancer (29). MammaPrint has recently been approved by the U.S. Food and Drug Administration to assess the 10-year mortality risk from breast cancer (30). The study of epigenetics, such as hypermethylation to silence transcription of BRCA1 in sporadic ovarian cancer, is rapidly expanding and will be applied to prognostics and therapeutics (31).

References

1. Robles-Diaz L, Goldfrank DJ, Kauff ND, Robson M, Offit K. Hereditary ovarian cancer in Ashkenazi Jews. Fam Cancer 2004;3:259–64.

2. Antoniou A, Pharoah PD, Narod S, Risch HA, Eyfjord JE, Hopper JL, et al. Average risks of breast and ovarian cancer associated with BRCA1 or BRCA2 mutations detected in case series unselected for family history: a combined analysis of 22 studies [published erratum appears in Am J Hum Genet 2003;73:709]. Am J Hum Genet 2003;72:1117–30.

3. Lavie O, Hornreich G, Ben-Arie A, Rennert G, Cohen Y, Keidar R, et al. BRCA germline mutations in Jewish women with uterine serous papillary carcinoma. Gynecol Oncol 2004;92:521–4.

4. Lakhani SR, Reis-Filho JS, Filford L, Penault-Llorca F, van der Vijver M, Parry S, et al. Prediction of BRCA1 status in patients with breast cancer using estrogen receptor and basal phenotype. Breast Cancer Linkage Consortium. Clin Cancer Res 2005;11:5175–80.

5. Kandel MJ, Stadler Z, Masciari S, Collins L, Schnitt S, Harris L, et al. Prevalence of BRCA1 mutations in triple negative breast cancer (BC) [abstract]. J Clin Oncol 2006; 24(suppl):5s.

6. Cass I, Baldwin RL, Varkey T, Mosiehi R, Narod SA, Karlan BY. Improved survival in women with BRCA-associated ovarian carcinoma. Cancer 2003;97:2187–95.

7. Levine DA, Argenta PA, Yee CJ, Marshall DS, Olvera N, Bogomolniy F, et al. Fallopian tube and primary peritoneal carcinomas associated with BRCA mutations. J Clin Oncol 2003;21:4222–7.

8. Bandera CA, Muto MG, Schorge JO, Berkowitz RS, Rubin SC, Mok SC. *BRCA1* gene mutations in women with papillary serous carcinoma of the peritoneum. Obstet Gynecol 1998;92:596–600.

9. Frank TS, Deffenbaugh AM, Reid JE, Hulick M, Ward BE, Lingenfelter B, et al. Clinical characteristics of individuals with germline mutations in *BRCA1* and *BRCA2*: analysis of 10,000 individuals. J Clin Oncol 2002;20:1480–90.

10. Kriege M, Brekelmans CT, Boetes C, Besnard PE, Zonderland HM, Obdeijn IM, et al. Efficacy of MRI and mammography for breast-cancer screening in women with a familial or genetic predisposition. Magnetic Resonance Imaging Screening Study Group. N Engl J Med 2004; 351:427–37.

11. Scheuer L, Kauff N, Robson M, Kelly B, Barakat R, Satagopan J, et al. Outcome of preventive surgery and screening for breast and ovarian cancer in *BRCA* mutation carriers. J Clin Oncol 2002;20:1260–8.

12. Frost MH, Schaid DJ, Sellers TA, Slezak JM, Arnold PG, Woods JE, et al. Long-term satisfaction and psychological and social function following bilateral prophylactic mastectomy. JAMA 2000;284:319–24.

13. Kauff ND, Satagopan JM, Robson ME, Scheuer L, Hensley M, Hudis CA, et al. Risk-reducing salpingo-oophorectomy in women with a *BRCA1* or *BRCA2* mutation. N Engl J Med 2002;346:1609–15.

14. Domchek SM, Friebel TM, Neuhausen SL, Wagner T, Evans G, Isaacs C, et al. Mortality after bilateral salpingo-oophorectomy in *BRCA1* and *BRCA2* mutation carriers: a prospective cohort study. Lancet Oncol 2006;7:223–9.

15. Powell CB. Occult ovarian cancer at the time of risk-reducing salpingo-oophorectomy. Gynecol Oncol 2006;100:1–2.

16. Rebbeck TR, Lynch HT, Neuhausen SL, Narod SA, Van't Veer L, Garber JE, et al. Prophylactic oophorectomy in carriers of *BRCA1* or *BRCA2* mutations. Prevention and Observation of Surgical End Points Study Group. N Engl J Med 2002;346:1616–22.

17. Kauff ND, Domchek SM, Friebel TM, Lee JB, Roth R, Robson ME, et al. Multi-center prospective analysis of risk reducing salpingo-oophorectomy to prevent *BRCA*-associated breast and ovarian cancer [abstract]. J Clin Oncol 2006;24(suppl):49s.

18. Powell CB, Kenley E, Chen LM, Crawford, B, McLennan J, Zaloudek C, et al. Risk-reducing salpingo-oophorectomy in *BRCA* mutation carriers: role of serial sectioning in the detection of occult malignancy. J Clin Oncol 2005; 23:127–32.

19. Claes E, Evers-Kiebooms G, Boogaerts A, Decruyenaere M, Denayer L, Legius E. Diagnostic genetic testing for hereditary breast and ovarian cancer in cancer patients: women's looking back on the pre-test period and a psychological evaluation. Genet Test 2004;8:13–21.

20. Armstrong K, Schwartz JS, Randall T, Rubin SC, Weber B. Hormone replacement therapy and life expectancy after prophylactic oophorectomy in women with *BRCA*1/2 mutations: a decision analysis. J Clin Oncol 2004;22: 1045–54.

21. Gronwald J, Tung N. Foulkes WD, Offit K, Gershoni R, Daly M, et al. Tamoxifen and contralateral breast cancer in *BRCA1* and *BRCA2* carriers: an update. Hereditary Breast Cancer Clinical Study Group. Int J Cancer 2006;118: 2281–4.

22. McLaughlin JR, Risch HA, Lubinski J, Moller P, Ghadirian P, Lynch H, et al. Reproductive risk factors for ovarian cancer in carriers of *BRCA1* or *BRCA2* mutations: a case-control study. Hereditary Ovarian Cancer Clinical Study Group. Lancet Oncol 2007;8:26–34.

23. McCabe N, Turner NC, Lord CJ, Kluzek K, Bialkowska A, Swift S, et al. Deficiency in the repair of DNA damage by homologous recombination and sensitivity to poly(ADP-ribose) polymerase inhibition. Cancer Res 2006;66: 8109–15.

24. Lynch HT, de la Chapelle A. Hereditary colorectal cancer. N Engl J Med 2003;348:919–32.

25. Schmeler KM, Lynch HT, Chen LM, Munsell MF, Soliman PT, Clark MB, et al. Prophylactic surgery to reduce the risk of gynecologic cancers in the Lynch syndrome. N Engl J Med 2006;354:261–9.

26. Umar A, Boland CR, Terdiman JP, Syngal S, de la Chapelle A, Ruschoff J, et al. Revised Bethesda Guidelines for hereditary nonpolyposis colorectal cancer (Lynch syndrome) and microsatellite instability. J Natl Cancer Inst 2004;96:261–8.

27. Jarvinen HJ, Aarnio M, Mustonen H, Aktan-Collan K, Aaltonen LA, Peltomaki P, et al. Controlled 15-year trial on screening for colorectal cancer in families with hereditary nonpolyposis colorectal cancer. Gastroenterology 2000; 118:829–34.

28. Miller KD. E2100: a phase III trial of paclitaxel versus paclitaxel/bevacizumab for metastatic breast cancer. Clin Breast Cancer 2003;3:421–2.

29. Paik S, Shak S, Tang G, Kim C, Baker J, Cronin M, et al. A multigene assay to predict recurrence of tamoxifen-treated, node-negative breast cancer. N Engl J Med 2004;351: 2817–26.

30. van de Vijver MJ, He YD, van't Veer LJ, Dai H, Hart AA, Voskuil DW, et al. A gene-expression signature as a predictor of survival in breast cancer. N Engl J Med 2002;347: 1999–2009.

31. Chan KY, Ozcelik H, Cheung AN, Hgan HY, Khoo US. Epigenetic factors controlling the *BRCA1* and *BRCA2* genes in sporadic ovarian cancer. Cancer Res 2002;62: 4151–6.

Cancer of the Breast

Mary Louise Gemignani, MD

Breast cancer remains the most common type of cancer in women and is second only to lung cancer as the leading cause of cancer-related death in the United States. It is estimated that in 2008 there will be 182,460 new cases of breast cancer diagnosed in women, along with 40,480 cancer-related deaths (1). For women, the lifetime risk of developing breast cancer is 13.2% (Table 5), and the lifetime risk of dying of breast cancer is 3.6% (1 in 28). Although breast cancer remains a serious health concern, breast cancer mortality is declining in the United States and in other industrialized countries. This decline is thought to be caused by increased use of mammographic screening, early detection of breast cancer, and improved therapies.

RISK FACTORS

Patients often overestimate their own risk of developing breast cancer. Many studies report on relative risk, a ratio that depicts the likelihood over time of an event's occurrence in a study population relative to that in a reference population. It often is used to quantify risk factors for breast cancer. Absolute risk is a percentage that depicts the likelihood over time of the occurrence of an event. Several models exist to estimate a woman's risk of breast cancer. The Gail model, developed for use in the National Surgical Adjuvant Breast and Bowel Project (NSABP) Breast Cancer Prevention Trial, NSABP P-1, is available from the National Cancer Institute and measures absolute risk over time for breast cancer. However, in familial-type hereditary cases, the Gail model underestimates the risk of breast cancer by overlooking age at onset, bilaterality of disease among affected family members, and breast cancer in non–first-degree relatives. Discussion of risks with patients should be based on absolute risk assessment, not relative risk (2).

TABLE 5. Probability of Developing Breast Cancer by U.S. Women in 2001–2003

Age (years)	Risk
0–39	1 in 210
40–59	1 in 25
60–69	1 in 27
70 and older	1 in 15

Data from American Cancer Society. Cancer facts and figures 2007. Atlanta (GA): ACS; 2007. Available at: http://www.cancer.org/downloads/STT/CAFF2007PWSecured.pdf. Retrieved September 19, 2007.

Age and Family History

The incidence of breast cancer increases with age; age is the most significant risk factor (Box 5). Family history also is a significant risk factor. Hereditary types of breast cancer account for 5–10% of all types of breast cancer. Two tumor suppressor genes, *BRCA1* and *BRCA2*, have been well characterized and are thought to account for 84% of hereditary breast cancer. These genes have a high penetrance and are inherited in an autosomal dominant manner. (For a detailed discussion of hereditary breast cancer, refer to "Genetics and Gynecologic Cancer.")

History of Breast Biopsy

The number of breast biopsies a woman has undergone does not increase her risk of developing breast cancer. In contrast to the number of biopsies, the results of those biopsies may be significant. Patients with a biopsy finding of atypical ductal or lobular hyperplasia or lobular carcinoma in situ have an increased risk of developing invasive breast cancer over their lifetime.

Personal History of Breast Cancer

Women treated for breast cancer are at risk for the development of a contralateral breast cancer. Various studies have shown this risk to be between 0.5% and 1.0% per year. In addition, patients treated with breast conservation (lumpectomy and radiation therapy) are at risk for recurrence in their treated breast. In these women, this risk could be 10% or greater 10 years after treatment.

Reproductive History

Early menarche, late menopause, and nulliparity are thought to be risk factors for breast cancer. Age at first pregnancy also is thought to be a relative risk factor. Early

---

BOX 5

Factors That Affect the Risk of Breast Cancer in Women

Personal and Family History Factors With Relative Risk Greater Than 4.0
- Certain inherited genetic mutations for breast cancer
- Two or more first-degree relatives with breast cancer diagnosis received at an early age
- Personal history of breast cancer
- Age (65 years and older versus younger than 65 years, although risk increases across all ages until age 80 years)

Personal and Family History Factors With Relative Risk of 2.1–4.0
- One first-degree relative with breast cancer
- Nodular densities seen on mammogram (more than 75% of breast volume)
- Atypical hyperplasia
- High-dose ionizing radiation administered to the chest
- Ovaries not surgically removed before age 40 years

Personal and Family History Factors With Relative Risk of 1.1–2.0
- High socioeconomic status
- Urban residence
- Northern U.S. residence

Reproductive Factors That Increase Relative Risk
- Early menarche (younger than 12 years)
- Late menopause (older than 55 years)
- No full-term pregnancies (for breast cancer diagnosed at age 40 years or older)
- Late age at first full-term pregnancy (30 years or older)
- Absence of breast-feeding a child

Other Factors That Affect Circulating Hormones or Genetic Susceptibility
- Postmenopausal obesity
- Alcohol consumption
- Recent use of hormone therapy
- Recent oral contraceptive use
- Being tall
- Personal history of cancer of the endometrium, ovary, or colon
- Jewish heritage

Data from American Cancer Society. Breast cancer facts and figures 2005–2006. Atlanta (GA): ACS; 2005. Available at: http://www.cancer.org/downloads/STT/CAFF2005BrF.pdf. Retrieved September 19, 2007.

---

age at first pregnancy often is associated with a lower risk of breast cancer; pregnancy in an individual's third decade of life may reduce risk by as much as 30%. Some studies have reported breast-feeding to be protective.

It is estimated that the risk is increased by 2.8% for each additional year that a woman remains premenopausal after age 50 years (3). Bilateral oophorectomy before natural menopause has been reported to reduce the risk of breast cancer. Two recent studies reported on bilateral salpingo-oophorectomy in carriers of *BRCA1* or *BRCA2* mutations. Both studies noted the effectiveness of prophylactic oophorectomy in preventing ovarian cancer. Breast cancer risk was reduced 25–50% in the patients undergoing bilateral salpingo-oophorectomy before natural menopause (4, 5).

Exogenous Hormone Use

HORMONE THERAPY

Studies of hormone therapy (HT; combination estrogen plus progesterone therapy) have indicated an increased risk of invasive breast cancer, particularly with long duration of use (more than 10 years). Women who have received HT in the past but are not currently taking it are not at increased risk. Long-term (more than 10 years) use of HT has been associated with a relative increase in breast cancer risk, and the highest risk was noted in patients using HT with progestin (relative risk 1.41). It is thought that breast cancer that develops in HT users has a better prognosis than breast cancer that develops in postmenopausal nonusers. The tumors tend to be smaller and better differentiated with negative lymph nodes, and overall survival is better.

The results of The Women's Health Initiative were reported in 2002 (6). This trial was conducted between 1993 and 1998 and included a total of 16,609 women with an intact uterus who were randomized to receive combination HT (conjugated equine estrogen, 0.625 mg/d and medroxyprogesterone acetate, 2.5 mg/d) or placebo. The planned duration of the trial was 8.5 years; however, after a mean of 5.2 years of follow-up, the data and safety monitoring board of the committee recommended halting the trial because the incidence of invasive breast cancer had exceeded the stopping boundary that had been set at the initiation of the trial. The annual increased risk for an individual woman is still relatively small. The increased risk of breast cancer is apparent after 4 years of HT use.

ORAL CONTRACEPTIVES

Recent studies regarding oral contraceptive use and breast cancer risk have demonstrated little association with breast cancer incidence rates. One such study also found no association between women who have used oral contraceptives in the past or current users of oral contraceptives and breast cancer. The relative risk did not increase with longer periods of use or with higher doses of estrogen. Also, the use of oral contraceptives by women with a family history of breast cancer was not associated with an increased risk of breast cancer. Initiation of the use of oral contraceptives at a young age (younger than age 20 years) also did not increase the risk of developing breast cancer later in life (7). Women with significant risk of developing hereditary breast and ovarian cancer often may be advised to use oral contraceptives based on the demonstration of a protective effect (8).

Prior Exposure to Radiation Therapy

Exposure to ionizing radiation, such as in mantle irradiation to manage Hodgkin disease, poses a risk of breast cancer. This effect is noted 7–10 years after completion of radiation therapy. The cumulative probability of breast cancer at age 40 years in these women approaches 35%. The risk of breast cancer associated with radiation exposure decreases with increasing age at exposure.

Radiation therapy, however, may be used in the management of breast cancer. In conjunction with lumpectomy it is used in patients opting for breast conservation. Chest-wall irradiation after mastectomy is used with increasing frequency. Patients with large tumors (T3 lesions) and more than four positive nodes are offered chest-wall irradiation because they are at risk for local or regional failure. Chest-wall irradiation involves 50 Gy administered over the course of 5 weeks, with a 10-Gy boost to the mastectomy scar. For patients with a chest-wall recurrence, surgical debulking is followed by chest-wall irradiation.

Radiation therapy also can be used in the palliative setting. It can be used to manage metastatic lesions to the bone or brain and can help alleviate the patient's symptoms.

Ethnicity and Diet

Women of Ashkenazi Jewish descent have an increased incidence of mutation in the BRCA1 and BRCA2 genes. The incidence of carrying one of these genes is approximately 2.5% (1 in 40) in this population. These genes have an associated increase in risk of development of breast and ovarian cancer overall. (For a detailed discussion of hereditary breast cancer, see "Genetics and Gynecologic Cancer.")

Asian women have a low incidence of breast cancer. Although postmenopausal breast cancer is less common in Japanese women who have migrated to Western countries than among the general populations of these countries, after two or three generations, the incidence of breast cancer in these women approaches that of white women in the United States. The Western diet, with its increased intake of animal fat, has been implicated in studies as a risk factor. Reports have indicated that race and socioeconomic status have an adverse effect on breast cancer survival after controlling for age, stage, histology, and type of treatment. Obesity may increase the risk of developing breast cancer, particularly in postmenopausal women. A possible mechanism is the increase in endogenous estrogen caused by peripheral adipose conversion. Exercise and avoiding excessive weight gain, particularly in the postmenopausal period, is of benefit for breast cancer risk reduction.

Alcohol consumption has been reported to increase breast cancer risk in a dose-related manner. Women who ingest approximately one drink of alcohol per day have a slightly elevated risk of breast cancer over women who are nondrinkers. This risk is appreciably higher with moderate to high alcohol consumption (two to five drinks per day).

Analysis of published reports suggests that increased physical activity may reduce the risk of breast cancer. Hypothesized biologic mechanisms for this possible association include modulation of endogenous hormones, energy balance, and the immune system (9).

DOCUMENTATION

If no abnormal findings are noted on examination, it is critical to document the normal findings. The date of the last mammography, discussion of cancer screening, and plan for follow-up also should be recorded. Hormone prescriptions (for HT or oral contraceptives) should not be renewed without a documented annual breast examination and mammography, if indicated.

A great deal of litigation results from failure to diagnose breast cancer and usually involves physicians in primary care (family medicine, internal medicine, and obstetrics and gynecology). Documentation is important and should include details of procedures, the treatment plan, referrals, and follow-up (10).

MAMMOGRAPHY

The primary goal of mammography is to screen asymptomatic women to help detect breast cancer at an early stage. In general, routine screening mammography consists of a mediolateral oblique view and a craniocaudal view of each breast. With modern low-dose screening, the dose is less than 0.001 Gy (0.1 rad) per study. The effectiveness of screening varies depending on the density of the breast. Breast composition may be one of four patterns of increasing density, from almost entirely fat to extremely dense. The greater the breast density, the lower the sensitivity of mammography. It is important to note that the false-negative detection rate for mammography is 10–15% and that normal results of a mammogram do not eliminate the need for further evaluation of a breast mass.

Mammographic screening in women aged at least 40 years has reduced mortality by 20–30%. Many studies have demonstrated the efficacy of screening mammography in lowering breast cancer mortality rates. Eight large randomized trials on mammographic screening have been conducted to date. Six of the eight trials revealed a statistically significant reduction in mortality with mammographic screening. The reduction in mortality was not as evident among women aged 40–49 years as it was among women older than 50 years. The relative mortality reduction appears later in women aged 40–49 years at randomization than in women aged 50 years or older. It also is likely that the small numbers of women aged 40–49 years in the existing randomized trials may have contributed to this difference.

A published reanalysis excluded six of the eight studies because of issues related to randomization methods used and other factors in these trials (11). This reanalysis questioned the risk reduction offered by mammography. However, this review also has been criticized for the criteria used for exclusion. Much controversy resulted, and the risk reduction associated with mammography is an area of continued debate within the medical community. There are no new compelling data that would merit a change in current screening guidelines.

Screening Guidelines

For several years, the appropriate age at which to start mammographic screening has been the subject of significant debate. In 1997, the American Cancer Society (ACS) and the National Cancer Institute (NCI) modified the guidelines for mammographic screening for women aged 40–49 years, recommending regular mammography for women in this age group. The recommended intervals differ: The ACS recommends yearly mammography starting at 40 years, whereas the NCI recommends mammography every 1 or 2 years. The American College of Obstetricians and Gynecologists recommends mammography every 1–2 years for women aged 40–49 years, and annually thereafter. Annual screening mammography may start when women are younger than 40 years in a few special circumstances (Table 6).

Breast Imaging Reporting and Data System

The American College of Radiology (ACR) uses a terminology and lexicon system called the Breast Imaging Reporting and Data System (BI-RADS). This lexicon was developed in 1995 as a response to a lack of uniformity in prior mammographic terminology and to confusion regarding the probability of a malignant finding. It reports abnormalities seen on mammography with a standardized

TABLE 6. Screening Mammography Guidelines for Women Younger than 40 Years

Condition	Timing of Annual Mammography
Lobular cancer in situ or breast cancer diagnosis	At time of diagnosis
First-degree relative with premenopausal breast cancer	10 years earlier than relative's age at diagnosis, but not younger than 25 years
Mantle irradiation for Hodgkin disease*	8 years after completion of radiation therapy; consider additional screening with magnetic resonance imaging
BRCA1 or BRCA2 mutation*	Age 25–35 years; specific age chosen based on adequacy of mammographic imaging in the first study and patient choice; consider additional screening with magnetic resonance imaging

*Saslow D, Boetes C, Burke W, Harms S, Leach MO, Lehman CD, et al. American Cancer Society guidelines for breast screening with magnetic resonance imaging as an adjunct to mammography. CA Cancer J Clin 2007;57:75–89.

reporting system that leads to a fixed assessment and specific management recommendations (Table 7).

The predictors of malignancy for the BI-RADS categories are 0–2% for category 3 and approximately 98% or greater for category 5. Category 4 is less predictable. Investigators have placed the risk of malignancy for this category at approximately 30%. The ACR Task Force published a new edition of the BI-RADS classification system

TABLE 7. American College of Radiology BI-RADS Assessment Categories

BI-RADS Category	Assessment
0	Need additional imaging evaluation; assessment is incomplete
1	Negative
2	Benign finding(s)
3	Probably benign finding; initial short-interval follow-up suggested
4*	Suspicious abnormality; biopsy should be considered
5	Highly suggestive of malignancy; appropriate action should be taken
6	Known biopsy; proven malignancy; appropriate action should be taken

Abbreviation: BI-RADS indicates Breast Imaging Reporting and Data System.

*Subdividing Category 4 into 4a, 4b, and 4c encourages the indication of relevant probabilities for malignancy within this category so the patient and her physician can make an informed decision on the ultimate course of action.

Modified from American College of Radiology. Breast imaging atlas: mammography, breast ultrasound, magnetic resonance imaging: BI-RADS. 4th ed. Reston (VA): ACR; 2003. Reprinted with permission of the American College of Radiology. No other representation of this material is authorized without expressed, written permission from the American College of Radiology.

that, in particular, will attempt to provide data on category 4 in terms of risk of malignancy. In the new edition of BI-RADS, category 4 is divided into three parts (12) based on the prebiopsy risk of malignancy of the lesion—4a (small), 4b (low, medium, and high), and 4c (substantial)—in an effort to better guide clinicians and to collect meaningful data about this category. By subdividing the category, the ACR hopes to provide better communication to the referring physician about the prebiopsy risk of malignancy. Additionally, the fourth edition of the lexicon also addresses the assignment of categories to ultrasound and magnetic resonance imaging (MRI) findings. One recent retrospective study evaluated interobserver variability and positive predictive value of BI-RADS categories 4a, 4b, and 4c. The risk of malignancy was found to be 6%, 15%, and 53%, respectively (13).

Diagnostic Mammography

Abnormalities found on mammographic screening may need further evaluation with additional mammography or other imaging modalities, such as ultrasonography or MRI. In some screening programs, the radiologist reviews mammograms as the test is being performed, and if additional views are needed, they are obtained the same day. In several studies, the frequency of calling for additional views has ranged from 5% to 11%.

Lesions Identified on Mammography

A description of the shape and margins of a lesion seen on a mammogram is important (Figure 4). The highest frequency of carcinoma is found in lesions with an irregular shape or spiculated borders, and carcinoma often is associated with pleomorphic calcifications that appear discontinuous and linear. This discontinuous linear pattern suggests the irregular filling of a duct with malignant cells.

Microcalcifications are described on the basis of morphology and distribution. They may be scattered or clus-

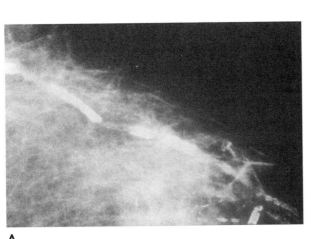 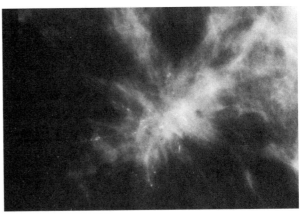

A   B

■ **FIG. 4.** Microcalcifications. **A.** Vascular calcifications. **B.** Pleomorphic microcalcifications associated with architectural distortion.

tered, coarse or fine, old or new. Microcalcifications can appear benign if they are large, coarse, vascular, like milk of calcium (calcium in cysts), or popcornlike (as seen with fibroadenomas). Intermediate calcifications usually are round or shaped like snowflakes and small or hazy. The calcifications with a higher probability of malignancy are pleomorphic or heterogeneous, varying in size and shape. They usually are fine (smaller than 0.5 mm) and may appear linear, branching, and discontinuous (Table 8). Other associated findings also are reported:

- Skin or nipple retraction
- Skin or trabecular thickening
- Skin lesions
- Axillary adenopathy

BREAST ULTRASONOGRAPHY AND MAGNETIC RESONANCE IMAGING

Breast ultrasonography can be used to distinguish between solid and cystic masses in the breast. It can be used to evaluate a focal mass identified on a mammogram or a palpable mass. It also is used as an adjuvant for biopsy. Because of its low specificity, breast ultrasonography is not thought to be a good modality for screening. It cannot replace mammography, as it has no ability to detect microcalcifications. Ultrasonography can complement mammography in young women with dense breasts (which limits the accuracy of mammography).

Magnetic resonance imaging has a high sensitivity (86–100%) in the diagnosis of breast cancer, but a relatively low specificity (37–97%). It is an expensive test that requires an intravenous contrast medium, and the technology for performing biopsy under MRI guidance is not widely available. Current uses include evaluation of breast implants for rupture, evaluation of pectoralis involvement with extensive breast cancer, and evaluation of postlumpectomy bed fibrosis. The use of MRI also may include evaluation of occult breast cancers and evaluation of multifocal disease in patients considering breast conservation.

Studies on the use of MRI for surveillance of women at high risk for hereditary breast cancer have been published recently. In one study, the authors compared breast MRI results with the results of mammographic, screening ultrasound, and physical examination in 196 women at high risk for developing breast cancer (those with proven mutations in the *BRCA* genes or strong family histories of breast cancer, ovarian cancer, or both). Six cases of invasive cancer were found, including two cases of cancer not identified through other modalities (ie, mammography, ultrasonography, or physical examination) (14). A study of 236 women with *BRCA* mutations and MRI in conjunction with mammographic screening and clinical breast examination detected 22 cases of cancer; 77% were detected by MRI, with 32% detected by MRI alone (15).

Women at high risk of developing breast cancer may benefit from additional screening modalities in conjunction with mammographic screening. Women who are deemed to be at high risk of developing breast cancer, such as women with *BRCA* mutations or a strong family history of breast cancer, ovarian cancer, or both, have been shown to benefit from MRI screening. Recently, the ACS issued guidelines for the use of MRI screening in addition to mammography for high-risk patients. The ACS recommended MRI screening for women with an approximately 20–25% or greater lifetime risk of breast cancer. It included women with a strong family history of breast or ovarian cancer, women who were treated for Hodgkin disease, and *BRCA* mutation carriers as those who would benefit from MRI screening. For other subgroups of women, such as women with a personal history of breast cancer, lobular carcinoma in situ, atypical hyperplasia, or extremely dense breasts on mammography, the panel felt the existing evidence was not sufficient to recommend for or against MRI screening (16).

Digital Mammography

In 1991, the NCI convened a panel of experts on breast imaging. The panel placed high priority on the development of digital mammography. Four full-field systems were developed and underwent U.S. Food and Drug Administration testing. The benefits of digital mammography over traditional film mammography concern image acquisition and facilitation of storage. In addition, digital image processing allows manipulation of image contrast and may enhance subtle contrast differences.

Pilot studies and U.S. Department of Defense full-field digital mammography screening trials of digital mammography compared with conventional film mammography have found that the two modalities are similar in terms of the number of cancers diagnosed. The investigators noted that although the diagnostic accuracy of digital and

TABLE 8. Lesions Identified on Mammography

Mammographic Lesion	Description
Mass	Space-occupying lesion in two views; shape and density important
Microcalcification	Presence of calcium; shape, number, and distribution important
Asymmetry	Comparative differences in breast density
Architectural distortion	Spicules with no central mass visible

film mammography was similar, the accuracy of digital mammography was better in women younger than 50 years, women with radiographically dense breasts, and premenopausal or perimenopausal women (17). Thus, in women who met these criteria, the investigators recommended digital mammography. When both technologies are available, the use of digital mammography can be tailored to the individual (18).

With ongoing research into this new technology, new adjuvant technologies may be developed. For example, telemammography will make telemedicine consultations possible. Computer-aided diagnosis may facilitate second opinions for digital mammographic studies.

DIAGNOSTIC EVALUATION

All patients with a mass should undergo bilateral mammography. Besides providing valuable information about the characteristics of the mass, mammography will screen the normal surrounding breast and the contralateral breast for nonpalpable mammographic abnormalities (densities or calcifications). Evaluation of a palpable mass is important to determine whether it is cancerous, even if the mammography results are normal.

Fine-Needle Aspiration or Biopsy

Fine-needle aspiration can be extremely useful in the evaluation of a palpable breast mass. It can differentiate between solid and cystic masses.

If the lesion is not cystic or is suspected of being solid, fine-needle aspiration can be performed. The procedure requires a cytopathologist experienced in breast pathology. The false-negative rate can range from 3% to 35%, depending on the expertise of the aspirator and the cytopathologist, the size of the lesion, the location within the breast, and the cellular composition of the lesion. Normal findings of fine-needle aspiration in the presence of a mass suggestive of abnormalities should not preclude further diagnostic evaluation. A finding of atypical cells on fine-needle aspiration warrants a surgical biopsy.

The false-positive rate of fine-needle aspiration is less than 1%. In the United States, however, definitive surgical treatment is not performed on the basis of a fine-needle aspiration alone; tissue diagnosis is preferred before definitive surgery.

Image-Guided Percutaneous Breast Biopsy

Image-guided percutaneous breast biopsy increasingly is being used as an alternative to surgical biopsy. This technique is less invasive than surgical excision, and because less tissue is removed, the method results in less scarring seen on subsequent mammograms. Regardless of whether the lesion is diagnosed as benign or malignant, patients who have percutaneous biopsies undergo fewer operations, and management can be streamlined.

The choice of which image-guided modality to use depends on the lesion. Stereotactic biopsy is best for calcifications. If a lesion is seen on ultrasonography, it is best to use that modality, as it is easier to use and has been reported to be less costly. Available tissue-acquisition devices include fine needles, automated core needles, directional vacuum-assisted probes, and biopsy cannulas. Most centers use larger (14-gauge) tissue-acquisition devices instead of fine needles because tissue diagnosis is more accurate when a larger volume of tissue is obtained.

Accurate placement of a localizing clip through the biopsy probe is necessary to facilitate any needed subsequent localization. If atypia is noted on a core biopsy, a surgical excision of the area is recommended because it is thought that there is a 50% chance of finding a coexistent carcinoma.

Surgical Excision for Breast Biopsy

A biopsy can be performed on an outpatient basis using local anesthesia in most patients. It is important to choose the appropriate incision and location. Unless the lesion is close to the nipple or suspected of being a fibroadenoma, the incision should be made in proximity to the mass and not be circumareolar. The surgeon should keep in mind the possibility of subsequent mastectomy when making the incision. Many times, the biopsy is part of the treatment. The specimen should be adequately oriented for margin analysis by the pathologist and tested for the appropriate markers, such as estrogen receptor status, progesterone receptor status, and *HER-2/neu*.

PATHOLOGIC EVALUATION

Ductal Carcinoma In Situ

Ductal carcinoma in situ is an abnormal proliferation of malignant epithelial cells within the mammary ductal–lobular system without invasion into the surrounding stroma (Fig. 5). It is classified as a heterogenous group of lesions with different growth patterns and cytologic features. Classification of ductal carcinoma in situ traditionally has been based on architectural patterns. The most common types are comedo, cribriform, micropapillary, papillary, and solid.

Paget disease is involvement of the nipple with intraductal carcinoma. In the absence of a palpable mass, invasive carcinoma occurs in less than 40% of cases. The diagnosis is determined by a nipple biopsy.

Lobular Carcinoma In Situ

Lobular carcinoma in situ (Fig. 6) is a noninvasive lesion characterized by a solid proliferation of small cells with round to oval nuclei that distorts the involved spaces in the

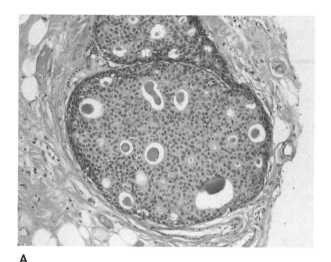

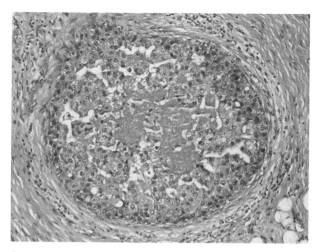

A   **B**

■ **FIG. 5.** Ductal carcinoma in situ. **A**. Low grade. **B**. High grade.

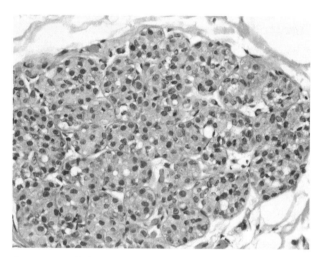

■ **FIG. 6.** Lobular carcinoma in situ.

terminal duct–lobular units. It is usually an incidental microscopic finding that is not detected clinically or by gross pathologic examination. It often is multicentric, and it is a risk factor for breast cancer. The cancer that develops may be ductal or lobular, and the risk is the same for both breasts.

Invasive Cancer

There are two types of invasive cancer of the breast: ductal and lobular. Invasive ductal carcinoma is the most common group and makes up 65–80% of all mammary carcinomas. Included in this group are special subtypes: tubular, medullary, metaplastic, mucinous (colloid) papillary, and adenoid cystic carcinoma. Infiltrating lobular carcinoma has been reported to constitute 10–14% of invasive carcinomas. The cells tend to grow circumferentially around ducts and lobules and have a linear arrangement referred to as "Indian file."

INFLAMMATORY CARCINOMA

Inflammatory carcinoma is characterized by cutaneous findings present with an underlying invasive carcinoma. Usually the invasive tumor is a poorly differentiated infiltrating ductal carcinoma. Upon microscopic evaluation, skin involvement often reveals tumor emboli in dermal lymphatics with an associated lymphocytic reaction in the dermis. Often this diagnosis is clinical.

METASTASES FROM EXTRAMAMMARY TUMORS

The most common primary site of an occult extramammary tumor is the lung. Other primary sites include the ovaries, uterus, kidneys, and stomach. The most common sites of previously diagnosed extramammary tumors are melanomas and the prostate, cervix, uterus, and urinary bladder. Often, identification of an in situ component helps provide definitive evidence of a mammary origin (19).

BIOLOGIC MARKERS AND PROGNOSTIC FACTORS

Axillary Lymph Node Status

The most important prognostic factor is nodal status. The presence of metastasis to the lymph nodes, as well as the number of lymph nodes involved, is significant and correlates with local failure and distant metastases. Nodal status is predictive of overall survival. Patients with positive nodes have a worse prognosis than patients with negative nodes. The highest risk of local and distant disease recurrence exists in patients with more than three positive nodes. However, patients with one to three positive nodes may be at an increased risk for local recurrence. Current trials in the use of adjuvant irradiation in these patients, particularly patients who underwent mastectomy, are under way (20).

Tumor Size and Histologic Grade

Tumor size correlates with the incidence of lymph node metastasis. The size of the tumor is important even in the absence of lymph node involvement, however. Patients with tumors smaller than 1 cm or with tumors with good histologic types that measure less than 3 cm do well. Histologic grade also correlates with breast cancer outcome. Poorly differentiated tumors have been associated with more aggressive behavior.

Estrogen and Progesterone Receptors

Hormone receptors can be measured by immunohistochemical studies using monoclonal antibodies directed against them. Positivity correlates with response to antihormonal agents. Two thirds of breast cancer cases are hormone receptor positive, a characteristic that correlates with an overall better prognosis. Recently genomic tests, such as Oncotype DX, are used to predict recurrence, prognosis, and therapeutic response in node-negative, estrogen receptor–positive breast cancers (21).

In patients with metastatic disease, antihormonal therapy, including tamoxifen or aromatase inhibitors, provides 20% response rates. Antihormonal therapy is less toxic than chemotherapy and provides excellent first-line agents for patients with metastatic disease in whom disease stabilization is the goal of therapy. Additionally, in young women with metastatic estrogen receptor–positive cancer, estrogen blockade—either surgical (bilateral oophorectomy) or medical—can offer disease stabilization.

HER-2/neu

HER-2/neu is an oncogene whose protein product may function as a growth factor receptor. It can be detected by an immunohistochemical demonstration of the protein product or by gene amplification. Overexpression or amplification has been shown to correlate with a poor prognosis; however, the studies differ with regard to the method of detection used, as well as the interpretation of results.

p53 Protein

The protein product of the tumor suppressor gene p53 is a nuclear transcription factor with many functions, including regulation of the cell cycle and apoptosis. Most clinical studies have used immunohistochemistry to study protein expression. An accumulation of p53 protein has been reported to correlate with reduced survival in some studies.

STAGING

Staging of breast cancer uses the tumor–node–metastasis system. The American Joint Committee on Cancer determines staging using a clinical and pathologic staging system based on the tumor–node–metastasis system. The 1997 version allows the inclusion of all information available before the first definitive treatment, including operative findings and pathologic information (Table 9).

TREATMENT

Surgical Treatment

Mastectomy encompasses removal of the breast, and in the case of the modified radical mastectomy, removal of the axillary nodal contents. The improvement in irradiation techniques and interest in preservation of the breast led to breast-conservation therapy. Six randomized trials in patients with stage I and stage II carcinoma of the breast have compared breast-conservation therapy with radical or modified radical mastectomy.

In breast-conserving surgery, a wide local excision is performed, along with excision of the tumor and a 1–2-cm rim of normal tissue (a lumpectomy). This procedure differs from a quadrantectomy, which involves a resection of the tumor with the overlying skin and the involved quadrant of the breast. In the trials, there was comparable disease-free survival in patients undergoing mastectomy and breast conservation; the only difference was in local recurrence. Many other nonrandomized trials report results similar to the randomized trials.

In 1990, a consensus development conference on early-stage breast cancer convened by the NCI concluded that breast-conservation therapy is equivalent to mastectomy and provides similar overall survival. It stated that breast-conservation therapy is preferable because it preserves the breast (22).

Cosmetic results should be considered when deciding whether to offer breast-conserving surgery; tumor size in relation to breast size is an important consideration. In addition, consideration must be given to other factors that may affect the ability to receive radiation therapy (eg, history of prior breast or chest irradiation, concurrent pregnancy, or autoimmune connective tissue disease). Women with multiple cancer in the breast are not candidates for this approach and require a mastectomy. In addition, when mammography has detected extensive calcifications suggesting a diffuse process, the patient may be better treated with mastectomy.

The status of negative margins at the time of lumpectomy remains controversial. Generally, a re-excision should be performed if the margins are not negative. An extensive intraductal component exists when more than 25% of the tumor is associated with ductal carcinoma in situ. In these cases, the invasive component may be outside the area of the intraductal carcinoma. This finding has been reported to be associated with a higher relapse rate with breast-conservation therapy; however, this higher relapse rate is thought to be secondary to the difficulty in obtaining clear margins and may indicate the presence of residual intraductal carcinoma in patients with involved margins (23).

TABLE 9. Tumor–Node–Metastasis Staging of Breast Cancer

Classification	Clinical Characteristics
Primary Tumor (T)	

Definitions for classifying the primary tumor (T) are the same for clinical and pathologic classification. If the measurement is made by physical examination, the examiner will use the major headings (T1, T2, or T3). If other measurements, such as mammographic or pathologic measurements, are used, the subsets of T1 can be used. Tumors should be measured to the nearest 0.1-cm increment.

Classification	Clinical Characteristics
TX	Primary tumor cannot be assessed
T0	No evidence of primary tumor
Tis	Carcinoma in situ
Tis (DCIS)	Ductal carcinoma in situ
Tis (LCIS)	Lobular carcinoma in situ
Tis (Paget)	Paget disease of the nipple with no tumor

Note: Paget disease associated with a tumor is classified according to the size of the tumor.

Classification	Clinical Characteristics
T1	Tumor 2 cm or less in greatest dimension
T1mic	Microinvasion 0.1 cm or less in greatest dimension
T1a	Tumor more than 0.1 cm but not more than 0.5 cm in greatest dimension
T1b	Tumor more than 0.5 cm but not more than 1 cm in greatest dimension
T1c	Tumor more than 1 cm but not more than 2 cm in greatest dimension
T2	Tumor more than 2 cm but not more than 5 cm in greatest dimension
T3	Tumor more than 5 cm in greatest dimension
T4	Tumor of any size with direct extension to a) chest wall or b) skin, only as described below
T4a	Extension to chest wall, not including pectoralis muscle
T4b	Edema (including *peau d'orange*) or ulceration of the skin of the breast, or satellite skin nodules confined to the same breast
T4c	Both T4a and T4b
T4d	Inflammatory carcinoma

Regional Lymph Nodes (N)
Clinical

Classification	Clinical Characteristics
NX	Regional lymph nodes cannot be assessed (for example, they were previously removed)
N0	No regional lymph node metastasis
N1	Metastasis to movable ipsilateral axillary lymph node(s)

Regional Lymph Nodes (N) (continued)

Classification	Clinical Characteristics
N2	Metastasis in ipsilateral axillary lymph nodes fixed or matted, or in clinically apparent* ipsilateral mammary nodes in the absence of clinically evident axillary lymph node metastasis
N2a	Metastasis in ipsilateral axillary lymph nodes fixed to one another (matted) or to other structures
N2b	Metastasis only in clinically apparent* ipsilateral internal mammary nodes and in the absence of clinically evident axillary lymph node metastasis
N3	Metastasis in ipsilateral infraclavicular lymph node(s) with or without axillary lymph node involvement, or in clinically apparent* ipsilateral internal mammary/lymph node(s) and in the presence of clinically evident axillary lymph node metastasis; or metastasis in ipsilateral supraclavicular lymph node(s) with or without axillary or internal mammary involvement
N3a	Metastasis in ipsilateral infraclavicular lymph node(s)
N3b	Metastasis in ipsilateral internal mammary lymph node(s) and axillary lymph node(s)
N3c	Metastasis in ipsilateral supraclavicular lymph node(s)

Pathologic (pN)†

Classification	Clinical Characteristics
pNX	Regional lymph nodes cannot be assessed (for example, they were previously removed, or not removed for pathologic study)
pN0	No regional lymph node metastasis histologically; no additional examination for isolated tumor cells

Note: Isolated tumor cells are defined as single tumor cells or small cell clusters not greater than 0.2 mm that usually are detected only by immunohistochemical or molecular methods but that may be verified on hematoxylineosin stains. Isolated tumor cells do not usually show evidence of malignant activity (for example, proliferation or stromal reaction).

Classification	Clinical Characteristics
pN0(i–)	No regional lymph node metastasis determined histologically, negative immunohistochemistry findings
pN0(i+)	No regional lymph node metastasis determined histologically, positive immunohistochemistry findings, no immunohistochemistry cluster greater than 0.2 mm

(continued)

TABLE 9. Tumor–Node–Metastasis Staging of Breast Cancer (continued)

Classification	Clinical Characteristics	Classification	Clinical Characteristics
			of axillary lymph node metastasis
Pathologic (pN)† (continued)		pN2a	Metastasis in four to nine axillary lymph nodes (at least one tumor deposit greater than 2 mm)
pN0(mol–)	No regional lymph node metastasis determined histologically, negative molecular findings (RT-PCR)	pN2b	Metastasis in clinically apparent* internal mammary lymph nodes in the absence of axillary lymph node metastasis
pN0(mol+)	No regional lymph node metastasis determined histologically, positive molecular findings (RT-PCR)	pN3	Metastasis in 10 or more axillary lymph nodes, or in infraclavicular lymph nodes, or in clinically apparent* ipsilateral internal mammary lymph nodes in the presence of one or more positive axillary lymph nodes; or in more than three axillary lymph nodes with clinically negative microscopic metastasis in internal mammary lymph nodes; or in ipsilateral supraclavicular lymph nodes
pN1	Metastasis in one to three axillary lymph nodes or in internal mammary nodes or both with microscopic disease detected by sentinel lymph node dissection but not clinically apparent‡		
pN1mi	Micrometastasis (greater than 0.2 mm, none greater than 2 mm)		
pN1a	Metastasis in one to three axillary lymph nodes		
pN1b	Metastasis in internal mammary nodes with microscopic disease detected by sentinel lymph node dissection but not clinically apparent‡	pN3a	Metastasis in 10 or more axillary lymph nodes (at least one tumor deposit greater than 2 mm) or metastasis to the infraclavicular lymph nodes
pN1c	Metastasis in one to three axillary lymph nodes and in internal mammary lymph nodes with microscopic disease detected by sentinel lymph node dissection but not clinically apparent‡ (if associated with more than three positive axillary lymph nodes, the internal mammary nodes are classified as pN3b to reflect increased tumor burden)	pN3b	Metastasis in clinically apparent* ipsilateral internal mammary lymph nodes in the presence of one or more positive axillary lymph nodes or in more than three axillary lymph nodes and in internal mammary lymph nodes with microscopic disease detected by sentinel lymph node dissection but not clinically apparent‡
		pN3c	Metastasis in ipsilateral supraclavicular lymph nodes
		Distant Metastasis (M)	
pN2	Metastasis in four to nine axillary lymph nodes, or in clinically apparent* internal mammary lymph nodes in the absence	MX	Distant metastasis cannot be assessed
		M0	No distant metastasis

Abbreviations: RT-PCR indicates reverse transcriptase/polymerase chain reaction.

*Clinically apparent is defined as detected by imaging studies (excluding lymphoscintigraphy) or by clinical examination or grossly visible pathologically.

†Classification is based on axillary lymph node dissection with or without sentinel lymph node dissection. Classification based solely on sentinel lymph node dissection without subsequent axillary lymph node dissection is designated (sn) for "sentinel node;" for example, pN0(i+)(sn).

‡Not clinically apparent is defined as not detected by imaging studies (excluding lymphoscintigraphy) or by clinical examination.

Singletary, S.E., et al. Breast. In: Greene, F.L., Page, D.L., Fleming, I.D., et al., editors. AJCC Cancer Staging Manual, Sixth Edition. New York: Springer, 2002: 227–228. Used with the permission of the American Joint Committee on Cancer (AJCC), Chicago, Illinois. The original source for this material is the AJCC Cancer Staging Manual, Sixth Edition (2002) published by Springer Science and Business Media LLC, www.springerlink.com.

Interest in partial-breast irradiation for early-stage breast cancers has prompted single-institution studies on the use of brachytherapy catheters, the MammoSite Balloon (Proxima Co, Alpharetta, GA), and three-dimensional external-beam partial-breast treatment. These approaches may be an alternative to the standard 5–6-week whole-breast irradiation treatment. To shorten the irradiation course, the proportion of breast tissue to be irradiated is significantly less. Data on local recurrences after irradiation show that most recurrences after lumpectomy and whole-breast irradiation occur in the same quadrant—thus the reason to consider partial-breast irradiation. The National Surgical Adjuvant Breast and Bowel Project and Radiation Therapy Oncology Group cooperative groups are conducting a phase 3 trial comparing whole-breast radiation therapy to some form of partial-breast irradiation.

Axillary Lymphadenectomy

The status of the axilla is the most important prognostic factor for patients with breast cancer. Metastatic involvement of lymph nodes usually occurs in a stepwise manner. The incidence of "skip metastasis" is less than 2%. The use of axillary lymphadenectomy has been demonstrated to decrease local recurrence significantly, which ultimately may translate into a survival advantage. The National Surgical Adjuvant Breast and Bowel Project B-04 trial randomized patients with clinically negative nodes to one of three groups: radical mastectomy, total mastectomy with nodal irradiation, or total mastectomy alone. If recurrence occurred, survival was lower overall among patients who had no axillary nodal therapy (24).

The morbidity associated with axillary lymphadenectomy is not inconsequential. Approximately 10–15% of patients will develop lymphedema. In addition, numbness, pain, and weakness contribute to a significant decrease in the quality of life in these patients. Clinical examination of the axilla is inaccurate, because even in patients with a T1 lesion, there is a 10% risk of lymph node metastasis. Before the use of sentinel lymph node biopsy, there was no accurate method to stage the axilla adequately without an axillary lymphadenectomy.

Sentinel Lymph Node Biopsy

Sentinel lymph node biopsy in patients with breast cancer evolved from efforts to minimize the morbidity associated with axillary lymphadenectomy while still providing important staging information. In most studies, successful identification of the sentinel lymph node occurs between 92% and 98% of the time. The combination of blue dye and isotope has been reported to be better for identification of the sentinel lymph node; when used in combination, the positive predictive value of the technique approaches 100%, with a negative predictive value close to 95%. The false-negative rate is approximately 5–10% in most studies.

Greater scrutiny must be paid to sentinel lymph nodes through serial sectioning and immunohistochemical stains. This scrutiny is possible because only a few sentinel lymph nodes are obtained at the time of the procedure. It would not be cost-effective in a standard axillary lymphadenectomy, which yields an average of 20 nodes. Generally, a completion axillary lymphadenectomy is performed in patients who have positive sentinel nodes. There is considerable controversy as to whether a completion axillary lymphadenectomy should be performed in patients with micrometastatic disease (less than 2 mm in size) in the sentinel node.

Systemic Treatment

Multiple randomized studies have demonstrated that the addition of chemotherapy improves overall survival in patients with breast cancer. The decision to use adjuvant chemotherapy or hormone therapy depends on factors such as the size of the primary tumor, the expression or lack of expression of estrogen receptors or progesterone receptors, lymph node status, and the presence or absence of metastatic disease.

Adjuvant chemotherapy is standard treatment for patients with positive nodes or large tumors. The question of whether to use the combination of cyclophosphamide, methotrexate, and 5-fluorouracil or the combination of 5-fluorouracil, doxorubicin, and cyclophosphamide in high-risk patients (patients with tumors that are at least 2 cm or that are estrogen receptor negative or progesterone receptor negative with receptor-negative nodes) has been addressed. Although the anthracycline regimen is more toxic than the combination of cyclophosphamide, methotrexate, and 5-fluorouracil, recent trials have demonstrated its superiority. Determining whether to use fluorouracil, doxorubicin, and cyclophosphamide also is based on other factors. Tumors with *HER-2/neu* overexpression have an associated increased response rate with an anthracycline-based therapy.

The use of taxanes such as docetaxel and paclitaxel as adjuvant treatment, in combination with anthracycline-based chemotherapy, is being investigated. Several randomized trials have been conducted to test the feasibility and effectiveness of anthracycline or taxanes administered in a dose-dense fashion. Dose density refers to the frequency of administration of a drug or regimen compared with standard regimens. These trials have resulted in an overall modest, beneficial impact on disease recurrence in patients with early breast cancer (25). The most benefit was seen in patients with node-positive disease or hormone receptor–negative tumors and *HER-2/neu* overexpression. The Cancer and Leukemia Group B trial 9741 compared concurrent and sequential regimens in patients with node-positive breast cancer. In the trial's 2×2 factorial design, the regimens consisted of four concurrent cycles of doxorubicin and cyclophosphamide, followed by four cycles of paclitaxel in regimens given every 2 weeks and every 3 weeks. This treatment was compared with sequential treatment consisting of four cycles of doxorubicin, followed by four cycles of paclitaxel and four cycles of cyclophosphamide in regimens given every 2 weeks and every 3 weeks. The dose-dense (biweekly) treatment significantly improved disease-free survival and overall survival compared with the every-3-weeks regimen. There was no difference between sequential and concurrent schedules (26).

The use of trastuzumab in addition to combination chemotherapy also has been shown to cause a decrease in relapse in *HER-2/neu*–positive breast cancer cases. Recently, *HER-2/neu* has been used as a predictor of response to certain chemotherapeutic agents (ie, doxorubicin-based therapy). Trastuzumab is a humanized anti-*HER-2* antibody against the extracellular domain of the

2-neu oncoprotein. Its use in the metastatic setting has been reported to demonstrate an increase in response rate and a prolongation of disease-free and overall survival (27).

Four major trials—Herceptin Adjuvant, National Surgical Adjuvant Breast and Bowel Project B-31, North Central Cancer Treatment Group N9831, and Breast Cancer International Research Group 006—have investigated the use of trastuzumab in the adjuvant setting. These trials have shown that trastuzumab reduces the 3-year risk of recurrence by approximately 50% in this population. More than 13,000 women with *HER-2/neu*–positive breast cancers were enrolled and received 1 year of adjuvant treatment with trastuzumab. These trials used different chemotherapy regimens, but they had similar improvements in recurrence-free survival. Cardiac events were at an acceptable level; however, the trials did note a slightly higher (0.6–3.3%) incidence of congestive heart failure that was responsive to treatment. There was an overall survival benefit in the National Surgical Adjuvant Breast and Bowel Project B-31 and the North Central Cancer Treatment Group N9831 trials, and a trend toward an overall survival benefit in the Herceptin Adjuvant and the Breast Cancer International Research Group trials (28).

Recently, lapatinib in combination with capecitabine was approved by the U.S. Food and Drug Administration for the treatment of patients with advanced or metastatic breast cancer whose tumors overexpress *HER-2* and who have received previous therapy, including an anthracycline, a taxane, and trastuzumab.

Postmenopausal women with negative nodes and estrogen receptor–negative tumors larger than 1 cm also are considered for chemotherapy. In these patients, the combination of cyclophosphamide, methotrexate, and 5-fluorouracil usually is the treatment chosen.

Neoadjuvant Chemotherapy

Preoperative or neoadjuvant chemotherapy is attractive because it may reduce the amount of disease present and thereby help obtain surgical clean margins when the disease is still confined to the breast. Thus, in inflammatory breast cancer or N2 disease, neoadjuvant chemotherapy may improve surgical resectability. A significant response of 50–90% has been seen with this approach.

There was no difference in overall survival, however, between patients who received preoperative chemotherapy and patients who received postoperative chemotherapy. Several subsequent trials have reported a higher local recurrence rate for patients treated with neoadjuvant chemotherapy and breast conserving therapy.

Adjuvant Therapy

At the November 2000 National Institutes of Health Consensus Development Conference for Adjuvant Therapy for Breast Cancer, a consensus was reached regarding the use of adjuvant therapy in breast cancer. The published conclusions are listed in Box 6.

Tamoxifen is used as adjuvant hormonal treatment in premenopausal women with breast cancers that are estrogen receptor positive and progesterone receptor positive. Aromatase inhibitors are used as an alternative to tamoxifen in the adjuvant setting in postmenopausal, hormone-positive patients. Three double-blind, randomized, prospective studies—the Arimidex, Tamoxifen, Alone or in Combination Trial (ATAC); the Intergroup Exemestane Study; and the MA-17 trial—have confirmed the superiority of aromatase inhibitors over tamoxifen in the management of early-stage cancer in postmenopausal women (29–31). All three studies have demonstrated an increase

BOX 6

Guidelines for the Use of Adjuvant Therapy for Breast Cancer

- The use of adjuvant hormone therapy should be based on the presence of hormone-receptor protein in tumor tissues.
- Adjuvant polychemotherapy should be recommended to women with localized breast cancer regardless of lymph node, menopausal, or hormone-receptor status, because it improves survival.
- The inclusion of anthracycline chemotherapy in adjuvant chemotherapy has an associated small, but statistically significant, improvement in survival compared with regimens that do not contain anthracycline.
- Available data are inconclusive regarding the use of taxanes in node-positive disease.
- The use of adjuvant dose-intensive chemotherapy regimens in patients with high-risk breast cancer, and of taxanes in patients with lymph node–negative breast cancer, should be restricted to randomized studies.
- Women with a high risk of local recurrence will benefit from radiation therapy after mastectomy. This finding applies to women with four or more positive nodes or advanced primary cancer. In women with one to three positive nodes, the benefits of the use of postmastectomy irradiation are uncertain and should be tested in randomized controlled trials.
- Quality of life should be evaluated in selected randomized trials to examine the impact of the major short- and long-term adverse effects of adjuvant treatments.

The National Institutes of Health Consensus Development Conference: Adjuvant Therapy for Breast Cancer. Bethesda, Maryland, USA. November 1–3, 2000. Proceedings. J Natl Cancer Inst Monogr. 2001;30:1–152.

in disease-free survival. Short-term adverse effects were acceptable, but all had a negative impact on bone health. Based on the results of these trials, patients who are postmenopausal have the option of starting anastrozole as first-line therapy after initial diagnosis. Patients who have used tamoxifen for 2–3 years can start taking an aromatase inhibitor to complete a total of 5 years of therapy. Patients who have completed 5 years of tamoxifen have the option of receiving no further therapy or taking letrozole. The optimal duration of letrozole in this setting has not been defined.

Breast Reconstruction

Breast reconstruction represents a major advance in cancer rehabilitation for patients undergoing a mastectomy. Immediate reconstruction has not interfered with disease detection and has the advantage of combining the two procedures into one. A delayed reconstruction can be performed if the patient is ambivalent about the reconstruction or if prolonged anesthesia would increase operative risk. It also is considered in patients with locally advanced disease if the reconstruction would delay adjuvant radiation therapy or chemotherapy.

Reconstruction options include expandable breast prostheses (implants) and autologous tissue transfer. Tissue transfer operations may yield the greatest symmetry between breasts, especially in patients with larger breasts; however, they take longer, require greater surgical expertise, involve a longer recovery, and create another scar at the donor site (the latissimus dorsi, transverse rectus abdominis, or gluteal muscle).

Special Issues

Patients with a genetic predisposition to breast cancer often ask about risk reduction. Many of these patients are young women. Appropriate counseling is important, because these women often experience regret after pro-

phylactic mastectomy. This procedure has been reported to have a risk reduction rate of approximately 90% in larger studies. However, this reduction often relates to the type of mastectomy performed (for example, subcutaneous mastectomy may not remove all breast tissue).

Participation in a screening program is another option. Many women considering prophylactic mastectomy are young and have dense breasts on mammography. The use of additional screening modalities, such as bilateral breast ultrasonography or MRI, should be considered. Breast self-examination and clinical breast examinations are other options (Table 10).

These women also are at risk of developing ovarian cancer, and prophylactic oophorectomy at approximately age 40 years is a risk-reducing option. In addition, prophylactic oophorectomy in women younger than 40 years has been reported to decrease the risk of breast cancer significantly. Even prophylactic risk-reducing salpingo-oophorectomy, however, does not exclude the risk of primary peritoneal cancer, which is estimated at 2% (5). Ovarian cancer screening programs now use serum CA 125 measurements and pelvic ultrasonography. Ovarian cancer screening is not recommended for the general population, however, because of the low specificity of the available tools. Women with a genetic predisposition to breast cancer also are candidates for chemoprevention (see "Genetics and Gynecologic Cancer").

References

1. American Cancer Society. Cancer facts and figures 2008. Atlanta (GA): ACS; 2008. Available at: http://www.cancer.org/downloads/STT/2008CAFFfinalsecured.pdf. Retrieved February 20, 2008.

2. Gail MH, Brinton LA, Byar DP, Corle DK, Green SB, Schairer C, et al. Projecting individualized probabilities of developing breast cancer for white females who are being examined annually. J Natl Cancer Inst 1989;81:1879–86.

TABLE 10. Options for Breast Cancer Surveillance for Carriers of BRCA1 and BRCA2 Mutations

Intervention	Provisional Recommendation	Quality of Evidence*	Cautionary Issues
Breast self-examination	Education regarding monthly self-examination	III, expert opinion only	Benefit not proven
Clinical breast examination	Annually or semiannually, beginning at age 25–35 years	III, expert opinion only	Benefit not proven
Mammography	Annually, beginning at age 25–35 years	III, expert opinion only (I, randomized trial, women of average risk aged 50–69 years)	Risks and benefits not established for women younger than 50 years

*I indicates highest quality (randomized controlled trials); III, lowest quality (expert opinion and case reports).

Modified from Burke W, Daly M, Garber J, Botkin J, Kahn MJ, Lynch P, et al. Recommendations for follow-up care of individuals with an inherited predisposition to cancer. II. BRCA1 and BRCA2. Cancer Genetics Studies Consortium. JAMA 1997;277:997–1003. Copyrighted 1997, American Medical Association.

3. Colditz GA, Hankinson SE, Hunter DJ, Willett WC, Manson JE, Stampfer MJ, et al. The use of estrogens and progestins and the risk of breast cancer in postmenopausal women. N Engl J Med 1995;332:1589–93.

4. Rebbeck TR, Levin AM, Eisen A, Snyder C, Watson P, Cannon-Albright L, et al. Breast cancer risk after bilateral prophylactic oophorectomy in BRCA1 mutation carriers. J Natl Cancer Inst 1999;91:1475–9.

5. Kauff ND, Satagopan JM, Robson ME, Scheuer L, Hensley M, Hudis CA, et al. Risk-reducing salpingo-oophorectomy in women with a BRCA1 or BRCA2 mutation. N Engl J Med 2002;346:1609–15.

6. Rossouw JE, Anderson GL, Prentice RL, LaCroix AZ, Kooperberg C, Stefanick ML, et al. Risks and benefits of estrogen plus progestin in healthy postmenopausal women: principal results from the Women's Health Initiative randomized controlled trial. Writing Group for the Women's Health Initiative Investigators. JAMA 2002;288:321–33.

7. Marchbanks PA, McDonald JA, Wilson HG, Folger SG, Mandel MG, Daling JR, et al. Oral contraceptives and the risk of breast cancer. N Engl J Med 2002;346:2025–32.

8. Narod SA, Risch H, Moslehi R, Dorum A, Neuhausen S, Olsson H, et al. Oral contraceptives and the risk of hereditary ovarian cancer. Hereditary Ovarian Cancer Clinical Study Group. N Engl J Med 1998;339:424–8.

9. Friedenreich CM, Thune I, Brinton LA, Albanes D. Epidemiologic issues related to the association between physical activity and breast cancer. Cancer 1998;83 (suppl):600–10.

10. Role of the obstetrician-gynecologist in the screening and diagnosis of breast masses. ACOG Committee Opinion No. 334. American College of Obstetricians and Gynecologists. Obstet Gynecol 2006;107:1213–4.

11. Gotzsche PC, Olsen O. Is screening for breast cancer with mammography justifiable? Lancet 2000;355:129–34.

12. American College of Radiology. Breast imaging atlas: mammography, breast ultrasound, magnetic resonance imaging: BI-RADS. 4th ed. Reston (VA): ACR; 2003.

13. Lazarus E, Mainiero MB, Schepps B, Koelliker SL, Livingston LS. BI-RADS lexicon for US and mammography: interobserver variability and positive predictive value. Radiology 2006;239:385–91.

14. Warner E, Plewes DB, Shumak RS, Catzavelos GC, Di Prospero LS, Yaffe MJ, et al. Comparison of breast magnetic resonance imaging, mammography, and ultrasound for surveillance of women at high risk for hereditary breast cancer. J Clin Oncol 2001;19:3524–31.

15. Warner E, Plewes DB, Hill KA, Causer PA, Zubovits JT, Jong RA, et al. Surveillance of BRCA1 and BRCA2 mutation carriers with magnetic resonance imaging, ultrasound, mammography, and clinical breast examination. JAMA 2004;292:1317–25.

16. Saslow D, Boetes C, Burke W, Harms S, Leach MO, Lehman CD, et al. American Cancer Society guidelines for breast screening with magnetic resonance imaging as an adjunct to mammography. CA Cancer J Clin 2007;57: 75–89.

17. Pisano ED, Gatsonis C, Hendrick E, Yaffe M, Baum JK, Acharyya S, et al. Diagnostic performance of digital versus film mammography for breast-cancer screening. Digital Mammographic Imaging Screening Trial (DMIST) Investigators Group [published erratum appears in N Engl J Med 2006;355:1840]. N Engl J Med 2005;353:1773–83.

18. Fenton JJ, Taplin SH, Carney PA, Abraham L, Sickles EA, D'Orsi C, et al. Influence of computer-aided detection on performance of screening mammography. N Engl J Med 2007;356:1399–409.

19. Gemignani ML. Breast cancer. In: Barakat RR, Bevers MW, Gershenson DM, Hoskins WJ, editors. Handbook of gynecologic oncology. 2nd ed. London: Martin Dunitz; 2002. p. 297–301.

20. Cheng JC, Chen CM, Liu MC, Tsou MH, Yang PS, Jian JJ, et al. Locoregional failure of postmastectomy patients with 1–3 positive axillary lymph nodes without adjuvant radiotherapy. Int J Radiat Oncol Biol Phys 2002;52:980–8.

21. Cronin M, Sangli C, Liu ML, Pho M, Dutta D, Nguyen A, et al. Analytical validation of the oncotype DX genomic diagnostic test for recurrence prognosis and therapeutic response prediction in node-negative, estrogen receptor–positive breast cancer. Clin Chem 2007;53:1084–91.

22. Bonadonna G. Adjuvant chemotherapy in node-negative breast cancer. NCI consensus conference. Eur J Cancer 1990;26:844–5.

23. Silverstein MJ, Lagios MD, Groshen S, Waisman JR, Lewinsky BS, Martino S, et al. The influence of margin width on local control of ductal carcinoma in situ of the breast. N Engl J Med 1999;340:1455–61.

24. Fisher ER, Palekar A, Rockette H, Redmond C, Fisher B. Pathologic findings from the National Surgical Adjuvant Breast Project (Protocol No. 4), V: Significance of axillary nodal micro- and macrometastases. Cancer 1978;42:2032–8.

25. Kummel S, Rezai M, Kimmig R, Schmid P. Dose-dense chemotherapy for primary breast cancer. Curr Opin Obstet Gynecol. 2007;19:75–81.

26. Citron ML, Berry DA, Cirrincione C, Hudis C, Winer EP, Gradishar WJ, et al. Randomized trial of dose-dense versus conventionally scheduled and sequential versus concurrent combination chemotherapy as postoperative adjuvant treatment of node-positive primary breast cancer: first report of Intergroup Trial C9741/Cancer and Leukemia Group B Trial 9741 [published erratum appears in J Clin Oncol 2003;21:2226]. J Clin Oncol 2003;21:1431–9.

27. Muss HB, Thor AD, Berry DA, Kute T, Liu ET, Koerner F, et al. c-erbB-2 expression and response to adjuvant therapy in women with node-positive early breast cancer [published erratum appears in N Engl J Med 1994;331:211]. N Engl J Med 1994;330:1260–6.

28. Baselga J, Perez EA, Pienkowski T, Bell R. Adjuvant trastuzumab: a milestone in the treatment of HER-2-positive early breast cancer. Oncologist 2006;11(suppl):4–12.

29. Baum M, Budzar AU, Cuzick J, Forbes J, Houghton JH, Klijn JG, et al. Anastrozole alone or in combination with tamoxifen versus tamoxifen alone for adjuvant treatment of postmenopausal women with early breast cancer: first results of the ATAC randomised trial. ATAC Trialists' Group [published erratum appears in Lancet 2002;360: 1520]. Lancet 2002;359:2131–9.

30. Coombes RC, Hall E, Gibson LJ, Paridaens R, Jassem J, Delozier T, et al. A randomized trial of exemestane after two to three years of tamoxifen therapy in postmenopausal women with primary breast cancer. Intergroup Exemestane Study [published errata appear in N Engl J Med 2004;351:2461, N Engl J Med;355:1746]. N Engl J Med 2004;350:1081–92.

31. Goss PE, Ingle JN, Martino S, Robert NJ, Muss HB, Piccart MJ, et al. A randomized trial of letrozole in postmenopausal women after five years of tamoxifen therapy for early-stage breast cancer. N Engl J Med 2003;349:1793–802.

Cancer of the Vulva

R. Wendel Naumann, MD

EPIDEMIOLOGY

Cancer of the vulva includes any malignancy that arises in the skin, glands, or underlying stroma of the vulva or perineum, including the mons pubis, labia minora, labia majora, Bartholin glands, or clitoris. Approximately 3,460 new cases of cancer of the vulva are expected to be identified in 2008, and 870 women are expected to die of this form of cancer (1). Approximately 90% of vulvar cancer cases are squamous cell cancer and arise from the keratinized skin covering the vulva and perineum. Melanoma is the second most common type of vulvar malignancy; sarcoma is the third. The most common sarcomas found in the vulva and perineum include leiomyosarcoma, malignant fibrous histiocytoma, and epithelioid sarcoma. However, a sarcoma can arise from any structure in the vulva, including blood vessels, skeletal muscle, and fat. Less common types of carcinoma of the vulva include basal cell carcinoma and verrucous carcinoma. Adenocarcinoma of the vulva can arise in the Bartholin's gland or in the apocrine sweat glands. Breast carcinoma has been reported in the vulva and is thought to develop from ectopic breast tissue contained within the milk line that extends down into the perineum.

The incidence of invasive squamous cell vulvar cancer increased 20% between 1973 and 2000. In that same period, analysis of the Surveillance, Epidemiology, and End Results database showed that the incidence of in situ carcinomas of the vulva increased by more than 400%. The peak incidence of in situ carcinoma of the vulva is between ages 40 years and 49 years, which is approximately 20 years younger than for vulvar cancer (2).

Premalignant lesions of the vulva are collectively known as vulvar intraepithelial neoplasia (VIN). Exposure to human papillomavirus (HPV) has been linked to more than 70% of vulvar intraepithelial lesions (3). However, the link between HPV and vulvar cancer is not as well established as it is for cervical cancer. Whereas almost all cervical cancers arise from HPV-related precursor lesions, that does not appear to be the case for vulvar cancer. Molecular analysis has detected HPV DNA in only approximately 40% of vulvar cancers. Cases not associated with HPV infection often are associated with vulvar dystrophies such as lichen sclerosus and squamous cell hyperplasia (4) (Box 7).

PRESENTATION AND SCREENING

Most VIN lesions are asymptomatic and are detected on examination. The most common symptoms of VIN include pruritus or vulvar discomfort. Patients with vulvar cancer can have symptoms similar to those of VIN, or they may present with an asymptomatic mass, bleeding, or discharge. A delay in the diagnosis of vulvar carcinoma is common. At the time of presentation, most women with vulvar cancer have had symptoms for more than 6 months, and many have had previous medical consultations in that period (5). This delay can occur because patients do not seek care or because persistent vulvar lesions were being treated without a biopsy. The diagnosis of any persistent lesion on the vulva should be confirmed by histology.

VULVAR INTRAEPITHELIAL NEOPLASIA

Diagnosis

There are two separate histologic subtypes of VIN. The most common type of VIN, known as *warty basaloid*, is related to HPV infection. These lesions often are seen in younger women. Although traditionally, warty basaloid VIN had been graded in a three-level system, the International Society for the Study of Vulvovaginal Disease voted not to use a grading system for VIN in 2004. This system eliminated VIN 1 and combined VIN 2 and VIN 3

BOX 7

Risk Factors of Squamous Carcinoma of the Vulva

- Sexual activity
- Genital condylomata
- Smoking
- Preinvasive or invasive genital tract neoplasms
- Immunosuppression
- Chronic vulvar conditions (for example, lichen sclerosus) with atypia

into a single VIN category. This was based on the fact that the diagnosis of VIN 1 is not reproducible and that VIN 1 is likely due to uncomplicated HPV infection (6, 7). The high-grade vulvar dysplasias were combined because VIN 2 is uncommon and carries a similar risk of progression to malignancy similar to that of VIN 3 (8).

The other variant of VIN is known as *simplex* or *differentiated VIN*. This subtype is associated with epidermal thickening and parakeratosis with elongated rete ridges. The cell nucleus can be enlarged or have a vesicular pattern. The cells may show abundant eosinophilic cytoplasm with prominent intercellular bridging and keratin pearls. This type of premalignant change does not appear to be related to HPV infection and may have a higher risk of progression to malignancy (8).

Superficially invasive vulvar cancers often are associated with adjacent VIN, suggesting that tumors arising from VIN may have a better prognosis (9). Lichen sclerosus also is found in association with vulvar cancers in as many as 40% of cases and is also considered a risk factor for the development of malignancy (10).

Screening for VIN or vulvar cancer in the general population currently is not recommended. In women with a history of vulvar cancer or VIN, careful regular inspection of the vulva should be undertaken at intervals appropriate for the risk of recurrence. For others with risk factors, a complete examination of the vulva should be performed at least once per year, and women should be cautioned to seek care if symptoms arise.

In women with VIN, the entire vulva should be carefully inspected because this process often is multifocal, especially with VIN related to HPV infection. Cervical cytologic studies, vaginal cytologic studies, or both also should be obtained, and the perianal area should be inspected. Colposcopy of the vulva can be performed, but it is more difficult than colposcopy of the cervix because of the large surface area and the variability in appearance of premalignant lesions. The appearance of VIN is varied and can be hyperpigmented, white, brown, or red. Because of the heavily keratinized skin, acetic acid may take up to 5 minutes to highlight abnormal areas. A biopsy should be performed on all suspicious lesions to ensure that a cancer is not missed when multiple dysplastic lesions are present. To facilitate biopsy, EMLA cream may be applied to ameliorate the pain from lidocaine injection. A punch biopsy is ideal to obtain a representative sample of the vulva.

Treatment

If the biopsy results report VIN 1, close observation is appropriate to see if the lesion will regress spontaneously. For VIN 2, the biopsy results should be reviewed to see if treatment is necessary. For VIN 3, management usually is surgical; however, other approaches have been used. In the case of a single focal lesion, either a wide excision of the dermal tissues can be performed or the tissue can be ablat-

ed with a laser. Excision is preferred if there is a possibility that the lesion could represent an early invasive carcinoma. Surgery should remove the entire dermal layer with at least 5-mm clinical margins and primary closure with minimal tension. Often an elliptical incision following Langer's lines can be performed. Even with good surgical technique, wound breakdown is common on the vulva. If the margins of excision are positive, most women can be monitored unless the specimen reveals invasive disease. At the time of the surgery, the specimen can be marked to aid in identifying sites at high risk of recurrence if the margins of resection are microscopically positive. For lesions involving the clitoris or for multifocal lesions, laser ablation is the preferred method of treatment after biopsies have been obtained to exclude malignant disease.

A variety of nonsurgical treatments for patients with VIN have been reported, including corticosteroids, 5-fluorouracil, interferons, imidazoquinolines (particularly imiquimod), photodynamic therapy, cidovir, retinoids, and vaccination (11). The results to date are based on small series and often are suboptimal.

PAGET DISEASE

Patients with Paget disease of the vulva often have symptoms of itching and irritation that often are made worse by topical irritants such as urine. Paget disease of the vulva, also known as *extramammary Paget disease*, is an intraepithelial neoplastic skin condition that is clinically manifested as a red, raised, pruritic lesion. Although not cancer per se, histologically the lesion is noted to contain cells with prominent nuclei and an increased amount of cytoplasm.

The treatment of patients with Paget disease of the vulva is wide excision. Histologic changes can extend past the gross extent on the skin, and there is a high rate of local recurrence. In addition, the process can be multifocal, leading to a high local recurrence rate even after a successful surgery with negative margins. Thus, women should report symptoms of a possible recurrence to the physician in a timely fashion. The treatment of patients with recurrence is reexcision. The use of a frozen section to determine margin status is controversial because of the high recurrence rate of this disease with negative margins, as well as the difficulty of determining margin status on frozen section.

INVASIVE CARCINOMA OF THE VULVA

Histologic Types

MELANOMA

Malignant melanoma is the second most frequent malignancy of the vulva, accounting for approximately 6% of vulvar malignancies. Melanomas of the vulva have the same characteristics as melanomas of other parts of the body (12). They occur most frequently in individuals with light skin. Subclassifications include superficial spreading melanoma, nodular melanoma, and lentigo maligna melanoma (acral–lentiginous melanoma). The mean decade of occurrence is the seventh.

Presenting symptoms include vulvar irritation and pruritus, vulvar mass, and bleeding and irritation associated with the mass. There is no screening for vulvar melanoma other than observation of the vulva during examination. Areas that are pigmented, thickened, or raised should be evaluated by full-thickness punch biopsy. The classification of melanoma is based on levels of invasion, determined either by skin characteristics or by depth of invasion. The prognosis for patients with melanoma of the vulva is directly related to the depth of invasion and the presence of metastatic disease in lymph nodes.

BARTHOLIN GLAND CARCINOMA

The Bartholin gland, also known as the *greater vestibular gland*, is found deep in the bulbocavernosus muscle in the ischial rectal fossa. It is recommended that a Bartholin gland be removed because of the risk of neoplastic growth if the gland enlarges in a postmenopausal patient or if gland enlargement recurs in a premenopausal patient, especially if there is a solid component. Epithelial malignancies of the Bartholin gland may be divided into four histologic groups: squamous cell carcinoma, transitional cell carcinoma, adenocarcinoma, and adenoid cystic carcinoma (13). Depending on the portion of the gland involved and its size, lymphatic spread can bypass the groin and go directly to the deep pelvic nodes. Imaging evaluation of the groin and the deep pelvic nodes before surgical removal is appropriate. Bartholin gland carcinomas are rarely bilateral.

OTHER ADENOCARCINOMAS

Adenocarcinoma of the sweat glands and other glands of the vulva is uncommon. A small proportion (1–4%) of cases of Paget disease have been associated with underlying adenocarcinoma in the sweat glands. Rarely, Paget disease also has been associated with underlying adenocarcinoma of the colon, and patients with this condition should undergo colonoscopy to exclude an occult cancer. These patients need ongoing surveillance to detect other possible types of cancer.

BASAL CELL CARCINOMA

Basal cell carcinoma can develop in squamous areas of the body, including the vulva. Basal cell carcinoma of the vulva is rare, accounting for fewer than 2% of all vulvar neoplasms. Usually, it occurs in patients in their sixth, seventh, and eighth decades of life. It is a slowly growing, ulcerative type of lesion with a raised border and a necrotic center. The histologic study shows a palisading series of squamous cells at the edge of the tumor that is growing in an orderly, aligned fashion.

These tumors rarely metastasize but are locally destructive. Usually, there is no lymph–vascular involvement.

VERRUCOUS CARCINOMA

Verrucous carcinoma, a variant of invasive squamous cell cancer of the vulva, often presents as an exophytic growth resembling a condyloma. On histologic analysis, the margin of this low-grade cancer is characterized by a pushing border rather than an infiltrating border. A variant of verrucous carcinoma is known as Buschke–Löwenstein giant condyloma and is related to HPV genotype 6. This local growth rarely metastasizes.

VULVAR SARCOMA

Vulvar sarcoma is cancer of mesenchymal elements of the vulva and is the third most common type of malignancy arising in the vulva. The most common types include leiomyosarcomas, which have the same characteristics and histologic definitions in the vulva as in the uterus. Leiomyosarcomas may be overtly malignant or low grade.

Staging

Carcinoma of the vulva is staged surgically. The stage is dependent on the size and depth of the lesion, as well as the nodal status. The cancer staging systems of the International Federation of Gynecology and Obstetrics and the American Joint Commission are shown in Tables 11 and 12. For staging purposes, the depth of invasion in vulvar carcinoma is generally measured from the deepest part of the tumor to the most superficial dermal papilla (14). Sometimes, the tumor thickness is reported as the distance from the deepest part of the tumor to the surface of the lesion. It is important to note which of these measurements is used. Tumor thickness can be several millimeters greater than the depth of invasion but has been reported to be more consistent (15).

Anatomy

The vulva includes all external genital structures—the mons pubis, labia majora, labia minora, clitoris, vaginal vestibule, and superficial muscles of the perineum—as well as the supporting structures exterior to the urogenital diaphragm. The superficial muscles in the vulva include the bulbocavernosus muscle, which is just lateral to the vagina under the labia majora, and the ischiocavernosus muscle, which runs from the tuberosity of the ischium to meet the bulbocavernosus muscle just lateral to the clitoris. The superficial transverse perineal muscle runs at the base of the triangle created by the ischiocavernosus

TABLE 11. The International Federation of Gynecology and Obstetrics 1995 Staging of Vulvar Cancer

Stage	Description
0	Carcinoma in situ
I	Lesions 2 cm or less confined to the vulva or perineum, no lymph node metastases
IA	Lesions 2 cm or less confined to the vulva or perineum with stromal invasion no greater than 1 mm*, no nodal metastases
IB	Lesions 2 cm or less confined to the vulva or perineum with stromal invasion greater than 1 mm, no nodal metastases
II	Tumor confined to the vulva, perineum, or both of more than 2 cm in the greatest dimension with no nodal metastases
III	Tumor of any size arising on the vulva, perineum, or both with 1) adjacent spread to the lower urethra, vagina, anus, or all and 2) unilateral lymph node metastases
IV	
IVA	Tumor invading any of the following: upper urethra, bladder mucosa, rectal mucosa, pelvic bone, or bilateral regional nodal metastases
IVB	Any distant metastasis, including pelvic lymph nodes

*The depth of invasion is determined by measurement of the tumor from the epithelial stromal junction of the adjacent most superficial dermal papilla to the deepest point of invasion.

Shepherd JH. Cervical and vulva cancer: changes in FIGO definitions of staging. Br J Obstet Gynaecol 1996;103:405–6.

TABLE 12. American Joint Commission on Cancer Staging of Vulvar Carcinoma

Stage Grouping	T	N	M
Stage I	T1	N0	M0
Stage II	T2	N0	M0
Stage III	T1	N1	M0
	T2	N1	M0
	T3	N0	M0
Stage IVA	T1	N2	M0
	T2	N2	M0
	T3	N2	M0
	T4	Any N	M0
Stage IVB	Any T	Any N	M1

Abbreviations:

Primary tumor (T)

TX—Primary tumor cannot be assessed

T0—No evidence of primary tumor

Tis—Carcinoma in situ

T1—Tumor confined to the vulva or to the vulva and perineum, less than or equal to 2 cm in greatest dimension

T2—Tumor confined to the vulva and perineum, greater than 2 cm in greatest dimension

T3—Tumor invasion into lower two thirds of the urethra, vagina, or anus

T4—Tumor invades bladder mucosa, upper urethral mucosa, or rectal mucosa, or is fixed to the pelvic bone

Regional lymph nodes (N)

NX—Regional lymph nodes cannot be assessed

N0—No regional lymph node metastasis

N1—Unilateral regional lymph node metastasis

N2—Bilateral regional lymph node metastasis

Distant metastasis (M)

MX—Distant metastasis cannot be assessed

M0—No distant metastasis

M1—Distant metastasis (including pelvic lymph nodes)

Used with permission of the American Joint Committee on Cancer (AJCC), Chicago, Illinois. The original source for this material is the AJCC Cancer Staging Manual, Sixth Edition (2002) published by Springer Science and Business Media LLC, www.springerlink.com.

muscle from the tuberosity of the ischium and the bulbocavernous muscle, where it inserts in the central tendinous point of the perineum. These muscles are covered by Colles fascia and make up the superficial genitourinary diaphragm, which is covered by subcutaneous fat and the skin of the vulva.

The groin triangle is bounded by the inguinal ligament superiorly, the adductor longus medially, and the sartorius laterally. The superficial groin nodes lie above the cribriform fascia in the groin triangle (Fig. 7). There are five vessels in the groin triangle above the cribriform fascia, the largest of which is the saphenous vein (Fig. 8). Often, a lateral accessory saphenous vein can be identified. The other vessels include the superficial circumflex, the superficial epigastric, and the external pudendal.

The lymphatics of the vulva and distal third of the vagina drain into the superficial inguinal node group. Most lymphatic flow then travels through the cribriform fascia to the deep inguinal nodes (Fig. 9). This group consists of three to four nodes that can be found medial to the femoral vein. The most superior of these nodes is the sentinel node to the pelvic lymphatics and is known as *the*

node of Cloquet. Direct spread to the deep nodal group without metastasis to the superficial group has been documented using lymphatic mapping (16). This type of direct spread is uncommon and represents approximately 3% of cases. Lymphatic mapping studies also have demonstrated that 10–20% of the lymphatic flow from the superficial node group travels directly to the pelvis without passage through the deep inguinal nodes or the node of Cloquet (16). A direct pathway from the clitoris or vulva to the pelvic nodes without passage through either the superficial or deep inguinal groups has not been identified.

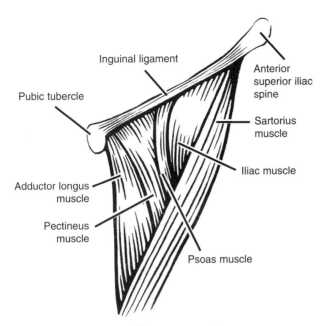

FIG. 7. Boundaries of the groin triangle.

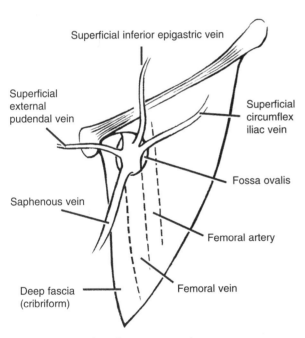

FIG. 8. Vessels in the groin triangle.

Surgical Treatment

Early attempts at resection of cancer developing on the vulva had a high failure rate, with recurrences both at the primary site and in the groin lymph nodes. At the beginning of the 20th century the survival rate for women with vulvar cancer was less than 25% (17). To counter this high mortality, en bloc resection of the vulva and the superficial and deep inguinal nodes through a single butterfly-shaped incision was introduced; it included at least 2-cm margins around the tumor and deep resection to the genitourinary diaphragm (18). With this technique, the cure rate for vul-

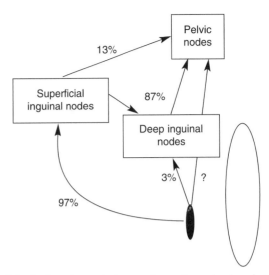

FIG. 9. Lymphatic drainage of a unilateral vulvar lesion. Data from Iversen T, Aas M. Lymph drainage from the vulva. Gynecol Oncol 1983;16:179–89.

var cancer increased dramatically. Even though this technique was later modified to remove less skin through a longhorn-shaped incision, the breakdown rate still exceeded 50%.

Modern efforts have focused on decreasing the extent of surgery while maintaining a high cure rate. Recent refinements to decrease the morbidity of surgery include 1) a definition for microinvasive carcinoma that does not require inguinal lymphadenectomy, 2) unilateral lymphadenectomy in early unilateral tumors, 3) the use of a triple-incision technique instead of an en bloc approach, 4) the use of radical local resection with 1-cm margins instead of complete vulvectomy, and 5) sparing of the saphenous vein in an attempt to prevent lymphedema.

RADICAL VULVECTOMY

The classic radical vulvectomy in the tradition of Way (19) applying the Halstead principles of breast cancer surgery is rarely indicated because it has been surpassed by the more conservative surgical modalities in the management of low-stage disease and the use of chemoradiation therapy in higher-stage disease. This ultraradical surgery is used only in selected cases for management of massive lesions and when chemoradiation therapy is not an option. (See the discussion of chemoradiation therapy.) As noted, in the past these operations were performed by extending the incision to include the groin lymphadenectomy—without leaving skin bridges and without separate groin lymphadenectomy. These operations have a high rate of incisional breakdown and morbidity.

MODIFICATIONS OF RADICAL VULVECTOMY

The modifications of radical vulvectomy are radical local (deep) excision and modified radical vulvectomy. For most low-stage carcinomas (stages I and II), less than a full radical vulvectomy—ie, radical local excision or modified radical vulvectomy (hemivulvectomy)—are sufficient treatments. The goal of these modifications of radical vulvectomy is to preserve as much of the vulva and other structures (including the clitoris, urethra, and anal tissue) as possible while achieving excellent local control of the primary vulvar malignancy. The necessary size of the vulvar carcinoma surgical specimen margin is 1 cm to achieve a low risk of local recurrence risk (20). Groin lymphadenectomy is performed through a separate incision. The proper resection of the vulvar tumor requires adequate skin, mucosal, and deep margins. In contrast to a superficial vulvectomy used to manage extensive VIN, dissection is carried to the deep fascia of the genitourinary diaphragm, but most of the vulva can be spared if the primary lesion is small. Once the lesion is removed, the vagina and vulvar skin can be mobilized and carefully reapproximated in a primary closure to reduce the tension on the incision.

The radical local (deep) excision is the most conservative modified radical vulvectomy and preserves as much normal vulvar tissues as possible. It is used for the surgical removal of small, T1, primary vulvar tumors (stage I). Such treatment has been shown to be as effective in handling local disease as more radical surgery, yet less morbid (21). Modified radical vulvectomy includes radical hemivulvectomy and any vulvectomy involving less-than-radical removal of the entire vulva.

Inguinal–Femoral Lymphadenectomy

The inguinal–femoral lymphadenectomy is carried out through an incision approximately at the level of the inguinal ligament and down through Scarpa fascia. This fascia is then undermined, and the lymph node–containing tissue above the cribriform fascia is dissected from the lateral aspect of the groin toward the medial aspect while the surgeon carefully identifies the vessels in the superficial groin triangle. This dissection is taken inferiorly approximately 4–6 cm below the inguinal ligament in the groin triangle and medially to the adductor longus border. The cribriform fascia is opened laterally and is taken as part of the specimen. The femoral vein then is dissected free, and the deep nodes from the medial portion of the femoral vein are removed. A closed suction drain is placed in the groin bed through a separate incision. The purpose of drainage is to decrease the risk of lymphocyst formation. Scarpa fascia is then closed, and the skin then closed.

The triple-incision technique was developed in response to the high wound breakdown rate of Way en bloc dissection (19). Concern was raised over the triple-incision technique because of the possibility of residual disease in the skin bridges due to cancer cells in the lymphatics between the primary tumor and the lymph nodes. However, isolated skin bridge metastases are rare. The triple-incision technique significantly improved primary healing rates

and was associated with significantly shorter operative time, less blood loss, and a shorter hospital stay without a difference in the overall recurrence rate (22, 23).

Ideally, a full lymphadenectomy would be performed only in women who have positive lymph nodes. According to studies on melanoma, cutaneous sentinel lymph node mapping can be highly accurate in detecting lymph node metastases. A review of 12 studies looking at sentinel node identification in vulvar cancer involving more than 350 women indicated that the technique of combining isosulfan blue with a radionuclide was successful in identifying a sentinel node in 92% of cases, with an overall negative predictive value of 99% (24). Sentinel lymphadenectomy may eventually replace routine inguinal–femoral lymphadenectomy (25).

Women with less than 1 mm of invasion are at low risk of lymph node metastasis. The inguinal–femoral lymphadenectomy may be omitted in these cases (26). Because the risk of nodal metastasis is low in women with 1–2 mm of invasion with well-differentiated tumors, inguinal–femoral lymphadenectomy might be omitted in these women if they are at high risk of sequelae from surgery (27). Midline lesions still require bilateral lymphadenectomy. A unilateral lymphadenectomy can be performed in women with lateral cancers (28). In women with positive ipsilateral nodes, the contralateral groin nodes generally should be removed.

Although the approach is controversial, some surgeons have omitted removal of the deep inguinal lymph nodes because recurrence in the deep inguinal and pelvic lymph nodes is uncommon if the superficial lymph node group is negative. A great portion of the lymphatic drainage from the skin proceeds to the superficial lymph nodes, then to deep lymph nodes, and finally through Cloquet node to the medial pelvic lymph node chain. It has been noted that the rate of deep groin node metastasis is between 3% and 5% when the superficial lymph node group is negative.

Inguinal–femoral lymphadenectomy can lead to acute infectious morbidity, as well as lymphocyst formation and chronic lymphedema. Reduction in morbidity from lymphadenectomy has come from defining a population in whom the lymphadenectomy can be eliminated or performed unilaterally.

The traditional description of inguinal–femoral lymphadenectomy includes ligation of the saphenous vein during removal of the superficial groin lymphatics. However, sparing the saphenous vein when possible can significantly decrease morbidity with a decrease in the incidence of wound cellulitis and acute and chronic lymphedema (29).

Lymphocysts usually manifest as asymptomatic masses in the groin and are noted in 10–20% of patients after groin lymphadenectomy (29). Although cellulitis after vulvectomy has been associated with an increase in the incidence of lymphedema, it has not been associated with an increase in lymphocyst formation. The drains in the groin lymph node beds usually are left in place until the daily output of the drain is less than 30 mL. When a new lymphocyst occurs in a dissected groin, the fluid should be aspirated and sent for cytologic testing to exclude recurrence. Multiple aspirations often are required and may not be curative. If the mass is symptomatic, the lymphocyst can be removed surgically. However, in one small series, lymphocysts were treated successfully by placing a suction drain in the groin until the output was less than 25 mL/d. The drain then was removed, and a pressure dressing was placed to prevent reaccumulation of the fluid (30). Sclerosis of lymphocysts with the application of povidone–iodine solution also has been described.

Cellulitis and lymphangitis can occur after inguinal–femoral lymphadenectomy. The incidence of cellulitis requiring antibiotics ranges from 20% to 40% (29). Often, patients who develop lymphocysts are at increased risk of developing lymphangitis. The etiologic agent often is a streptococcal species, and treatment with penicillin is adequate. If drains are still in place, first-generation cephalosporins may be more appropriate to eliminate *Staphylococcus aureus*.

Chronic lymphedema has been reported in 10–20% of women after inguinal–femoral lymphadenectomy (31). This problem can be disabling and is more common if irradiation is required after lymphadenectomy. The use of graduated compression stockings after lymphadenectomy can help prevent lymphedema. If edema does develop, the use of compression stockings, massage therapy, and limb wraps can help control the accumulation of fluid. However, lymphedema can be chronic and disabling in severe cases. Most major centers offer comprehensive lymphedema treatment programs.

Postoperative Management

Postoperative care should include prophylaxis against deep vein thrombosis and appropriate wound care. Patients with periurethral lesions may require prolonged use of a urinary catheter. Local wound care includes keeping the wound clean and dry. Drains are usually placed in the groin lymph node beds and should be left intact to prevent lymphocyst formation until less than 30 mL of fluid per day drains out, which may take 7–14 days for most patients.

Vulvar surgery can have serious psychologic sequelae, even in the absence of a functional problem after surgery. Patients may require counseling and treatment of depression after surgery (32).

Radiation Therapy

RADIATION THERAPY WITH CONCURRENT CHEMOTHERAPY (CHEMORADIATION THERAPY)

A combination of radiation therapy and chemotherapy is an alternative to surgery for stages III and IV invasive vulvar cancer. It should be considered for management of extensive large tumors or tumors that manifest bowel or bladder involvement (33). The Gynecologic Oncology Group (GOG) reported its experience with a combination of cisplatin and 5-fluorouracil with hyperfractionated radiation for patients with stage III or stage IV squamous cell carcinoma of the vulva. After chemotherapy and radiation therapy, 95% of women were candidates for surgery, and almost one half of the women had no visible disease after the completion of the chemoradiation therapy. Urinary and fecal continence was preserved in all but 5% of these women (34). Preoperative irradiation significantly increased the wound breakdown rate.

RADIATION THERAPY FOR POSITIVE MARGINS

The ability to obtain a negative margin around a tumor may depend on the size of the lesion. Radiation therapy should be considered for patients with a positive margin, especially where reexcision is not desirable (for example, around the clitoris or rectal sphincter). However, if the margin is clinically negative, close observation could be considered in some cases.

RADIATION THERAPY FOR POSITIVE LYMPH NODE METASTASIS

Adjuvant radiation therapy is recommended for most women with positive inguinal lymph nodes. Standard radiation fields include the groin nodes and the pelvic lymph node groups. The inguinal radiation usually is administered in an anterior field only to minimize radiation doses to the femoral head. Fractions of 180 cGy are used for a total of 28 treatments (total of 5,040 cGy). The port extends 2 cm above and 8 cm below the inguinal ligament. The pelvic lymph nodes often are treated at the same time using both an anterior and a posterior field. The radiation port extends up to the mid–sacroiliac joint. The lateral extent of the port is 2 cm lateral to the true pelvis across to 2 cm from the midline. This arrangement generally spares the bladder and rectum from high doses of radiation.

Irradiation to the groin and pelvis usually is recommended in women who have positive lymph nodes. The GOG studied the use of pelvic node lymphadenectomy alone instead of pelvic and groin irradiation and found that irradiation was superior (35). Even though it has not been demonstrated that women with a single node conclusively benefit from irradiation, it usually is recommended, because groin recurrence almost always is fatal.

In one trial, women with vulvar cancer and clinically negative lymph nodes were randomized to receive either radiation therapy or surgery (27). This study was closed prematurely because an interim analysis demonstrated a significant decrease in survival in women receiving only groin irradiation. However, the irradiation technique used in the study has been severely criticized (36).

Chemotherapy combined with radiation therapy also has been evaluated in women with large, bulky lymph node metastases. The GOG conducted a phase 2 study of chemoradiation therapy in women with vulvar cancer and N2 or N3 lymph nodes. In this study, 95% of women completing the protocol had resectable lymph nodes (37). More than 40% of these women had negative lymph nodes on pathologic examination at the time of surgery. However, toxicity from this treatment was significant with a mortality of 5%, and the overall risk of recurrence in the groin nodes was 50%.

Treatment of Uncommon Vulvar Malignancies

MELANOMA

The management of vulvar melanoma conforms to the recommendations for management of melanomas in other parts of the body. A wide local excision with margins of 2 cm in width and depth is considered adequate therapy. Lymph node status is prognostic and, as with other melanomas, can be evaluated by cutaneous sentinel lymph node biopsy. There is no proven therapeutic benefit to the removal of lymph nodes in women with vulvar melanoma. Results of chemotherapeutic and biologic treatments in women with high-risk melanoma have been disappointing. The length of remission may be increased with administration of interferon-α, but cure rates have been unaffected.

ADENOCARCINOMA AND BARTHOLIN GLAND CARCINOMA

Treatment for patients with adenocarcinoma and Bartholin gland carcinoma is the same as that for patients with squamous carcinoma. In addition, it should include ipsilateral inguinal–femoral lymphadenectomy, depending on the size of the tumor and its depth of involvement.

BASAL CELL CARCINOMA

Treatment of patients with basal cell carcinoma involves wide local excision. Because the tumors have a relatively wide base, care must be taken to ensure that excision margins are negative.

VERRUCOUS CARCINOMA

Management of this squamous carcinoma is surgical excision rather than irradiation or chemoradiation therapy, even if the lesion is large. The surgery is followed by appropriate reconstruction of the affected area. Inguinal–femoral lymphadenectomy is not considered necessary in this type of lesion. Reconstruction of the area with myocutaneous skin flaps and other plastic surgery techniques is appropriate. Early descriptions of this lesion on the vulva, as well as on the vagina and the cervix, included an anaplastic transformation if radiation therapy was used. It

is not clear whether the anaplasia represented inaccurate initial diagnosis or malignant transformation.

VULVAR SARCOMA

Management of vulvar sarcoma is surgical removal with wide margins. Although leiomyosarcoma may respond to radiation therapy, it spreads hematogenously, so radiation therapy is appropriate only for local control. Adjuvant chemotherapy has not been shown to be effective in managing leiomyosarcoma. Low-grade stromal sarcoma can be managed with surgical removal alone. Recurrences usually are local, and they are managed with wider reexcision. Even though sarcomas of the vulva are rare, the clinician should not ignore a solid or expanding lesion in the vulva, even if the skin over it is intact.

Follow-up and Prognosis

Patients should be monitored closely after treatment for vulvar carcinoma. Examinations are recommended every 6 months for as many as 5 years after treatment. Risk factors for recurrence include International Federation of Gynecology and Obstetrics stage, lymph–vascular space involvement, tumor size, nodal status, and age (Box 8). The preoperative risk of lymph node metastasis can be estimated by the size of the primary lesion and the depth of tumor invasion.

BOX 8

Vulvar Cancer: Treatment, Prognosis, and Risk of Relapse

- **Stage IA:** 99–100% 5-year survival rate with radical local excision

- **Stage IB:** 90% 5-year survival rate with radical local excision, modified radical vulvectomy, and unilateral inguinal–femoral lymphadenectomy

- **Stage II:** 80% 5-year survival rate with modified radical vulvectomy and unilateral or bilateral inguinal–femoral lymphadenectomy

- **Stage III:** 60–70% 5-year survival rate with radical vulvectomy and bilateral inguinal–femoral lymphadenectomy or chemoradiation therapy and surgery to resect residual disease as needed

- **Stage IVA:** 20–50% 5-year survival rate with chemoradiation therapy followed by surgery to resect residual disease as necessary

- **Stage IVB:** Less than 1% 5-year survival rate with chemotherapy for metastatic disease and radiation therapy followed by surgery in selected cases to achieve local control

Local recurrence can occur many years after surgery. In a GOG series, it was noted that the median time to local recurrence was 36 months (38). A report from the Mayo Clinic showed that as many as 10% of patients treated for vulvar cancer had a local recurrence more than 5 years after the original diagnosis (39). However, it could be argued that some of these late local recurrences could represent new primary cancer cases (40).

Detection of local recurrence of vulvar carcinoma is important because most women are candidates for a second surgical excision. The long-term survival rate after radical excision of a vulvar recurrence has been reported as 50–60% (40). Survival is better in women who originally presented with early-stage disease. Other factors that diminish the cure rate after local recurrence include disease at sites other than the vulva and a short interval from initial treatment to recurrence (41). For a large recurrence, an exenterative procedure can be attempted. A long-term survival rate of 38% has been reported after exenterative surgery in this situation (42).

Whereas local recurrences can present late and have a good prognosis, recurrence in the groin often presents early and has a dismal prognosis, with a mortality of more than 90%. Metastatic disease in the groin nodes at the time of initial surgery increases the risk of recurrence in the groin in the first 2 years. After the first 2 years, the risk of groin recurrence is low, regardless of the status of the nodes at the time of the initial surgery. Resection of a groin recurrence should be undertaken with caution but may have a limited role in the management of vulvar cancer, especially in the subset of patients who have not received groin irradiation (43). After groin irradiation, this area heals slowly, and infection can compromise the femoral vessels.

Chemotherapy for Metastatic Disease

Chemotherapy for metastatic vulvar cancer is the same as that for metastatic cervical cancer, ie, is platinum based (see "Invasive Cervical Neoplasia"). The initial management of locally advanced disease is similar to that of advanced or bulky cervical cancer. The regimens include carboplatin, cisplatin, paclitaxel, and topotecan. Chemotherapy for metastatic vulvar carcinoma is palliative.

References

1. American Cancer Society. Cancer facts and figures 2008. Atlanta (GA): ACS; 2008. Available at: http://www.cancer.org/downloads/STT/2008CAFFfinalsecured.pdf. Retrieved February 20, 2008.
2. Judson PL, Habermann EB, Baxter NN, Durham SB, Virnig BA. Trends in the incidence of invasive and in situ vulvar carcinoma. Obstet Gynecol 2006;107:1018–22.
3. Madeleine MM, Daling JR, Carter JJ, Wipf GC, Schwartz SM, McKnight B, et al. Cofactors with human papillomavirus in a population-based study of vulvar cancer [published erratum appears in J Natl Cancer Inst 1997;89:1896]. J Natl Cancer Inst 1997;89:1516–23.
4. Scurry J, Wilkinson EJ. Review of terminology of precursors of vulvar squamous cell carcinoma. J Low Genit Tract Dis 2006;10:161–9.
5. Jones RW, Joura EA. Analyzing prior clinical events at presentation in 102 women with vulvar carcinoma: evidence of diagnostic delays. J Reprod Med 1999;44:766–8.
6. Micheletti L, Barbero M, Preti M, Zanotto Valentino MC, Chiringhello B, Pippione M. Vulvar intraepithelial neoplasia of low grade: a challenging diagnosis. Eur J Gynaecol Oncol 1994;15:70–4.
7. Preti M, Mezzetti M, Robertson C, Sideri M. Inter-observer variation in histopathological diagnosis and grading of vulvar intraepithelial neoplasia: results of a European collaborative study. BJOG 2000;107:594–9.
8. Scurry J. International Society for the Study of Vulvovaginal Disease abandons grading of vulvar intraepithelial neoplasia. Australas J Dermatol 2006;47:146–8.
9. Dvoretsky PM, Bonfiglio TA, Helmkamp BF, Ramsey G, Chuang C, Beecham JB. The pathology of superficially invasive, thin vulvar squamous cell carcinoma. Int J Gynecol Pathol 1984;3:331–42.
10. Carli P, Cattaneo A, De Mgnis A, Biggeri A, Taddei G, Giannotti B. Squamous cell carcinoma arising in vulval lichen sclerosus: a longitudinal cohort study. Eur J Cancer Prev 1995;4:491–5.
11. Todd RW, Luesley DM. Medical management of vulvar intraepithelial neoplasia. J Lower Genit Tract Dis 2005;9:206–12.
12. Phillips GL, Bundy BN, Okagaki T, Kucera PR, Stehman FB. Malignant melanoma of the vulva treated by radical hemivulvectomy: a prospective study of the Gynecologic Oncology Group. Cancer 1994;73:2626–32.
13. Cardosi RJ, Speights A, Fiorica JV, Grendys EC Jr, Hakam A, Hoffman MS. Bartholin's gland carcinoma: a 15-year experience. Gynecol Oncol 2001;82:247–51.
14. Wilkinson EJ. Superficial invasive carcinoma of the vulva. Clin Obstet Gynecol 1985;28:188–95.
15. Kurzl R, Messerer D, Baltzer J, Lohe KJ, Zander J. Comparative morphometric study on the depth of invasion in vulvar carcinoma. Gynecol Oncol 1988;29:12–25.
16. Iversen T, Aas M. Lymph drainage from the vulva. Gynecol Oncol 1983;16:179–89.
17. Basset, A. Traitement chirurgical operatoire de l'epithelioma primitif du clitoris indications-technique-resultats. Rev Chir Orthop 1912;46:546. [French]
18. Way S. Carcinoma of the vulva. Am J Obstet Gynecol 1960;79:692–7.
19. Taussig F. Cancer of the vulva: an analysis of 155 cases (1911–1940). Am J Obstet Gynecol 1940;40:764–79.
20. Heaps JM, Fu YS, Montz FJ, Hacker NF, Berek JS. Surgical-pathologic variables predictive of local recurrence

in squamous cell carcinoma of the vulva. Gynecol Oncol 1990;38:309–14.

21. Hacker NF, Van Der Velden J. Conservative management of early vulvar cancer. Cancer 1993;71(suppl 4):1673–7.

22. Hacker NF, Leuchter RS, Berek JS, Castaldo TW, Lagasse LD. Radical vulvectomy and bilateral inguinal lymphadenectomy through separate groin incisions. Obstet Gynecol 1981;58:574–9.

23. Helm CW, Hatch K, Austin JM, Partridge EE, Soong SJ, Elder JE, et al. A matched comparison of single and triple incision techniques for the surgical treatment of carcinoma of the vulva. Gynecol Oncol 1992:46:150–6.

24. Plante M, Renaud MC, Roy M. Sentinel node evaluation in gynecologic cancer. Oncology (Williston Park) 2004;18: 75–87; discussion 88–90, 95–6.

25. Van der Zee AG, Oonk MH, De Hullu JA, Ansink AC, Vergote I, Verheijen R, et al. On the safety of implementation of the sentinal node procedure in vulvar cancer: an observational study [abstract]. Internat J Gynecol Cancer 2006;16(suppl 3):608–9.

26. Kelley JL 3rd, Burke TW, Tornos C, Morris M, Gershenson DM, Silva EG, et al. Minimally invasive vulvar carcinoma: an indication for conservative surgical therapy. Gynecol Oncol 1992:44:240–4.

27. Sedlis A, Homesley H, Bundy BN, Marshall R, Yordan E, Hacker N, et al. Positive groin lymph nodes in superficial squamous cell vulvar cancer: a Gynecologic Oncology Group Study. Am J Obstet Gynecol 1987;156:1159–64.

28. Hacker NF, Berek JS, Lagasse LD, Nieberg RK, Leuchter RS. Individualization of treatment for stage I squamous cell vulvar carcinoma. Obstet Gynecol 1984;63:155–62.

29. Zhang SH, Sood AK, Sorosky JI, Anderson B, Buller RE. Preservation of the saphenous vein during inguinal lymphadenectomy decreases morbidity in patients with carcinoma of the vulva. Cancer 2000;89:1520–5.

30. Leminen A, Forss M, Paavonen J. Wound complications in patients with carcinoma of the vulva: comparison between radical and modified vulvectomies. Eur J Obstet Gynecol Reprod Biol 2000;93:193–7.

31. Rouzier R, Haddad B, Atallah D, Dubois P, Paniel BJ. Surgery for vulvar cancer. Clin Obstet Gynecol 2005;48: 869–78.

32. Green MS, Naumann RW, Elliot M, Hall JB, Higgins RV, Grigsby JH. Sexual dysfunction following vulvectomy. Gynecol Oncol 2000;77:73–7.

33. Berek JS, Heaps JM, Fu YS, Juillard GJ, Hacker NF. Concurrent cisplatin and 5-fluorouracil chemotherapy and radiation therapy for advanced-stage squamous carcinoma of the vulva. Gynecol Oncol 1991;42:192–201.

34. Moore DH, Thomas GM, Montana GS, Saxer A, Gallup DG, Olt G. Preoperative chemoradiation for advanced vulvar cancer: a phase II study of the Gynecologic Oncology Group. Int J Radiat Oncol Biol Phys 1998;42:79–85.

35. Homesley HD, Bundy BN, Sedlis A, Adcock L. Radiation therapy versus pelvic node resection for carcinoma of the vulva with positive groin nodes. Obstet Gynecol 1986;68: 733–40.

36. McCall AR, Olson MC, Potkul RK. The variation of inguinal lymph node depth in adult women and its importance in planning elective irradiation for vulvar cancer. Cancer 1995;75:2286–8.

37. Montana GS, Thomas GM, Moore DH, Saxer A, Mangan CE, Lentz SS, et al. Preoperative chemoradiation for carcinoma of the vulva with N2/N3 nodes: a Gynecologic Oncology Group study. Int J Radiat Oncol Biol Phys 2000; 48:1007–13.

38. Stehman FB, Bundy BN, Ball H, Calrke-Peasron DL. Sites of failure and times to failure in carcinoma of the vulva treated conservatively: a Gynecologic Oncology Group study. Am J Obstet Gynecol 1996;174:1128–32; discussion 1132–3.

39. Gonzales Bosquet J, Magrina JF, Gaffey TA, Hernandez JL, Webb MJ, Cliby WA, et al. Long-term survival and disease recurrence in patients with primary squamous cell carcinoma of the vulva. Gynecol Oncol 2005;97:828–33.

40. Podratz KC, Symmonds RE, Taylor WF. Carcinoma of the vulva: analysis of treatment failures. Am J Obstet Gynecol 1982:143:340–51.

41. Piura B, Masotina A, Murdoch J, Lopes A, Morgan P, Monaghan J. Recurrent squamous cell carcinoma of the vulva: a study of 73 cases. Gynecol Oncol 1993:48:189–95.

42. Miller B, Morris M, Levenback C, Burke TW, Gershenson DM. Pelvic exenteration for primary and recurrent vulvar cancer. Gynecol Oncol 1995;58:202–5.

43. Hopkins MP, Reid GC, Morley GW. The surgical management of recurrent squamous cell carcinoma of the vulva. Obstet Gynecol 1990;75:1001–5.

Vaginal Neoplasia

Jesus Gonzalez Bosquet, MD, PhD, and William A. Cliby, MD

Vaginal neoplasia is rare and usually is secondary to cervical or vulvar cancer that has spread to the vagina from the primary site. Vulvar and cervical cancer must be excluded before a primary vaginal cancer can be diagnosed (1). Because of the rarity of this type of cancer, there is little high-quality evidence in the literature concerning it, particularly with regard to therapy.

The American Cancer Society estimates that in the year 2008, approximately 2,210 new cases of vaginal cancer will be diagnosed in the United States, and 760 women will die of this cancer (2). Overall, it accounts for approximately 1% of gynecologic cancers (3).

There are important differences in management and prognosis between preinvasive and invasive neoplasias of the vagina. Thus, these entities will be discussed separately.

VAGINAL INTRAEPITHELIAL NEOPLASIA

The grading used for preinvasive lesions of the vagina is the same used for intraepithelial neoplasia of the cervix. There are three degrees, depending on the extension of epithelial involvement: vaginal intraepithelial neoplasia (VAIN) 1 involves the basal epithelial layers; VAIN 2 involves up to two thirds of the vaginal epithelium; and VAIN 3, or vaginal carcinoma in situ, involves most of the vaginal epithelium. Most commonly, VAIN is located in the upper third of the vagina, a finding that may be partly related to the association with the more common cervical lesions. It has been suggested that one half to two thirds of all patients with VAIN are individuals who have had either cervical or vulvar neoplasia. In those individuals who have been treated for cervical neoplasia, VAIN can appear many years later.

In the National Cancer Data Base, a large central registry of hospital-referred cancer cases (4), invasive carcinoma was the most common diagnosis for primary vaginal cancer, and carcinoma in situ accounted for 28% of all carcinoma cases (5). The percentage of VAIN 3 carcinomas decreases with age, ranging from 82% of VAIN 3 in patients younger than 20 years to only 11% in patients older than 80 years.

Diagnosis

An abnormal Pap test result from the vagina in a patient who underwent hysterectomy usually is the first indication of possible neoplasia in the vagina, although occasionally cervical intraepithelial neoplasia that extends into the vagina is identified during the workup for the abnormal Pap test result. It is uncommon to find lesions in the vagina in the presence of a normal cervix (1). Patients with vaginal bleeding, aside from expected bleeding in the postoperative period, should always undergo evaluation for possible vaginal neoplasia.

Once a patient has had an abnormal Pap test result, identification of a lesion or lesions in the vagina is important, because often VAIN can be multifocal. Colposcopy with directed biopsy is the preferred method of diagnosis. Lugol staining of the vagina may be helpful in identifying nonstaining lesions in the vagina. Colposcopically, the lesions are similar to those observed in cervical neoplasia. Adequate biopsy samples should be taken to avoid missing an early invasive lesion.

Current guidelines suggest that continued follow-up with Pap tests is indicated in individuals who have been treated previously for either an intraepithelial or invasive lesion of the cervix or vulva. There is no evidence that subsequent Pap test screening is of value in individuals who have had a hysterectomy for benign reasons (6).

Management

Patients with VAIN 1 and VAIN 2 can be monitored and typically will not require therapy. Many of these patients have a human papillomavirus infection or atrophic change of the vagina. Topical estrogen therapy may be useful in some women.

Patients with VAIN 3 generally require treatment. If there is a single, well-localized lesion, biopsy and local excision is probably the management of choice. In some instances, small lesions can be removed entirely with the biopsy forceps in the office. Again, if vaginal atrophy exists, the application of topical estrogen may be useful.

Other modalities that also are used in the management of cervical intraepithelial neoplasia have been suggested for the management of VAIN 3. These techniques include laser ablation and cryosurgical ablation. Because the vaginal epithelium is very thin, the use of these modalities is limited.

Topical application of 5-fluorouracil cream also has been used in the management of VAIN 3, and it may be considered in selected patients who do not respond to expectant management, topical estrogens, or local excision. This product essentially causes desquamation of the vaginal epithelium, which is expected to be replaced by normal epithelium. Weekly insertion of 5-fluorouracil cream deep in the vagina at bedtime for 8–10 consecutive weeks has been shown to be effective (7). However, overuse may lead to vaginal irritation or scalding that may result in scarring. One month to 6 weeks after completion of therapy, the vagina is reexamined to determine the effectiveness.

For patients who develop VAIN after receiving radiation therapy to the cervix, a definitive diagnosis must be obtained with biopsy to exclude invasive vaginal cancer. The management of VAIN in these patients is similar to that in nonirradiated individuals, although surgical excision is more difficult.

SQUAMOUS CELL CARCINOMA

When primary squamous cell carcinoma occurs in the vagina, it usually is in the upper third, similar to intraepithelial lesions. The disease occurs in women aged between 35 years and 90 years, with most cases occurring in women aged 60 years and 79 years. Depending on where the carcinoma is located, extension with regard to lymph node metastasis mimics the adjacent organ. If disease is in the upper vagina, it follows a spread pattern similar to that of cervical cancer, with metastasis to the pelvic lymph nodes. If the lesion is low in the vagina, extension is similar to that seen in vulvar cancer, with inguinal node extension followed by extension to the deep pelvic nodes.

The cause of primary squamous cell carcinoma of the vagina is unknown, although it is assumed to be related to many of the same factors as carcinoma of the cervix (8). Bleeding is the most common symptom, but when bleeding is present it usually indicates an advanced lesion. An earlier sign may be a vaginal discharge, which may be bloody. Other symptoms, such as urinary tract symptoms, are less common.

Once the diagnosis has been established, evaluation and clinical staging are performed based on the criteria of the International Federation of Gynecology and Obstetrics (Table 13). Location of the lesion may require cystoscopy or proctoscopy. Magnetic resonance imaging or computed tomography scanning of the pelvis may be helpful in identifying metastatic disease in patients with advanced lesions, a finding that can be confirmed with fine-needle aspiration.

The findings of the physical examination, staging procedure, and imaging studies as well as patient comorbidities and performance status influence treatment decisions. Because vaginal neoplasia is uncommon, physicians extrapolate management strategies from those for vulvar and cervical neoplasia. Improvements in response, sur-

vival, and local control of the disease associated with the use of chemoradiation therapy in patients with locally advanced cervical cancer have increased interest in using cisplatin concomitantly with radiation therapy for the management of vaginal squamous cell carcinoma. Although no trials have compared radiation therapy and chemoradiation therapy in patients with vaginal cancer, a number of institutions have considered the latter treatment as the first line for managing this neoplasia. In general, treatment is tailored to the extent of the disease. Large cancers are managed initially with chemoradiation therapy in an attempt to shrink the tumor so local therapy will be more effective.

Stage I Lesions

Most patients with stage I squamous cell carcinoma of the vagina are treated with radiation. Stage I lesions that are superficially invasive respond well to brachytherapy; as much as 100% of local control can be achieved with intracavitary and interstitial techniques. There are no well-established criteria for the use of external beam radiotherapy.

In selected patients with stage I lesions, surgery could be contemplated. Patients with small lesions close to the cervix may be treated with radical hysterectomy with upper vaginectomy and pelvic lymphadenectomy. Patients with smaller lesions close to the introitus may be treated with wide local excision and ipsilateral inguino–femoral lymphadenectomy. The long-term survival outcome in these selected patients ranges from 70% to 91% (9–11).

TABLE 13. Carcinoma of the Vagina: International Federation of Gynecology and Obstetrics Staging

Stage	Description
0	Carcinoma in situ: intraepithelial neoplasia grade 3
I	Carcinoma is limited to the vaginal wall
II	Carcinoma has involved the subvaginal tissue but has not extended to the pelvic sidewall
III	Carcinoma has extended to the pelvic sidewall
IV	Carcinoma has extended beyond the true pelvis or has involved the mucosa of the bladder or rectum; bullous edema as such does not permit a case to be allotted to stage IV
IVA	Tumor invades bladder, or rectal mucosa, or both, or direct extension beyond the true pelvis or all
IVB	Spread to distant organs

This table was published in International Journal of Gynecology and Obstetrics, volume 95, supplement, Beller U, Benedet JL, Creasman WT, Ngan HY, Quinn MA, Maisonneuve P, et al. Carcinoma of the vagina. International Federation of Gynecology and Obstetrics. FIGO annual report on the results of treatment in gynecological cancer, s29–42, copyright Elsevier 2006.

Fertility-sparing surgery for patients with early cervical cancer via vaginal radical trachelectomy and laparoscopic pelvic lymphadenectomy has been applied successfully in carefully selected patients (12). These techniques theoretically are applicable to early apical vaginal neoplasias in young patients who desire fertility. The decision to undertake this alternative approach should be made on an individual basis.

Stage IIA Lesions

In stage IIA disease, the tumor extends to subvaginal tissue without parametrial involvement. The recommended treatment is external beam radiation followed by intracavitary brachytherapy, interstitial brachytherapy, or both (13). Radical surgery has been suggested for patients with localized stage II vaginal cancer that meet criteria similar to those of the surgical candidates in stage I, although this approach remains controversial. The long-term survival outcome for patients with stage IIA lesions treated with radiation is approximately 55% and with 80% local tumor control (13).

Lesions of Stages IIB, III, and IV

In stages IIB, III, and IV vaginal cancer, the disease has spread outside the organ, with invasion to the parametrium (stage IIB), pelvic side wall (stage III), or proximal or distant organs (stage IV). In addition to the type of radiation delivered to patients in stage IIA, in some cases a boost of radiation to the parametrial area may be considered. Long-term survival rates of patients with stage IIB, III, and IV disease are 35%, 38%, and 0%, respectively, after treatment with radiation therapy (13).

Recurrent Squamous Cell Carcinoma

Patients who did not receive radiotherapy should be treated with external beam radiotherapy followed, when feasible, by brachytherapy. The same principles as those used for treating patients with advanced-stage disease should be applied (14).

In selected patients with persistent or recurrent cancer, some type of pelvic exenteration may be considered. Reasonable results may be obtained in patients with solitary central recurrences. However, even in experienced centers using well-rounded selection criteria, the procedure may be canceled in approximately one fourth of the cases because metastases are discovered at exploratory surgery (9). Chemotherapy could be used in medically fit patients who do not meet the aforementioned criteria, although the overall outcome generally is poor.

OTHER VAGINAL TUMORS

Verrucous Carcinoma

Verrucous carcinoma, a rare variant of well-differentiated squamous cell carcinoma, presents as a large, soft, cauliflowerlike mass. These tumors grow locally without deep invasion, and surgical treatment with complete local excision often is curative. No lymphatic assessment is needed. The neoplasia is resistant to radiation.

Malignant Melanoma

Although multiple therapies have been applied to malignant melanoma of the vagina, surgery remains the treatment of choice. The role of postoperative radiation therapy is unclear, but there is limited evidence to support its use (14). The use of systemic chemotherapy or immunotherapy in the management of cutaneous melanoma is being investigated, but more results are needed before these therapies can be applied to vaginal melanoma. Prognosis of patients with vaginal melanoma is poor.

Endodermal Sinus Tumor

Endodermal sinus tumor is very rare, is most likely of germ cell origin, and usually appears before an individual is aged 2 years. Before the introduction of chemotherapy as treatment, the survival was very poor. According to experience with endodermal sinus tumor of the ovary, it seems reasonable to manage these tumors with local excision and postoperative chemotherapy (15) followed by monitoring with alpha-fetoprotein.

Malignant Lymphoma

Malignant lymphoma of the vagina often represents spread from another primary site or, less likely, the primary site arising from an extranodal site. The mucosa usually remains intact, and the mass should undergo biopsy for definitive diagnosis. Management is radiation therapy and combination chemotherapy, not surgery. Radiation therapy is used to prevent local recurrences in bulky disease.

Clear Cell Adenocarcinoma

Clear cell adenocarcinoma of the cervix and vagina is associated with first-trimester in utero diethylstilbestrol (DES) exposure (16). Whereas there is a peak in the age incidence in the late teens and late 20s, a possible second peak after age 50 years has been reported (17). The increased risk of clear cell adenocarcinoma in women whose mothers began DES treatment in early pregnancy may be due in part to the larger area of ectopic glandular epithelium in the vagina of these patients. Increased areas of tuboendometrial-type epithelium in patients exposed to DES in early gestation may provide a greater opportunity for interaction with unidentified cocarcinogens.

Vaginal clear cell adenocarcinoma usually occurs in the upper third of the anterior vaginal wall. Ninety percent of cases are stage I or stage II at the time of diagnosis. These tumors vary greatly in size; most are exophytic and superficially invasive.

Therapy for vaginal adenocarcinoma is similar to that for squamous cell carcinoma. Patients with stage I disease treated with radiation therapy or surgery based on the criteria used for squamous cell carcinoma have an expected overall 5-year survival of 92% and an overall 10-year survival of 88%, respectively (18). For patients with stage II disease, a combination of external beam irradiation and brachytherapy, similar to that used for squamous cell carcinoma, had an overall 5- and 10-year survival of 83% and 65%, respectively (19). In selected cases, radical surgery could be considered.

References

1. Creasman WT. Vaginal cancers. Curr Opin Obstet Gynecol 2005;17:71–6.

2. American Cancer Society. Cancer facts and figures 2008. Atlanta (GA): ACS; 2008. Available at: http://www.cancer.org/downloads/STT/2008CAFFfinalsecured.pdf. Retrieved February 20, 2008.

3. Society of Gynecologic Oncologists Clinical Practice Guidelines. Practice guidelines: vaginal cancer. Oncology (Williston Park) 1998;12:449–52.

4. Jessup JM, Menck HR, Winchester DP, Hundahl SA, Murphy GP. The National Cancer Data Base report on patterns of hospital reporting. Cancer 1996;78:1829–37.

5. Creasman WT, Phillips JL, Menck HR. The National Cancer Data Base report on cancer of the vagina. Cancer 1998;83:1033–40.

6. Fetters MD, Fischer G, Reed BD. Effectiveness of vaginal Papanicolaou smear screening after total hysterectomy for benign disease. JAMA 1996;275:940–7.

7. Kirwan P, Naftalin NJ. Topical 5-fluorouracil in the treatment of vaginal intraepithelial neoplasia. Br J Obstet Gynaecol 1985;92:287–91.

8. Daling JR, Madeleine MM, Schwartz SM, Shera KA, Carter JJ, McKnight B, et al. A population-based study of squamous cell vaginal cancer: HPV and cofactors. Gynecol Oncol 2002;84:263–70.

9. Davis KP, Stanhope CR, Garton GR, Atkinson EJ, O'Brien PC. Invasive vaginal carcinoma: analysis of early-stage disease. Gynecol Oncol 1991;42:131–6.

10. Stock RG, Chen AS, Seski J. A 30-year experience in the management of primary carcinoma of the vagina: analysis of prognostic factors and treatment modalities. Gynecol Oncol 1995;56:45–52.

11. Tjalma WA, Monaghan JM, de Barros Lopes A, Naik R, Nordin AJ, Weyler JJ. The role of surgery in invasive squamous carcinoma of the vagina. Gynecol Oncol 2001;81:360–5.

12. Plante M, Renaud MC, Hoskins IA, Roy M. Vaginal radical trachelectomy: a valuable fertility-preserving option in the management of early-stage cervical cancer. A series of 50 pregnancies and review of the literature. Gynecol Oncol 2005;98:3–10.

13. Perez CA, Grigsby PW, Garipagaoglu M, Mutch DG, Lockett MA. Factors affecting long-term outcome of irradiation in carcinoma of the vagina. Int J Radiat Oncol Biol Phys 1999;44:37–45.

14. Cardenes H, Roth L, McGuire W, Look K. Vagina. In: Hoskins WJ, editor. Principles and practice of gynecologic oncology. 4th ed. Philadelphia (PA): Lippincott Williams & Wilkins; 2005. p. 707–42.

15. Williams S, Blessing JA, Liao SY, Ball H, Hanjani P. Adjuvant therapy of ovarian germ cell tumors with cisplatin, etoposide, and bleomycin: a trial of the Gynecologic Oncology Group. J Clin Oncol 1994;12:701–6.

16. Herbst AL, Ulfelder H, Poskanzer DC. Adenocarcinoma of the vagina: association of maternal stilbestrol therapy with tumor appearance in young women. N Engl J Med 1971;284:878–81.

17. Herbst AL. Behavior of estrogen-associated female genital tract cancer and its relation to neoplasia following intrauterine exposure to diethylstilbestrol (DES). Gynecol Oncol 2000;76:147–56.

18. Senekjian EK, Frey KW, Anderson D, Herbst AL. Local therapy in stage I clear cell adenocarcinoma of the vagina. Cancer 1987;60:1319–24.

19. Senekjian EK, Frey KW, Stone C, Herbst AL. An evaluation of stage II vaginal clear cell adenocarcinoma according to substages. Gynecol Oncol 1988;31:56–64.

Cervical Neoplasia

Mark Spitzer, MD, and David H. Moore, MD

PREINVASIVE CERVICAL NEOPLASIA

Cervical cancer and its precursors are caused by human papillomavirus (HPV). Oncogenic (high-risk) HPV genotypes have been identified in 99.7% of all cases of cervical cancer (1), and the mechanism by which persistent infection with oncogenic HPV genotypes initiates oncogenesis is well understood (2). However, virtually all HPV infections regress spontaneously. Therefore, HPV is essential to the development of cervical neoplasia, but it does not function independently (3).

Because of the relationship between HPV and cervical cancer, many modalities have been proposed and evaluated for HPV testing. These approaches include screening (in conjunction with the Pap test), triage of women with Pap tests results reported as "atypical squamous cells of undetermined significance" (ASC-US), and testing to assess the effectiveness of management of cervical intraepithelial neoplasia (CIN). In the past 5 years advances have been reported in all these areas.

Guidelines for the management of cervical cytologic abnormalities and cervical cancer precursors have been updated to reflect these advances (4, 5). The Bethesda System of reporting cervical cytologic studies is the most widely used system in the United States (Box 9).

Risk Factors

Most demographic and behavioral factors traditionally associated with cervical cancer, such as lower socioeconomic class, fewer years of education, more lifetime sexual partners, lower age at first intercourse, pregnancy, and parity, are indirect measures of HPV infection (6). Certain HPV genotypes, primarily genotypes 16 and 18, are most

---

RESOURCES

Cervical Neoplasia

American Society for Colposcopy and Cervical Pathology
http://www.asccp.org

CDC—National Breast and Cervical Cancer Early Detection Program
http://www.cdc.gov/cancer/nbccedp

National Cervical Cancer Coalition
http://www.nccc-online.org

BOX 9

The 2001 Bethesda System (Abridged)

Specimen Adequacy

Satisfactory for evaluation (note presence or absence of endocervical or transformation zone component)

Unsatisfactory for evaluation (specify reason)

 Specimen rejected or not processed (specify reason)

 Specimen processed and examined, but unsatisfactory for evaluation of epithelial abnormality because of (specify reason)

General Categorization (Optional)

Negative for intraepithelial lesion or malignancy

Epithelial cell abnormality

Other

Interpretation or Result

Negative for Intraepithelial Lesion or Malignancy

Organisms

 Trichomonas vaginalis

 Fungal organisms morphologically consistent with *Candida* species

 Shift in flora suggestive of bacterial vaginosis

 Bacteria morphologically consistent with *Actinomyces* species

 Cellular changes consistent with herpes simplex virus

Other nonneoplastic findings (optional to report; list not comprehensive)

 Reactive cellular changes associated with

 —inflammation (includes typical repair)

 —radiation

 —intrauterine contraceptive device

Glandular cells status after hysterectomy

Atrophy

Epithelial Cell Abnormalities

Squamous cell

 Atypical squamous cells

 —of undetermined significance

 —cannot exclude high-grade squamous intraepithelial lesion

(continued)

51

The 2001 Bethesda System (Abridged) (continued)

Interpretation or Result (continued)

Epithelial Cell Abnormalities (continued)

Squamous cell *(continued)*

Low-grade squamous intraepithelial lesion

—encompassing: human papillomavirus or mild dysplasia or CIN 1

High-grade squamous intraepithelial lesion

—encompassing: moderate and severe dysplasia, carcinoma in situ; CIN 2 and CIN 3

Squamous cell carcinoma

Glandular cell

—Atypical glandular cells (specify endocervical, endometrial, or not otherwise specified)

—Atypical glandular cells, favor neoplastic (specify endocervical or not otherwise specified)

—Endocervical adenocarcinoma in situ

—Adenocarcinoma

Other (List Not Comprehensive)

Endometrial cells in a woman aged 40 years or older

Automated Review and Ancillary Testing (Include as Appropriate)

Educational Notes and Suggestions (Optional)

Abbreviation: CIN indicates cervical intraepithelial neoplasia.

Modified from Solomon D, Davey D, Kurman R, Moriarty A, O'Connor D, Prey M, et al. The 2001 Bethesda System: terminology for reporting results of cervical cytology. Forum Group Members and the Bethesda 2001 Workshop. JAMA. 2002; 287:2114–9. Copyright © 2002, American Medical Association. All rights reserved.

highly associated with cervical neoplasia. Other HPV genotypes also are associated with cervical cancer (7). The persistence of an HPV infection is a risk factor for persistent or progressive cervical dysplasia (8), and HPV 16 infection is more likely to be persistent than infections caused by the other oncogenic HPV genotypes (9). Individuals may possess a genetic susceptibility to cervical cancer, but the relative risks are small (10). The risk of cervical cancer is 3.5 times greater among smokers than among nonsmokers; carcinogens from cigarette smoke have been found in high concentrations in the cervical mucus of smokers, suggesting a plausible biologic explanation for this association (11). However, other case–control studies have shown that this association can disappear after adjusting for HPV infection (6).

Etiology

All genotypes of HPV have five early (*E*) genes (*E1, E2, E5, E6,* and *E7*) that are required for viral replication or cellular transformation and two late (*L*) genes (*L1* and *L2*) that code for the viral capsid (12). The cellular p53 protein normally responds to DNA damage or cellular stress by activating the expression of genes involved in cell cycle arrest, apoptosis (programmed cell death), or both (13). This process kills damaged or mutated cells or prevents them from dividing until the damage is repaired. The gene *E6* in oncogenic HPV binds with *p53* and rapidly degrades it (14). Loss of *p53* function allows mutated and damaged cells to replicate (15).

In normal cells the retinoblastoma tumor suppressor protein (*pRb*) is hypophosphorylated early in the cell cycle. Hypophosphorylated *pRb* binds and inactivates the transcription factors that allow cell cycle progression. Normal cells produce growth factors that signal the phosphorylation of *pRb* and allow cell cycle progression (16). Damaged or mutated cells do not produce these signals, resulting in cell cycle arrest. The gene *E7* in oncogenic HPV binds with *pRb* and releases signals even in abnormal cells. This process allows damaged cells to survive rather than undergo apoptosis (17). Both processes can lead to uncontrolled replication of cells that results in cervical neoplasia.

Early in HPV infection, the HPV genomes exist as circular, extrachromosomal copies. However, some viral genomes can become inserted into the DNA of the host cell chromosomes. This process is called *integration*. The integration process has been correlated with the transition from low-grade to high-grade lesions (18). The gene *E2* suppresses the expression of the *E6* and *E7* oncogenes. During integration there is a loss, by break or deletion, of the viral *E2* gene that interferes with *E2* control of *E6* and *E7*, leading to increased levels of those gene products and further interference with the function of the tumor suppressor genes (19).

Angiogenesis is the acquisition of a new blood supply from the existing vasculature and is required for tumors to obtain nutrients and oxygen and to remove waste products. Recent data indicate that expression of *E6* and *E7* gene products (from oncogenic HPV types) in their target cell causes an increase in angiogenesis (20).

Screening

Most HPV infections in young women, including women with CIN 1 and mild dysplasia, are transient; 70% of oncogenic HPV types and 90% of low-risk types regress within 3 years (21). Regression rates of more than 90% within 2 years have been reported in college populations (22). Lesions also are more likely to regress in adolescents than in adults, possibly because a lesion in an adult is more likely to represent disease that has persisted since the individual's youth. The National Cancer Institute's Surveillance, Epidemiology, and End Results program reported that from 1995 to 1999, the incidence rate of invasive cervical cancer was 0 per 100,000 women per year for women aged 10–19 years and 1.7 per 100,000 women per year for women aged 20–24 years (23). Based on these data and the low risk of missing an important cervical lesion until 3–5 years after initial exposure to HPV, the American Cancer Society (24) and the American College of Obstetricians and Gynecologists (ACOG) (25) recommend that cervical cancer screening begin approximately 3 years after the initiation of sexual intercourse or age 21 years. Beginning screening early also may increase anxiety, morbidity, and expense from increased follow-up procedures.

The American College of Obstetricians and Gynecologists recommends that women younger than 30 years have annual cytologic screening. Women with certain risk factors, such as women with a history of CIN 2 or CIN 3, women infected with human immunodeficiency virus (HIV), immunocompromised women, or women who were exposed to diethylstilbestrol in utero, should continue to be screened annually after age 30 years. Low-risk women who have had three annual cytologic screenings with results of "negative for intraepithelial lesion or malignancy" may undergo Pap testing less frequently (every 2–3 years), depending on the discretion of the physician and the patient (25).

Human papillomavirus DNA testing in combination with cervical cytologic testing has been approved by the U. S. Food and Drug Administration as a screening tool for cervical neoplasia in women older than 30 years. The age cutoff of 30 years was selected because at younger ages, the prevalence of HPV infection is very high, whereas the prevalence of cervical cancer is relatively low. Screening young women leads to unnecessary testing and worry because most abnormal test results are likely to revert to normal spontaneously. Interim guidance on the use of dual screening was developed by the National Cancer Institute, the American Society for Colposcopy and Cervical Pathology, and the American Cancer Society at a joint workshop in 2003 (26) and was reaffirmed as part of the 2006 Consensus Conference (4). Studies using combined HPV–cervical cytologic testing reported a negative predictive value of 99–100% for CIN 2 and CIN 3 (27–29). Women with concurrent negative test results (normal cytologic findings and negative HPV DNA test results) can be reassured that their risk of unidentified CIN 2 and CIN 3 or cervical cancer is approximately 1 in 1,000 (7). Based on the natural history of the disease and the results of several large longitudinal studies (30) and health policy modeling studies (31), the risk for women with concurrent negative test results is comparable to, or less than, that of women with three consecutive negative conventional cytologic results.

The 2006 Consensus Guidelines, as well as the U.S. Food and Drug Administration, recommended that women with negative concurrent test results be rescreened no more frequently than every 3 years. For women who have negative cytology results but have positive oncogenic HPV DNA test results, both tests should be repeated in 12 months. If the oncogenic HPV test result persists on repeated testing, colposcopy is indicated regardless of the cytologic findings. The women with cytologic abnormalities should be managed according to published guidelines (Fig. 10).

It is difficult to set an upper age limit for cervical cancer screening. There is a consensus that the incidence of cervical cancer in older women is almost entirely confined to unscreened and underscreened women. Evidence suggests that there is very low risk of cervical cancer for women aged 50 years and older in countries with organized screening programs (32). In the United States, cervical cancer is rare among older women who have undergone screening (32). Furthermore, atrophy, cervical stenosis, false-positive cytologic results, and patient anxiety and discomfort suggest that Pap tests in well-screened older women may do more harm than good. The choice of an exact age at which to cease screening is arbitrary. The American Cancer Society recommends that screening may be discontinued in low-risk women aged 70 years (24). The U.S. Preventive Services Task Force has set age 65 years as the upper limit for screening but noted that efforts should be made to identify and screen elderly women who are underscreened (33). The American College of Obstetricians and Gynecologists noted that older women who are sexually active and have had multiple partners as well as women with a previous history of abnormal cytologic test results, may continue to be at some risk for cervical neoplasia. Women in both of these categories should continue to have routine cervical cytologic examinations (34).

Because primary vaginal cancer is so rare, women who have had a hysterectomy and have no history of high-grade CIN are at very low risk of developing vaginal cancer. Cytologic screening in this group has a low rate of detecting an abnormality and a very low positive predictive value. Continued routine vaginal cytologic examinations in such women are not cost-effective and may cause anxiety and overtreatment. Therefore, women who have had a total hysterectomy may discontinue screening if they have no history of high-grade CIN. The women who have a history of high-grade CIN may discontinue screening after three consecutive satisfactory normal annual examinations (24, 34).

Management Guidelines

Following is a summary of management guidelines. This summary points out the areas that have been affected by the 2006 update (4, 5).

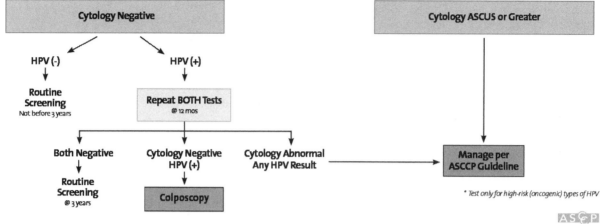

Use of HPV DNA Testing* as an Adjunct to Cytology for Cervical Cancer Screening in Women 30 Years and Older

■ **FIG. 10.** Use of human papillomavirus DNA testing as an adjunct to cytology for cervical cancer screening in women aged 30 years and older. Abbreviations: ASCCP indicates American Society for Colposcopy and Cervical Cytology; ASCUS, atypical squamous cells of undetermined significance; HPV, human papillomavirus. Wright TC. Management of cervical cytologic abnormalities. J Low Genit Tract Dis 2007;11:201–22. Reprinted from the Journal of Lower Genital Tract Disease Vol. 11 Issue 4, with the permission of ASCCP © American Society for Colposcopy and Cervical Pathology 2007. No copies of the algorithms may be made without the prior consent of ASCCP.

LOW-GRADE SQUAMOUS INTRAEPITHELIAL LESIONS AND ATYPICAL SQUAMOUS CELLS OF UNDETERMINED SIGNIFICANCE

Between 1996 and 2003, the rate of low-grade squamous intraepithelial lesions (LSIL) in the United States increased from 1.6% to 2.1% (35), whereas the rates for other cytologic categories did not change. This increase was probably caused by the widespread use of liquid-based cytologic testing, in which the rate of LSIL (2.4%) is almost twice the rate found with conventional cytologic testing (1.4%).

General Population

The 2006 Consensus Guidelines for the initial triage of ASC-US cytology are unchanged from the 2001 guidelines and are presented in Figure 11. After the initial triage, women who screen positive for HPV DNA and women with ASC-US results on two repeated tests should be managed in the same fashion as women with LSIL and be referred for colposcopic evaluation (Fig. 12). One significant change in the 2006 guidelines was an attempt to standardize follow-up after colposcopy. Follow-up with HPV DNA testing is almost always performed at 12 months, and follow-up with repeated cytologic testing is always performed at 6 months and 12 months. There is no recommendation for follow-up at 3 months. After a negative HPV DNA test result or two repeated "negative for intraepithelial lesion or malignancy" cytologic results are obtained, women can return to routine cytologic screening (4).

Data from the ASCUS/LSIL Triage Study for Cervical Cancer (ALTS) showed that the overall risk rate of CIN 2 or CIN 3 in women with LSIL and HPV-positive ASC-US was not affected by the referral cytology (36). When monitored for 24 months, women who originally presented with LSIL cytology and women with HPV-positive ASC-US had the same cumulative rates of CIN 2 and CIN 3 (27.6% and 26.7%, respectively). This finding supports uniformity in the management of women with HPV-positive ASC-US and LSIL cytologic results. In addition, recent studies have highlighted a negative impact on subsequent pregnancies after loop electrosurgical excision. Loop electrosurgical excision appears to approximately double the risk that a woman subsequently will have preterm delivery, a low birth weight infant, or premature rupture of membranes (37, 38). Therefore, a conservative approach to the management of these minimal lesions (follow-up rather than treatment) was favored except when a clear benefit of treatment was demonstrated.

A conservative follow-up protocol is more controversial for women with an unsatisfactory colposcopic examination because of the fear that they may have occult CIN 2 or CIN 3 or cancer within the endocervical canal. In a report on a subgroup of women with LSIL without previously identified CIN 2 or CIN 3 who underwent excisional procedures, the rate of detection of CIN 2 or CIN 3 in the excisional specimen was approximately 10% in women with unsatisfactory colposcopic results regardless of the results of endocervical sampling (39). This rate was lower than the rate of CIN 2 or CIN 3 among women in the same study who had satisfactory colposcopic results. No cases of cancer were

Management of Women with Atypical Squamous Cells of Undetermined Significance (ASC-US)

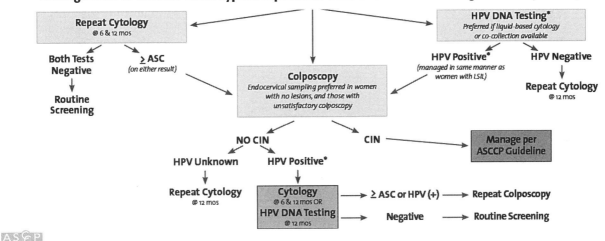

*Test only for high-risk (oncogenic) types of HPV

■ **FIG. 11.** Management of women with atypical squamous cells of undetermined significance. Abbreviations: ASC indicates atypical squamous cells; ASCCP, American Society for Colposcopy and Cervical Cytology; CIN, cervical intraepithelial neoplasia; HPV, human papillomavirus; LSIL, low-grade squamous intraepithelial lesion. Wright TC. Management of cervical cytologic abnormalities. J Low Genit Tract Dis 2007;11:201–22. Reprinted from the Journal of Lower Genital Tract Disease Vol. 11 Issue 4, with the permission of ASCCP © American Society for Colposcopy and Cervical Pathology 2007. No copies of the algorithms may be made without the prior consent of ASCCP.

Management of Women with Low-grade Squamous Intraepithelial Lesion (LSIL)*

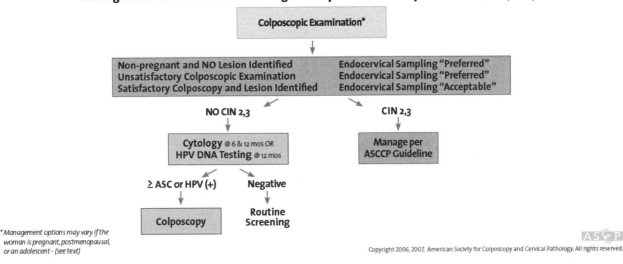

*Management options may vary if the woman is pregnant, postmenopausal, or an adolescent - (see text)

■ **FIG. 12.** Management of women with low-grade squamous intraepithelial lesion. Abbreviations: ASC indicates atypical squamous cells; ASCCP, American Society for Colposcopy and Cervical Pathology; CIN, cervical intraepithelial neoplasia; HPV, human papillomavirus. Wright TC. Management of cervical cytologic abnormalities. J Low Genit Tract Dis 2007;11:201–22. Reprinted from the Journal of Lower Genital Tract Disease Vol. 11 Issue 4, with the permission of ASCCP © American Society for Colposcopy and Cervical Pathology 2007. No copies of the algorithms may be made without the prior consent of ASCCP.

missed. Furthermore, the risk of CIN 2 or CIN 3 in ALTS did not vary significantly between women with LSIL or HPV-positive ASC-US whose initial biopsy report was positive for CIN 1 and women who had a negative biopsy or women who did not undergo biopsy (36). Therefore, the management of all these women should be similar.

Special Populations

As noted in the previous section, invasive cervical cancer is exceedingly rare in adolescent women (aged 20 years and younger). In contrast, minor-grade cytologic abnormalities (ASC and LSIL) are more common in women aged 15–19 years than in older women and are associated with minor cytologic abnormalities that are of little long-term clinical significance (40).

Human papillomavirus DNA positivity is much more prevalent in women aged 18–22 years (71%) than in those older than 29 years (31%) (41). Thus, using HPV DNA testing for triage in adolescents and young women with ASC-US would refer large numbers of women to colposcopy when there is low risk of having cervical cancer. In addition, many adolescents experience multiple sequential HPV infections, so repetitively positive HPV DNA test results in this age group may represent repeated transient infections rather than a persistent infection.

Although a small proportion of adolescents with LSIL may have underlying CIN 3, prospective follow-up studies of adolescents with LSIL show very high rates of regression to normal status—as high as 91% at 36 months (42). Moreover, it is not unusual for regression to take years to occur. Among adolescents with LSIL who had not experienced regression at 2 years, 60% regressed to normal status over the following 12 months (42). All CIN lesions, including CIN 3, may regress.

The management of pregnant women with ASC-US is identical to that of nonpregnant women except that endo-cervical curettage is unacceptable in pregnant women. Deferring the initial colposcopy until at least 6 weeks after delivery is acceptable. In pregnant women who have no cytologically, histologically, or colposcopically suspected CIN 2, CIN 3, or cancer at the initial colposcopy, follow-up after delivery is recommended. Additional colposcopic and cytologic examinations during pregnancy are unacceptable for these women (4).

Several studies (43) noted the very low rate of progression of LSIL during pregnancy and questioned the value of performing more that one colposcopy in the evaluation of LSIL during pregnancy. Therefore, the 2006 guidelines recommend that after an initial colposcopy, additional colposcopic and cytologic examinations during pregnancy are unacceptable.

The initial management of postmenopausal women with cytologic findings of LSIL follows a pattern identical to that of the initial management of ASC-US cytology (4). The risk of significant pathology in well-screened postmenopausal women with ASC-US is relatively low (32, 44). Human papillomavirus DNA testing is actually a more efficient triage tool in older women with ASC-US, because it refers a lower proportion to colposcopy (45). In ALTS, only 20% of women aged 40 years or older with ASC-US tested positive for HPV DNA (46). Similarly, some studies have found that the prevalence of both HPV DNA positivity and CIN 2 or CIN 3 are lower in older women with LSIL than in younger women (45). This finding suggests that postmenopausal women with LSIL can be managed less aggressively than premenopausal women.

The 2001 guidelines, citing expert opinion, recommended repeated cytologic screening after treatment with vaginal estrogen cream as a triage option in postmenopausal women with LSIL cytology. In the 2006 guidelines, citing lack of supporting data, this approach was eliminated as a triage option. According to the 2006 guidelines, postmenopausal women with ASC-US and LSIL should be managed in the same manner as women with ASC-US in the general population.

"Positive for ASC-US" is a common cytology result in women infected with HIV. Two recent follow-up studies reported that 60–78% of women infected with HIV have ASC-US during 4–5 years of follow-up (47). The 2001 guidelines recommended colposcopy for all immunosuppressed women with ASC-US. This recommendation was based on studies that reported a high prevalence of both HPV DNA positivity and of significant cervical pathology in this population (27). However, more recent studies have found a lower prevalence of CIN 2 or CIN 3 and HPV DNA positivity (46). The 2006 guidelines recommend that women infected with HIV and other immunosuppressed women with ASC-US be managed in the same manner as women with ASC-US in the general population.

HIGH-GRADE SQUAMOUS INTRAEPITHELIAL LESION AND ATYPICAL SQUAMOUS CELLS—CANNOT EXCLUDE HIGH-GRADE SQUAMOUS INTRAEPITHELIAL LESION

In the 2001 guidelines, all women with the cytologic finding of "atypical squamous cells—cannot exclude high-grade squamous intraepithelial lesion" (ASC-H) were referred for colposcopy. If no lesion was identified, a review of the cytology, colposcopy, and histology findings was recommended when possible. By 2006, it became evident that in the community at large, this review rarely resulted in a change of diagnosis. Therefore, the recommendation to review the cytology, colposcopy, and histology findings was made optional. Otherwise, the recommended management of women with ASC-H remains unchanged from the 2001 guidelines (4).

In the United States, approximately 0.5% of all Pap test results are reported as "high-grade squamous intraepithelial lesion" (HSIL) (35). The rate of HSIL varies with age, decreasing from 0.6% in women aged 20–29 years to 0.1% in women aged 50–59 years (44). The loop electrosurgical excision procedure (LEEP) identifies CIN 2, CIN 3, or cancer in 84–97% of women with HSIL Pap test results and in 53–66% of women with findings of HSIL after a single colposcopic examination (48). Approximately 2% of women with HSIL have invasive cancer (49). Because the rate of CIN 2 or CIN 3 is so high in adults with HSIL cytologic findings, "see and treat" may be an acceptable approach to management of these women. However, in women who are planning a future pregnancy, the risks of a LEEP procedure on their subsequent pregnancies should be explained. As with ASC-H cytologic findings, when no lesion is identified, the recommendation to review the cytology, colposcopy, and histology findings was made optional in 2006 (4).

In adolescents, when the histologic diagnosis is CIN 2 and CIN 3, CIN 2 is the most statistically likely diagnosis, and regression is more likely. Nearly 90% of adolescents undergoing see-and-treat LEEP because of HSIL cytologic findings have no CIN 2 or CIN 3 on the LEEP specimen, and the risk of adverse effects exceeds the potential benefit for patients without dysplasia (38). This finding argues against a see-and-treat approach in this population (4).

In adults, see-and-treat diagnostic excisional procedure (such as LEEP) is acceptable. When CIN 2 or CIN 3 is not identified histologically, colposcopy findings are satisfactory, and the endocervical curettage result is normal, observation with colposcopy and cytology at 6-month intervals for 1 year is acceptable as long as repeated cytology testing does not show HSIL. After 1 year of observation, women with two consecutive "negative for intraepithelial lesion or malignancy" results can return to routine cytologic screening. A diagnostic excisional procedure also is acceptable. The remaining HSIL guidelines are unchanged (Fig. 13) (4).

ATYPICAL GLANDULAR CELLS AND OTHER GLANDULAR ABNORMALITIES

The risk associated with atypical glandular cells (AGC) is dramatically higher than that seen with ASC. The risk associated with glandular abnormalities increases as the description in the Bethesda classification system advances from "AGC—not otherwise specified" (AGC-NOS) to "AGC, favor neoplasia" and finally to adenocarcinoma in situ (AIS). Recent series have reported that 9–38% of women with AGC have significant neoplasia (CIN 2 or CIN 3, AIS, or cancer), and 3–17% of women have invasive cancer (50–52). The rate and type of significant findings in women with AGC vary with age (51). Women younger than 35 years with AGC are more likely to have CIN and less likely to have cancer, whereas in older women the risk of glandular lesions, including malignancies, is higher (50). Human papillomavirus testing, cervical cytology, and colposcopy are all poor at detecting glandular disease (52). Because the risk of neoplasia (including invasive cancer) is high for women with "AGC, favor neoplasia," AIS, or repeated cytologic results of AGC and the sensitivity of available diagnostic tests is poor, diagnostic excisional procedures may be necessary for these women.

In premenopausal women, benign-appearing endometrial cells or the presence of endometrial stromal cells or histiocytes are rarely associated with significant pathology (53). However, in postmenopausal women they may be associated with significant endometrial pathology (54) and may be thought of as microscopic postmenopausal bleeding. Benign-appearing glandular cells derived from small accessory ducts, foci of benign adenosis, or prolapse of the fallopian tube into the vagina are sometimes seen in cytologic specimens after total hysterectomy and have no clinical significance.

The initial workup for women with glandular cytologic abnormalities is mostly unchanged (Fig. 14). Colposcopy with endocervical sampling is recommended for all these women, with the addition of endometrial sam-

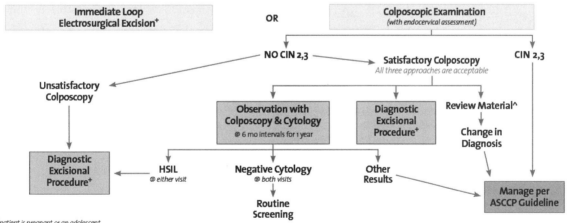

Management of Women with High-grade Squamous Intraepithelial Lesion (HSIL)*

+ Not if patient is pregnant or an adolescent
^ Includes referral cytology, colposcopic findings, and all biopsies
* Management options may vary if the woman is pregnant, postmenopausal, or an adolescent

■ **FIG. 13.** Management of women with high-grade squamous intraepithelial lesion. Abbreviations: ASCCP indicates American Society for Colposcopy and Cervical Pathology; CIN, cervical intraepithelial neoplasia; HSIL, high-grade squamous intraepithelial lesion. Wright TC. Management of cervical cytologic abnormalities. J Low Genit Tract Dis 2007;11:201–22. Reprinted from the Journal of Lower Genital Tract Disease Vol. 11 Issue 4, with the permission of ASCCP © American Society for Colposcopy and Cervical Pathology 2007. No copies of the algorithms may be made without the prior consent of ASCCP.

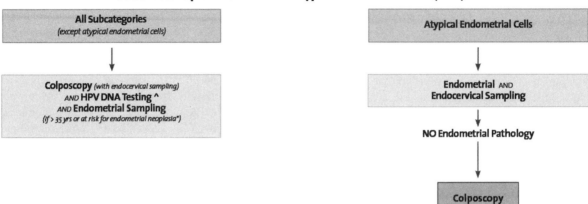

Initial Workup of Women with Atypical Glandular Cells (AGC)

^ If not already obtained. Test only for high-risk (oncogenic) types.
* Includes unexplained vaginal bleeding or conditions suggesting chronic anovulation.

■ **FIG. 14.** Initial workup of women with atypical glandular cells. Abbreviation: HPV indicates human papillomavirus. Wright TC. Management of cervical cytologic abnormalities. J Low Genit Tract Dis 2007;11:201–22. Reprinted from the Journal of Lower Genital Tract Disease Vol. 11 Issue 4, with the permission of ASCCP © American Society for Colposcopy and Cervical Pathology 2007. No copies of the algorithms may be made without the prior consent of ASCCP.

pling in women older than 35 years or women with clinical indications suggesting a risk of neoplastic endometrial lesions (for example, unexplained vaginal bleeding, chronic anovulation, or atypical endometrial cells). In the latter case, colposcopy can be deferred until the results of the initial biopsies are known. Although triage of these women using cytology or HPV testing continued to be unacceptable, the 2006 guidelines added that HPV DNA testing at the time of colposcopy is preferred in women with atypical endocervical, endometrial, or glandular cells NOS.

Knowledge of the HPV status in women with either atypical endocervical, endometrial, or glandular cells NOS who do not have CIN 2 or CIN 3 or glandular neoplasia identified histologically will allow expedited triage. Women who tested positive for HPV should have their Pap test and HPV test repeated at 6 months and those who tested negative for HPV, at 12 months. Women with a positive HPV test result or an abnormal Pap test result would be referred to colposcopy; women in whom both tests are negative can resume routine cytologic testing. In contrast, if the HPV status is unknown, the Pap test should be repeated every 6 months until there are four consecutive "negative for intraepithelial lesion or malignancy" results before the woman can resume routine cytologic testing (Fig. 15) (4).

In women with atypical endocervical, endometrial, or glandular cells NOS, the evaluation can be concluded and management according to the 2006 Consensus Guidelines can be initiated if CIN is identified histologically but no glandular neoplasia is present. In contrast, it is recommended that women with atypical endocervical or glandular cells that "favor neoplasia" or endocervical AIS

undergo a diagnostic excisional procedure unless invasive disease is identified during the initial colposcopic workup.

Endometrial assessment is recommended in postmenopausal women with benign endometrial cells regardless of symptoms. In premenopausal women and in women with a cytologic report of benign glandular cells after a hysterectomy, no further evaluation is required (4).

CERVICAL INTRAEPITHELIAL NEOPLASIA

One of the most important factors in the development of the 2006 Consensus Guidelines was the recognition that all management of CIN was associated with some increased risk of adverse pregnancy outcome (37, 38, 55). It has been long recognized that cervical conization increases a woman's risk of future preterm labor, delivery of low birth weight infants, and cesarean delivery (56), but other treatment methods were thought to have no adverse effects on future pregnancies. However, several large retrospective series have reported that after a LEEP or laser conization, women also are at increased risk for future preterm delivery, low birth weight infants, and premature rupture of membranes (37, 38). One study evaluated the effect of ablative methods and LEEP on pregnancy outcome. Results confirmed that all treatment modalities for CIN increase the risk of preterm delivery to some extent (55). In 2006, this potential adverse effect on pregnancy was taken into consideration in planning the management of women with CIN.

Another important consideration in the management of women with CIN is how long after treatment they remain at risk. A recent systematic review reported that women remain at increased risk of invasive cancer for at least 20

Subsequent Management of Women with Atypical Glandular Cells (AGC)

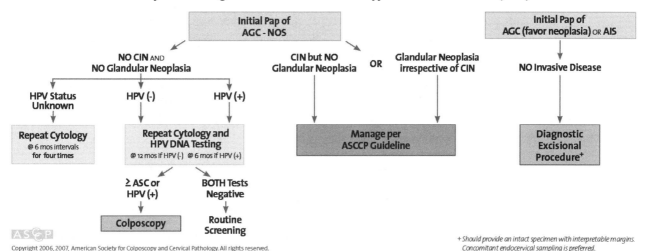

+ Should provide an intact specimen with interpretable margins.
Concomitant endocervical sampling is preferred.

■ **FIG. 15.** Subsequent management of women with atypical glandular cells. Abbreviations: AGC indicates atypical glandular cells; AGC-NOS, atypical glandular cells—not otherwise specified; AIS, adenocarcinoma in situ; ASC, atypical squamous cells; ASCCP, American Society for Colposcopy and Cervical Pathology; CIN, cervical intraepithelial neoplasia; HPV, human papillomavirus. Wright TC. Management of cervical cytologic abnormalities. J Low Genit Tract Dis 2007;11:201–22. Reprinted from the Journal of Lower Genital Tract Disease Vol. 11 Issue 4, with the permission of ASCCP © American Society for Colposcopy and Cervical Pathology 2007. No copies of the algorithms may be made without the prior consent of ASCCP.

years after treatment (56 per 100,000 women–years compared with 5.6 per 100,000 women–years for the general U.S. population) (57). Therefore, long-term follow-up is essential.

Special populations were identified for whom treatment would offer little benefit while adding significant risk. Adolescents (aged 20 years and younger) and young women have a very high incidence of CIN lesions, but the rate of spontaneous regression of these lesions also is very high (42), and the risk of invasive cervical cancer is very low (44). Pregnant women have a very low risk of progression of CIN 2 or CIN 3 to invasive cervical cancer during pregnancy, and the incidence of spontaneous regression after delivery is relatively high (58). Furthermore, the complications associated with management of CIN during pregnancy are significant, and there is a high rate of recurrent or persistent disease after treatment of these women (59). Therefore, management of CIN was drastically restricted in these women.

Cervical Intraepithelial Neoplasia Grade 1

Cervical intraepithelial neoplasia 1 represents a heterogeneous group of lesions, and the histologic diagnosis is poorly reproducible (60). Most CIN 1 will regress spontaneously, and CIN 1 uncommonly progresses to CIN 2 or CIN 3 (36).

CIN 1 Preceded by ASC-US, ASC-H, or LSIL Cytologic Findings. Patients with CIN 1 should not be treated initially. One very important change in the 2006 guidelines is the initial recommendation to monitor patients with CIN 1 without treatment, with no distinction between sat-

isfactory and unsatisfactory colposcopic results. The 2001 guidelines recommended that women with CIN 1 and unsatisfactory colposcopic results undergo an excisional procedure. The 2006 guidelines recommend follow-up regardless of the colposcopic results. The recommended initial management is the same for women with LSIL and HPV-positive ASC-US who do not have CIN 2 or CIN 3 on biopsy, regardless of the findings (CIN 1, normal biopsy, or normal colposcopy with no biopsy performed). The guidelines recommend follow-up with either HPV DNA testing every 12 months or repeated cervical cytologic testing every 6–12 months, with referral to colposcopy if the HPV DNA test result is positive or if repeated cytologic findings are reported as ASC-US or greater. After a negative HPV test or two consecutive normal cytology tests, the woman may return to routine cytologic screening. If CIN 1 persists for at least 2 years, continued follow-up remains an option. However, it is also acceptable to treat a woman with either excision or ablation if the colposcopic examination is satisfactory, or to treat her with a diagnostic excisional procedure if the colposcopic examination is unsatisfactory, the endocervical sampling contains CIN, or the patient has been previously treated (Fig. 13) (5).

CIN 1 Preceded by HSIL Cytologic Findings. Under the 2001 guidelines, CIN 1 preceded by an HSIL finding would have resulted in review of the cytologic and histologic results and a diagnostic excisional procedure if the diagnosis was confirmed. In the 2006 guidelines, however, the management changed in two ways. First, the review of the cytologic and histologic results was made optional (see the HSIL guidelines in this section). Furthermore, for women with satisfactory colposcopic findings and a normal endocervical curettage result, the option to monitor with colposcopy and cytology at 6-month intervals for 1 year was added to that of performing a diagnostic excisional procedure. In women with a repeated HSIL diagnosis or an unsatisfactory colposcopic result, a diagnostic excisional procedure is recommended. Women with two consecutive normal cytologic results can resume routine screening (Fig. 15) (5).

The management of adolescents with CIN 1 is the same as that for adolescents with LSIL (Fig. 16) (5). The recommended management of pregnant women with a histologic diagnosis of CIN 1 is follow-up without treatment. Treatment of pregnant women for CIN 1 is unacceptable (5).

Cervical Intraepithelial Neoplasia 2 and Cervical Intraepithelial Neoplasia 3

The initial management and posttreatment follow-up of women with CIN 2 or CIN 3 are essentially unchanged in the 2006 guidelines. One small change is that cytologic follow-up occurs at 6-month intervals (not 4- to 6-month intervals), and the woman can return to routine screening after two normal cytologic results (not three, as in the 2001 guidelines). Follow-up with HPV DNA testing at 6–12 months remains an option. Women who return to routine screening should continue follow-up for at least 20 years (5).

In the 2001 guidelines, observation was preferred, but treatment was acceptable for adolescents and young women with a histologic diagnosis of CIN 2. In the 2006 guidelines, the option to monitor (with colposcopy and cytology) women at 6-month intervals without treatment for up to 24 months was extended to adolescents with CIN 2-NOS or CIN 3-NOS, provided colposcopic findings are satisfactory. After two consecutive negative Pap test results, adolescents and young women with normal colposcopic results can return to routine cytologic screening. Treatment remains acceptable. When a histologic diagnosis of CIN 3 is specified, CIN 2-NOS or CIN 3-NOS persists for 24 months, or colposcopic findings are unsatisfactory, treatment is recommended (5). The management of pregnant women with CIN 2 or CIN 3 remains essentially unchanged in the 2006 guidelines (5).

ADENOCARCINOMA IN SITU

The 2001 guidelines did not address the management of histologic AIS. Management of women with AIS is challenging and controversial. One of the main problems with AIS is the unreliability of available screening (cytology) and diagnostic (colposcopy) tools in identifying these lesions. Also, unlike squamous lesions, AIS is frequently multifocal and frequently has skip lesions, so it is difficult to be sure that a conization with negative margins represents completely excised disease. For these reasons, hysterectomy was always a recommended management option for women with AIS. However, newer studies have shown that conization cures most of these patients (failure rate in patients with negative conization margins is less than 10%) (61). Margin status is one of the most clinically useful predictors of residual disease (62).

Management of Adolescent Women with Either Atypical Squamous Cells of Undetermined Significance (ASC-US) or Low-grade Squamous Intraepithelial Lesion (LSIL)

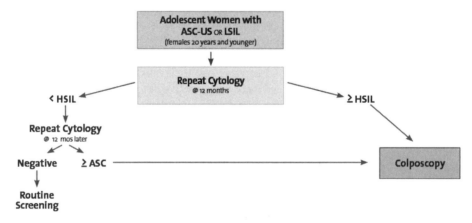

■ **FIG. 16.** Management of adolescent women with either atypical squamous cells of undetermined significance or low-grade squamous intraepithelial lesion. Abbreviations: ASC indicates atypical squamous cells; ASC-US; atypical squamous cells of undetermined significance; HSIL, high-grade squamous intraepithelial lesion; LSIL, low-grade squamous intraepithelial lesion. Wright TC. Management of cervical cytologic abnormalities. J Low Genit Tract Dis 2007;11:201–22. Reprinted from the Journal of Lower Genital Tract Disease Vol. 11 Issue 4, with the permission of ASCCP © American Society for Colposcopy and Cervical Pathology 2007. No copies of the algorithms may be made without the prior consent of ASCCP.

All women with AIS should have an ample diagnostic excisional procedure. Cervical conization may be preferred, because the failure rate may be higher with LEEP because the specimen is smaller. Hysterectomy is preferred for women who have no desire for future childbearing. Follow-up at 6-month intervals with cytology, HPV DNA testing, and colposcopy with endocervical sampling is acceptable if future fertility is desired. If conservative management is planned and the margins of the specimen are involved or endocervical sampling obtained at the time of excision contains CIN or AIS, reexcision to ensure negative margins is preferred (5).

INVASIVE CERVICAL NEOPLASIA

The lifetime risk of a woman's developing cervical cancer in the United States is 1 in 135. Approximately 11,070 new cases and 3,870 deaths due to cervical cancer are predicted to occur in 2008 (63). Worldwide, cervical cancer is the second-leading cause of cancer mortality in women. Among the approximately 500,000 new cases each year; three fourths occur in developing countries (64).

Approximately 80% of cases of cervical cancer are squamous cell carcinomas, and 15% are adenocarcinomas. Other histologic types are rare and include adenoid cystic carcinomas, neuroendocrine (large cell and small cell) carcinomas, lymphomas, melanomas, and sarcomas. Although concerns linger that patients with adenocarcinomas may have a worse prognosis, there are no convincing data showing that these patients should be managed differently.

The use of cervical cytologic testing has reduced the incidence of cervical cancer by approximately 70% in every country where it is readily available. Unfortunately, screening has not been able to eliminate the disease, even in countries where screening is mandated. Human papillomavirus vaccination has the potential to eradicate cervical cancer by eliminating infection with HPV, but the currently available vaccines protect only against genotypes 16 and 18, which account for 70% of cervical cancer.

Diagnosis and Staging

Women with early-stage cervical cancer often have no symptoms. When symptoms are present, they include vaginal discharge, abnormal bleeding, or pain. Abnormal bleeding may occur in the form of postcoital bleeding, abnormal menses, or postmenopausal bleeding. Although most women with abnormal bleeding will eventually prove not to have malignant disease, cervical cancer initially must be considered in the differential diagnosis. Pelvic or lower back pain becomes more frequent with increasing tumor size. The presence of sciatica is of concern because it may suggest lateral extension or metastasis to the pelvic sidewall. With advancing disease, patients may have weight loss or symptoms of bowel or urinary

tract fistulae. Women with azotemia secondary to ureteral obstruction and a pelvic mass are more likely to have cervical carcinoma than primary cancer of the bladder.

The diagnosis of cervical cancer is confirmed by a positive tissue biopsy result. When a tumor is clinically evident, an office punch biopsy usually is sufficient to establish the diagnosis of invasive cervical cancer. However, if the biopsy shows only intraepithelial disease of either squamous or adenomatous type, or invasion is 3 mm or less, a cervical cone biopsy is indicated. A cervical cone biopsy should be performed with caution in the presence of a visible or palpable tumor because of the risk of hemorrhage.

Cancer staging is important for treatment planning and outcomes reporting. The International Federation of Gynecology and Obstetrics (FIGO) staging system for cervical carcinoma is based exclusively on clinical evaluation (Table 14). Furthermore, clinical staging of cervical cancer may be performed where medical resources are scarce. This system acknowledges the prognostic importance of tumor size in stage IB disease and distinguishes clinically occult tumors with negligible risk of extracervical metastasis (stage IA1) from microscopically larger lesions with some risk (approximately 5%) for lymph node involvement (65). Except for pelvic examination and tissue biopsy, allowable clinical staging procedures are uninformative for most patients with stage IA1–IB1 disease but often provide important clinical information to guide treatment planning for patients presenting with larger tumors (Table 15).

Critics of the FIGO staging system point out that several important prognostic factors, such as lymph node metastasis, cannot be assessed with allowable staging procedures. Several modalities can better assess disease extent than those allowed by the FIGO staging; they include computed tomography (CT), magnetic resonance imaging (MRI), positron emission tomography (PET), and surgical staging.

Computed tomography can assess the status of the ureters, retroperitoneal lymph nodes, and abdominal viscera. However, CT does not accurately visualize cervical tumors or the extent of paracervical infiltration. Magnetic resonance imaging is superior to CT in defining the extent of disease in the cervix and parametria and can be particularly useful to radiation oncologists planning intracavitary brachytherapy. Neither CT nor MRI is accurate in assessing lymph nodes for the presence of microscopic metastasis. These summary statements are largely derived from retrospective studies. The American College of Radiology Imaging Network conducted a prospective comparison of MRI, CT, and FIGO staging in patients scheduled for surgical management of stage IB (or greater) cervical cancer. Computed tomography and MRI performed similarly and had lower staging accuracy than in previous single-institution studies (66). In a subsequent analysis, the American College of Radiology Imaging Network noted that MRI was superior to CT for evaluat-

TABLE 14. International Federation of Gynecology and Obstetrics Staging Classification for Cervical Carcinoma

Stage	Classification
0	Carcinoma in situ, cervical intraepithelial neoplasia grade 3.
I	The carcinoma is strictly confined to the cervix (extension to the corpus would be disregarded).
IA	Invasive carcinoma that can be diagnosed only by microscopy. All macroscopically visible lesions—even with superficial invasion—are allotted to stage IB carcinomas. Invasion is limited to a measured stromal invasion with a maximal depth of 5 mm and a horizontal extension of no greater than 7 mm. Depth of invasion should not be greater than 5 mm taken from the base of the epithelium of the original tissue—superficial or glandular. The involvement of vascular spaces—venous or lymphatic—should not change the stage allotment.
IA1	Measured stromal invasion no greater than 3 mm in depth and extension no greater than 7 mm.
IA2	Measured stromal invasion greater than 3 mm and no greater than 5 mm, with an extension no greater than 7 mm.
IB	Clinically visible lesions limited to the cervix uteri or preclinical cancer greater than stage IA.
IB1	Clinically visible lesions no greater than 4 cm.
IB2	Clinically visible lesions greater than 4 cm.
II	Cervical carcinoma invades beyond uterus, but not to the pelvic wall or to the lower third of the vagina.
IIA	No obvious parametrial involvement.
IIB	Obvious parametrial involvement.
III	The carcinoma has extended to the pelvic wall. On rectal examination, there is no cancer-free space between the tumor and the pelvic wall. The tumor involves the lower third of the vagina. All cases with hydronephrosis or nonfunctioning kidney are included, unless they are known to be due to other causes.
IIIA	Tumor involves lower third of the vagina, with no extension to the pelvic wall.
IIIB	Extension to the pelvic wall, or hydronephrosis or both or nonfunctioning kidney.
IV	The carcinoma has extended beyond the true pelvis or has involved (biopsy proven) the mucosa of the bladder or rectum. A bullous enema, as such, does not permit a case to be allotted to stage IV.
IVA	Spread of the growth to adjacent organs.
IVB	Spread to distant organs.

This table was published in International Journal of Gynecology and Obstetrics, volume 95, supplement, Quinn MA, Benedet JL, Odicino F, Maisonneuve P, Beller U, Creasman WT, et al. Carcinoma of the cervix uteri. International Federation of Gynecology and Obstetrics. FIGO annual report on the results of treatment in gynecological cancer, s43, copyright Elsevier 2006.

ing uterine body involvement but that neither method was accurate for evaluating cervical stromal invasion (67).

Positron emission tomography has been compared with CT for assessing lymph node status. In a retrospective study of 101 consecutive patients with newly diagnosed cervical cancer, the use of CT resulted in detecting enlarged pelvic and aortic lymph nodes in 20% and 7% of patients, respectively. Positron emission tomography detected abnormal uptake in pelvic and aortic lymph nodes in 67% and 21% of patients, respectively. However, lymph node metastases were not always confirmed by tissue biopsy (68). Another study prospectively evaluated PET compared with MRI or CT staging of patients with newly diagnosed (35%) or recurrent (65%) cervical cancer. Lesions identified on imaging were verified with the use of surgical biopsy or clinical follow-up. All three modalities were equivalent in identifying the primary tumor; however, PET was superior to MRI and CT in

identifying metastatic disease (69). Therefore, PET was deemed "reasonable and necessary" for pretreatment management of cervical cancer by the Centers for Medicare and Medicaid Services.

Stages IA1 and IA2 Cervical Cancer

The diagnosis of stage IA1 cervical cancer must be established by cone biopsy. The prognosis for patients with stage IA1 cervical cancer is excellent, because they are at very low risk of lymph node metastasis, recurrence, and death. Provided surgical margins are negative, cervical conization alone is adequate treatment for patients desiring future childbearing (70, 71) (Fig. 17). Women who choose conservative therapy over hysterectomy should undergo cytologic surveillance at least every 6 months for several years before resuming annual follow-up. In one series with a median follow-up of 45 months, there were

TABLE 15. International Federation of Gynecology and Obstetrics Staging Procedures for Cervical Cancer

Procedure	Clinical Notes
Pelvic examination	Examination under anesthesia preferred but not required
Colposcopy	Rarely necessary when a tumor is grossly evident
Tissue biopsy	Punch biopsy Cervical cone biopsy (cold-knife, laser, or loop electrosurgical excision procedure)
Chest radiography	Lung metastasis rare in apparent stage I disease, but important for rare histologic types (sarcoma, melanoma, neuroendocrine tumors)
Cystourethroscopy	The presence of bullous edema alone is not sufficient for the diagnosis of bladder invasion; biopsy is required
Intravenous pyelogram	Assessment of ureter obstruction
Barium enema	Large bowel obstruction rare at any stage
Sigmoidoscopy or colonoscopy	Assessment of rectal invasion
Imaging modalities (computed tomography, magnetic resonance imaging, positron emission tomography)	Not permitted in assigning FIGO stage
Surgical staging	Not permitted in assigning FIGO stage

Abbreviation: FIGO indicates International Federation of Gynecology and Obstetrics.

This table was published in International Journal of Gynecology and Obstetrics, volume 95, supplement, Quinn MA, Benedet JL, Odicino F, Maisonneuve P, Beller U, Creasman WT, et al. Carcinoma of the cervix uteri. International Federation of Gynecology and Obstetrics. FIGO annual report on the results of treatment in gynecological cancer, s43, copyright Elsevier 2006.

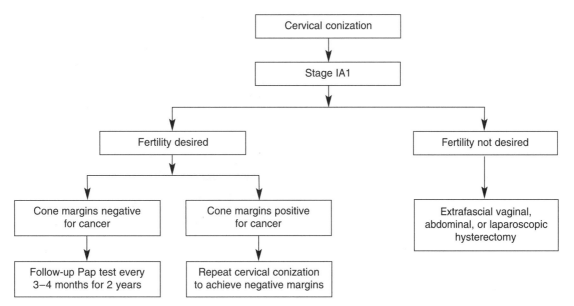

■ **FIG. 17.** Approach to management of stage IA1 cervical cancer.

no cases of cancer recurrence among 30 women treated with cone biopsy; however, three patients (10%) developed CIN 3 (72).

The diagnosis of stage IA2 cervical cancer also should be established by cone biopsy. Although the prognosis for these patients also is good, they are at higher risk for lymph node metastasis and treatment failure compared

with patients who have stage IA1 disease. Optimal therapy for these patients is more controversial; the patients' reproductive intentions should be taken into consideration (Figure 18). There are too few data regarding patients with stage IA2 cervical cancer treated with cervical conization alone. One study observed 22 patients with stage IA1 and 37 patients with stage IA2 cervical cancer (73). Forty-four

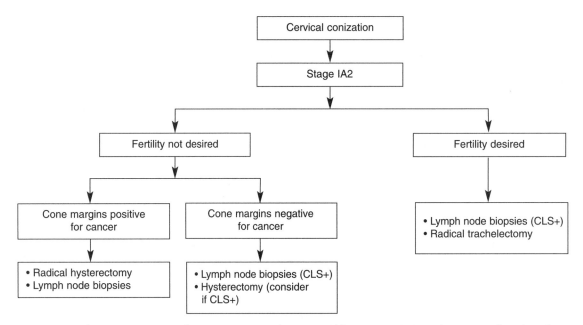

■ FIG. 18. Approach to management of stage IA2 cervical cancer. Abbreviation: CLS+ indicates capillary lymphatic space invasion.

patients initially underwent diagnostic (n=34) or therapeutic (n=10) conization, and 14 patients had involvement of the endocervical margin. Among the 10 patients who underwent cervical conization as definitive treatment, three patients later underwent radical hysterectomy because of cervical recurrence. Overall, seven patients in this series developed a recurrence. The mean age of patients with recurrence was 52.3 years, compared with the general mean age of 42.3 years ($P<.05$). Angiolymphatic invasion was positively correlated with recurrence and death ($P<.01$), as well as with the depth of invasion. The authors concluded that a cone specimen with an involved endocervical margin represented a high risk of recurrence and that this condition tended to occur in older patients; thus, age should be regarded as an important risk factor. Angiolymphatic invasion and greater depth of invasion also represented poor prognostic factors.

Most patients with stage IA2 cervical cancer have undergone either extrafascial or radical hysterectomy. In a review of the hospital records of 166 patients with microinvasive squamous cell carcinoma of the cervix, there were 143 cases of stage IA1 disease and 23 cases of stage IA2 disease (72). All patients treated conservatively had stage IA1 disease. Sixty-seven patients (stage IA1, 44; stage IA2, 23) underwent pelvic lymphadenectomy, and none had lymph node metastasis. Subsequently, 6% of the 143 patients with stage IA1 cervical cancer and 13% of the 23 patients with stage IA2 cervical cancer developed recurrent cervical neoplasia; however, only 4 patients (2.4%) in the entire series had a recurrence with invasive cancer. For patients with stage IA2 cervical cancer, the authors concluded that extrafascial hysterectomy might be an adequate therapy, and they questioned the need for lymphadenectomy. In a review of pathology

specimens from 394 patients with stage I squamous cell cervical carcinoma (depth of stromal invasion of 10 mm or less), none of the patients with depth of stromal invasion of less than 5 mm had pelvic lymph node metastasis (74). However, parametrial spread was found in one case of stage IA1 disease with marked lymphatic space involvement. There were no deaths due to disease in cases with depth of stromal invasion of less than 5 mm. Based on these observations, the authors recommended simple or modified radical hysterectomy with inguinal–femoral lymphadenectomy for stage IA2 cervical squamous cell carcinoma in the presence of lymph–vascular space involvement.

Early-Stage Adenocarcinoma

In a series of 32 patients with stage IA1–IA2 cervical adenocarcinoma, the patients underwent hysterectomy (n=29), radical trachelectomy (n=2), or cervical conization (n=1) (75). Postoperative radiation therapy was administered to one patient. Twenty-seven patients also underwent inguinal–femoral lymphadenectomy, and none had lymph node metastasis. With a mean follow-up of 54 months, no recurrences had been reported. Two patients developed chronic leg edema subsequent to lymphadenectomy. Given the excellent prognosis and the absence of lymph node metastases, the authors recommended less radical surgery for these patients. In another series, none of the 48 women with stage IA1 or stage IA2 cervical adenocarcinoma had parametrial disease or involved lymph nodes (76).

In another study, using the National Cancer Institute's Surveillance, Epidemiology, and End Results population database, 131 patients with stage IA1 cervical adenocarcinoma and 170 patients with stage IA2 cervical adeno-carcinoma were identified (77). Only 1 patient among the 140 who underwent lymph node biopsies had a positive lymph node. The tumor-related death rate was 0.76% for stage IA1 disease and 1.8% for stage IA2 disease. There was no difference in the death rate for patients treated with simple compared with radical hysterectomy. The authors stated that biopsy of the regional lymph nodes was warranted for women with stage IA2 disease.

In a subsequent review, the authors identified 560 cases of cervical adenocarcinoma (200 patients with stage IA1 disease, 286 patients with stage IA2 disease, and 74 patients with "localized" disease). Simple hysterectomy was performed in 272 patients (49%), and radical hysterectomy was performed in 210 patients (38%). Positive lymph nodes were found in 3 of the 197 patients (1.5%) who underwent lymphadenectomy, 2 of whom died. With mean follow-up of 51.6 months, there was no significant difference in survival for stage IA1 disease compared with stage IA2 disease (98.5% versus 98.6%, respectively). Combining these data with all other published series of early cervical adenocarcinoma, the authors identified 1,170 cases, including 585 patients with stage IA1 disease, 358 patients with stage IA2 disease, and 227 patients with forms of less defined early disease. Among 531 patients who underwent lymphadenectomy, 15 patients (1.3%) had one or more positive nodes; of these patients, 11 (73%) later developed recurrence or died. For IA1 disease compared with IA2 disease, there were no significant differences in the frequency of positive lymph nodes,

recurrence, or death. However, patients with forms of less defined early disease and patients with lesions larger than stage IA2 were at increased risk. The authors concluded that early invasive adenocarcinoma (stages IA1 and IA2) has an excellent prognosis and that conservative surgery may be appropriate (78). Others have suggested that fertility-preserving surgery (cone biopsy) may be sufficient therapy for patients with stage IA1 disease (62). These retrospective data suggest that the management of stage IA1 and stage IA2 cervical adenocarcinomas need not differ from that of squamous lesions.

Stage IB1–IIA Cervical Cancer

Approximately one half of all patients with cervical cancer receive an initial diagnosis of stage I disease. These patients have a number of acceptable treatment options that are largely based on surgery, radiation therapy, or both. Most retrospective analyses suggest that radical hysterectomy and pelvic radiation therapy are equally effective in the management of stage IB1 cervical cancer (Table 16). The choice of primary treatment can be influenced by a number of factors, including patient age, obesity status, coexisting medical problems, and physician bias. Younger and healthier patients have tended to undergo surgical treatment, and older and less healthy patients have tended to undergo radiation therapy. Therefore, important prognostic factors often are unbalanced between surgical and radiation therapy groups in retrospective comparisons.

In a comparison of outcome results of conventional surgery versus radiotherapy for 152 patients with cervical

TABLE 16. Surgery Compared With Radiation Therapy for Stages IB1 and IIA Cervical Cancer

Treatment	Advantages	Disadvantages
Radical hysterectomy with pelvic lymphadenectomy	Preserves ovarian function	Surgical morbidity and mortality
	Results in more functional vagina	Risk of general anesthesia
	Gives opportunity to obtain pathologic information with which to individualize treatment	Risk of bleeding and transfusion
		Long-term problems with bladder or rectal function
	Is preferred in women who have received radiation therapy	Possible need for postoperative radiation therapy
	Is preferred in women at risk for irradiation complications (pelvic kidney, extensive adhesions from previous surgery or infection, diverticular disease, tuboovarian abscess)	
External beam radiation therapy with either high-dose-rate or low-dose-rate intracavitary brachytherapy	Avoids risk of surgical morbidity, blood loss and transfusion, general anesthesia	Permanent ovarian failure
		Vaginal shortening and fibrosis
	Allows outpatient treatment	Long-term problems with bladder or rectal function
		Risk of bladder fistula
		Risk of bowel or rectal fistula or stricture

cancer treated with radical surgery or high-dose-rate intra-cavitary brachytherapy, the median follow-up time was 43.5 months (79). The median age was 53 years (range, 25–81 years). There were 13 patients (9%) with stage IA disease, 52 patients (34%) with stage IB disease, 24 patients (16%) with stage IIA disease, and 63 patients (41%) with stage IIB disease. The surgery group included 115 patients (76%) who underwent radical hysterectomy with inguinal–femoral lymphadenectomy. Of these patients, 72 patients (63%) received postoperative radio-therapy. Thirty-seven patients (24%) were assigned to the radiotherapy group. Of these patients, 14 patients (38%) received concurrent chemotherapy. With mean follow-up of 43 months, the 5-year cause-specific survival rates for patients in the surgery and radiotherapy groups were 80% and 82%, respectively. The differences in the survival rates between the two treatments for each of the stage I or stage II patients also were not statistically significant.

There have been few attempts to prospectively compare surgery with radiation therapy, and future prospects for overcoming clinician biases to allow for randomized trials in all but the patient populations at highest risk for treatment failure are limited. It is consistent with the previous discussion of stage IA disease that there do not appear to be differences in outcome for patients with stage IB squamous cell carcinoma or adenocarcinoma of the cervix. In a retrospective analysis of 521 patients treated with radical surgery, overall survival of 88% and 84%, respectively, was reported for patients with squamous cell carcinoma and adenocarcinoma (80). Age, tumor size, grade, depth of invasion, lymph–vascular space involvement, and lymph node metastasis were no different between the two cell types, although metastasis to more than three lymph nodes was significantly higher in patients with adenocarcinoma (80).

Two perceived advantages of surgery include preservation of ovarian function in younger women and fewer detrimental effects on vaginal function. These advantages can be lost if postoperative radiation therapy is administered. Despite bilateral ovarian transposition beyond the anticipated treatment field, permanent ovarian failure occurs in approximately one half of patients if postoperative pelvic radiation therapy is administered. Classic indications for radiation therapy after radical hysterectomy include a positive or close surgical margin, disease extension into parametrial tissues, and lymph node metastasis.

The Gynecologic Oncology Group (GOG) conducted a phase 3 study to determine the role of postoperative radiation therapy in patients with high-risk factors in the hysterectomy specimen but without the classic indications listed previously (81). Eligible patients had stage IB cervical cancer with negative lymph nodes and with two or more of the following features: more than one third (deep) stromal invasion, capillary lymphatic space involvement, and tumor diameter more than 4 cm. There were 137 patients randomized to receive pelvic irradiation and 140

patients randomized to observation. The administration of postoperative radiation therapy resulted in a significant reduction in risk of recurrence (hazard ratio, 0.54; 90% confidence interval, 0.35–0.81; P=.007) and a significant reduction in risk of progression or death (hazard ratio, 0.58; 90% confidence interval, 0.4–0.85; P=.009). Radiation therapy appeared to be particularly beneficial to patients with adenocarcinoma and adenosquamous histologies. However, after an extensive follow-up, the improvement in overall survival with radiation therapy did not reach statistical significance.

Stage IB2 Cervical Cancer

RADICAL HYSTERECTOMY

As tumor size increases, so do the risk of other poor prognostic factors, indications for postoperative therapy, and the risk of treatment failure. One study compared patients with stage IB1 and stage IB2 cervical cancer treated with radical hysterectomy to define predictors of lymph node status and recurrence (82). Radical hysterectomy was performed in 109 patients with stage IB1 disease and in 86 patients with stage IB2 disease. Mean age, estimated blood loss, and perioperative complication rates were similar. There were 38 patients (14 of 109 patients with stage IB1 disease compared with 24 of 86 patients with stage IB2 disease; P=0.01) with positive lymph nodes, including nine patients with positive aortic nodes (two patients with stage IB1 disease and seven patients with stage IB2 disease). Parametrial involvement and outer-two thirds depth of invasion also were significantly more common among patients with stage IB2 tumors. Predictably, patients with stage IB2 disease received adjuvant radiation therapy more frequently than patients with stage IB1 disease (52% versus 37%; P=.04). With a median follow-up of 35 months, estimates of disease-free survival revealed tumor size (P=.008), nodal status (P=.0004), lymph–vascular space involvement (P=.002), parametrial involvement (P=.004), and depth of invasion (P=.0004) as significant univariate predictors. Neither tumor size nor nodal status was a significant predictor of outcome. The authors concluded that prognosis in patients with stage IB cervical cancer seems to be most influenced by factors other than tumor size, and that these factors are best determined pathologically after radical hysterectomy.

Radical hysterectomy is an appropriate treatment of stage IB2 cervical cancer and, according to one decision analysis, may be the most cost-effective strategy (83). Nonetheless, patients with bulky cervical tumors are more likely to have indications for postoperative radiation therapy. A National Cancer Institute consensus conference concluded that "primary therapy should avoid the routine use of radical surgery and radiation therapy" (84). If clinical evaluation reveals risk factors that would likely require postoperative treatment after radical hysterectomy, an alternative treatment approach should be considered. This area is one in which the use of an imaging modality such as PET may lead to a better selection of patients for primary operative intervention.

RADIATION THERAPY FOLLOWED BY ADJUVANT HYSTERECTOMY

The knowledge that adverse prognostic factors are more common among patients with larger tumors has prompted the study of radiation therapy followed by nonradical hysterectomy as a means of improving survival and perhaps reducing treatment-related complications. Retrospective studies of patients with bulky cervical tumors treated with radiation therapy followed by nonradical hysterectomy—compared with those who received radiation therapy alone—usually reported a lower pelvic recurrence rate for the surgical group.

The GOG conducted a randomized trial of radiation therapy with or without extrafascial hysterectomy for patients with stage IB2 cervical cancer. Although there was a lower incidence of local relapse, extrafascial hysterectomy after radiation therapy did not improve the overall survival rate. While awaiting the results of this study, the GOG initiated another phase 3 trial of concurrent chemotherapy and radiation therapy compared with radiation therapy alone in patients with stage IB2 cervical cancer. All patients underwent extrafascial hysterectomy 3–6 weeks after the completion of radiation therapy. Pretreatment CT, lymphangiography, or surgical staging confirming negative aortic lymph nodes was required for all patients. Chemotherapy consisted of a cisplatin dose of 40 mg/m^2 administered weekly during radiation therapy. Rates of progression-free and overall survival were significantly higher for patients who received weekly cisplatin (85). These studies showed that chemotherapy administered concurrently with radiation therapy is more important than adjuvant hysterectomy in the treatment of patients with bulky cervical cancer.

In a related context, the GOG, Southwest Oncology Group, and Radiation Therapy Oncology Group conducted a phase 3 study of radiation therapy compared with radiation therapy and chemotherapy for patients who had undergone radical hysterectomy and had either positive pelvic lymph nodes, parametrial involvement, or positive surgical margins. Eligible patients were randomized to receive pelvic radiation therapy alone compared with pelvic radiation therapy plus concurrent chemotherapy (cisplatin, 70 mg/m^2, plus fluorouracil, 1,000 mg/m^2, every 3 weeks for four cycles). There were 268 patients, and median follow-up was 42 months. The concurrent administration of chemotherapy resulted in improved progress-free and overall survival, and pelvic and extrapelvic recurrences were less frequent. The benefit of chemotherapy was not strongly associated with patient age, histologic type, or tumor grade. The absolute improvement in

5-year survival for radiation therapy and concurrent chemotherapy compared with radiation therapy alone in patients with tumors smaller than 2 cm was only 5% (82% versus 77%, respectively), whereas for patients with tumors larger than 2 cm it was 19% (77% versus 58%, respectively). Similarly, the absolute 5-year survival benefit was less evident among patients with one nodal metastasis (83% compared with 79%, respectively) than among patients with at least two positive nodes (75% compared with 55%, respectively) (86).

NEOADJUVANT CHEMOTHERAPY

Neoadjuvant chemotherapy (administered before surgery or radiation therapy) has proved effective against other solid tumors and has been studied in cervical carcinoma. This approach has several theoretical advantages. Chemotherapy may be more effective if given before tumor blood flow is altered by surgery or radiation therapy, may be less toxic when given before the bone marrow is exposed to radiation, and may effectively manage metastatic disease not appreciated by clinical staging procedures. Finally, neoadjuvant chemotherapy may reduce cervical tumor bulk and render radiation therapy more effective or surgery more feasible.

Several randomized trials have suggested improved outcome with neoadjuvant chemotherapy before radical pelvic surgery (87–89). A meta-analysis of 15 published trials indicated that there is no apparent survival advantage at 2-year and 3-year follow-up for neoadjuvant chemotherapy compared with standard therapy (90). Another meta-analysis, incorporating data from 21 randomized trials, indicated a highly significant reduction in the risk of death with neoadjuvant chemotherapy (91). A comparative study reported on 60 patients with stage IB–IIB bulky cervical cancer treated with preoperative external beam radiation therapy plus weekly cisplatin, 50 mg/m^2, or preoperative neoadjuvant chemotherapy (cisplatin, 50 mg/m^2, plus vincristine, 1 mg/m^2, every 7–10 days, for three courses) (92). Surgery was performed 4–6 weeks after the completion of preoperative treatment. Both groups were well balanced with respect to prognostic factors. After the completion of preoperative treatment, there was no significant difference in complete and partial clinical responses between the two groups. At surgery, there was no significant difference in lymph node status and parametrial involvement between the two groups. Pathologic complete response was significantly higher in the chemoradiation group ($P=.004$). The authors did not report recurrence or survival data.

No clinical trials to date have compared neoadjuvant chemotherapy with an acceptable control arm receiving radiation therapy plus concurrent chemotherapy. Until such studies have been conducted, neoadjuvant chemotherapy should be considered an investigational treatment for patients with cervical cancer.

Minimally Invasive Surgery and Fertility-Conserving Surgery

Alternative surgical approaches to managing cervical cancer are available. Laparoscopic radical hysterectomy and laparoscopically assisted radical vaginal hysterectomy techniques have been used to manage cervical cancer. In a prospective study of various approaches to pelvic lymphadenectomy, consecutive patients scheduled for radical surgery were randomly assigned to transperitoneal, extraperitoneal, or laparoscopic pelvic lymphadenectomy. Extraperitoneal and laparoscopic approaches were feasible, as effective as transperitoneal lymphadenectomy, and performed with a reasonable complication rate. Laparoscopic pelvic lymphadenectomy showed a significantly longer operative time; however, extraperitoneal and laparoscopic approaches minimized some postoperative complications, reducing length of stay (93).

A retrospective analysis was performed to evaluate the records of 35 consecutive patients undergoing laparoscopically assisted radical vaginal hysterectomy (N=27) for early cervical cancer and 32 consecutive patients who underwent abdominal radical hysterectomy (N=28) (94). Cohorts were similar in age, weight, previous abdominal surgery, histologic subtype, FIGO stage, resection margins, lymph node count and status, length of follow-up, and recurrence. There were significant differences between laparoscopic and abdominal approaches for duration of surgery (mean, 160 minutes versus 132 minutes), blood loss (479 mL versus 715 mL), hospital stay (mean, 5 days versus 9 days), postoperative complications (6 patients versus 20 patients), and duration of bladder catheterization (mean, 4 days versus 9 days). Four laparoscopic patients and no abdominal patients required repair of urinary tract injuries; no patients had long-term sequelae.

In another study, patients who underwent laparoscopic-assisted radical vaginal hysterectomy (N=71) and patients who underwent radical abdominal hysterectomy (N=205) for stage IA–IB cervical carcinoma were retrospectively compared (95). Both groups were similar with respect to age and Quetelet index. There were no differences in tumor size or grade, histology, depth of invasion, lymph node metastasis, or surgical margins. All laparoscopic procedures were completed successfully, with no conversions to laparotomy. Differences in intraoperative morbidity (laparoscopic versus abdominal) included blood loss (300 mL versus 500 mL; $P<.001$), operative time (3.5 hours versus 2.5 hours; $P<.001$), and intraoperative complications (13% versus 4%; $P<.03$). Intraoperative complications in the laparoscopy group included cystotomy (seven patients), ureteric injury (one patient), and bowel injury (one patient). The median time to normal urine residual was 10 days compared with 5 days ($P<.001$), and the median length of hospital stay was 1 day compared with 5 days ($P<.001$). The overall 2-year recurrence-free survival was 94% in both groups. These data showed that early cervical cancer can be managed successfully with laparoscopically assisted radical vaginal hysterectomy, with similar efficacy and recurrence rates as radical abdominal hysterectomy. The major benefits are less blood loss and shorter hospital stay. However, laparoscopic surgery is associated with an increase in intraoperative complications and an increased time to return to normal bladder function. Too few gynecologic surgeons have expertise in these procedures. The notion that laparoscopic procedures result in less morbidity, better cosmetic results, shorter recuperation, or equivalent survival should be verified in prospective comparative trials.

Approximately 10–15% of cervical cancers occur in women during their reproductive years, and some of these patients may be reluctant to undergo treatments that result in permanent loss of fertility. The techniques of laparoscopic inguinal–femoral lymphadenectomy and radical vaginal trachelectomy with placement of a cerclage around the lower uterine segment that is sutured to the vaginal cuff were first described more than a decade ago. One study reported on a series of 80 women who had undergone radical trachelectomy (96). There were 39 women who subsequently attempted pregnancy, resulting in a total of 22 pregnancies among 18 patients. In another study, authors planned radical vaginal trachelectomy in 82 patients with early-stage cervical cancer (stages IA, IB, and IIA), preceded by a complete laparoscopic inguinal–femoral lymphadenectomy and laparoscopic parametrectomy (97). The planned procedure was abandoned in 10 cases (12%) either because of positive nodes discovered at the time of surgery (4 patients), positive endocervical margins (5 patients), or extensive tubal adhesions (1 patient). The median age of the remaining 72 patients was 31 years, and most patients (75%) were nulliparous. Most lesions were stage IA2 (32%) or IB1 (60%). In terms of histology, 58% of lesions were squamous cell and 42% of lesions were adenocarcinomas. Vascular space invasion was present in 20% of cases and 90% of the lesions measured less than 2 cm. The mean follow-up was 60 months (6–156 months). The intraoperative complication rate was low (6%), and there were no bladder or ureteral injuries. The average hospital stay was 3 days. Excluding one patient with small cell neuroendocrine carcinoma who had a rapid recurrence and died, there were two recurrences (2.8%) and one death (1.4%). The actuarial recurrence-free survival was 95%. Tumor size greater than 2 cm was statistically significantly associated with a higher risk of recurrence ($P=.03$).

The technique of radical abdominal trachelectomy has been described in the literature (98). Some clinicians prefer the abdominal approach, in part because most gynecologic oncologists do not routinely perform radical vaginal hysterectomy, and the abdominal operation may be easier to perform. At present, there are no data comparing the radical abdominal trachelectomy and the radical vaginal trachelectomy.

Gynecologic oncologists generally do not offer radical trachelectomy to patients with tumors larger than 2 cm. It is more difficult to achieve negative surgical margins in patients with larger stage IB1 or stage IB2 tumors; furthermore, postoperative radiation therapy is more often needed, thereby negating fertility preservation. More data are needed regarding fertility outcome in patients undergoing radical trachelectomy. In this highly selected patient population, the cancer recurrence rate after these procedures appears to be comparable to that of women undergoing abdominal radical hysterectomy.

Stage IIB–IVA (Locally Advanced) Cervical Cancer

Patients presenting with more advanced pelvic tumors should undergo a thorough clinical evaluation before proceeding with treatment. Although it is not recognized in FIGO staging, prospective clinical trials often have required pretreatment imaging or surgical staging in this population at high risk for aortic lymph node metastasis or disease beyond the pelvis. Pretreatment assessment with MRI, CT, or PET is advised.

Radiation therapy is the mainstay of treatment for patients with stage IIB–IVA disease and obviates the need for gastrointestinal or urinary diversion (compared with primary pelvic exenteration). Results from several important clinical trials have changed the way in which locally advanced cervical cancer is managed. Although clinical trials in this patient population are ongoing and further advances are yet to be made, this area currently has the least controversy with respect to cervical cancer management.

If administered in combination with radiation therapy, chemotherapy theoretically could reduce local relapse (by way of drug–radiation interactions) and distant relapse (by way of cytotoxic effects)—and thus improve overall survival. Putative drug–radiation interactions include inhibition of sublethal damage repair; inhibition of recovery from potentially lethal damage; alterations in cellular kinetics shifting tumor cell populations to more radiosensitive phases of the cell cycle; and decreases in tumor bulk leading to improved blood supply, tissue oxygenation, and increased radiosensitivity.

These benefits remained largely theoretical until the results from five phase 3 trials conducted by National Cancer Institute–sponsored cooperative groups demonstrated appreciable survival advantages from the addition of cisplatin-based chemotherapy to primary radiation therapy. The relative risk of death in these five phase 3 trials was reduced by 30–50% with the addition of cisplatin or a cisplatin-containing regimen to radiation therapy. A subsequent meta-analysis of 19 randomized, controlled trials totaling 4,580 patients verified that the addition of chemotherapy to radiation therapy improved progression-free and overall survival (99). Although the search for the ideal "radiation sensitizer" is ongoing, external beam radiation therapy plus concurrent cisplatin (40 mg/m^2 per

week) chemotherapy followed by intracavitary brachytherapy is standard treatment for patients with locally advanced cervical cancer.

Recurrent and Metastatic Cervical Cancer

Clinicians have been overly cautious when applying more conservative management to cervical cancer because recurrent disease is rarely curable. A small number of patients with recurrent pelvic disease subsequent to primary surgery may be successfully treated with radiation therapy. Conversely, a small number of patients with recurrent pelvic disease after primary radiation therapy may be successfully treated with surgery. Pelvic exenteration is reserved for patients with a central pelvic recurrence. The triad of ureteral obstruction, sciatica, and lower extremity edema indicates pelvic sidewall involvement, and attempted surgical resection is not advised. Other poor prognostic factors include a short time interval between primary treatment and recurrence, poor nutritional status, and other patient factors (cardiovascular disease, pulmonary disease, and older patients with poor performance status). Improved outcome with pelvic exenteration has evolved through better patient selection and better operative techniques (100). Refinements in vaginal reconstruction, urinary diversion, and low rectal anastomosis have led to longer survival and better quality of life for many patients (101).

The prognosis is poor when curative radiation therapy or surgery is not feasible. For these patients, palliation is the primary goal of treatment. Cisplatin has long been considered the most active drug against cervical cancer. Clinical trials have attempted (without much success) to identify a chemotherapy agent or regimen yielding higher response rates and longer survival than does cisplatin alone. Single-agent cisplatin was compared with the combination of cisplatin plus paclitaxel in a prospective, controlled trial with quality-of-life assessments included among outcomes measures. The combination of cisplatin plus paclitaxel resulted in a higher objective response rate and longer progression-free survival, but no improvement in overall survival. Although toxicity was greater with combination therapy, this situation did not translate into any apparent decrement in patient-reported quality of life (102). Another GOG phase 3 study compared cisplatin versus cisplatin plus topotecan. Overall survival rates also were improved with a combination regimen (103). However, median survival rates with cisplatin plus topotecan were no greater than median survival rates with cisplatin plus paclitaxel in the previous study. An ongoing prospective clinical trial is comparing these regimens (cisplatin plus paclitaxel and cisplatin plus topotecan) with each other and with two other active cisplatin-containing combinations.

References

1. Walboomers JM, Jacobs MV, Manos MM, Bosch FX, Kummer JA, Shah KV, et al. Human papillomavirus is a necessary cause of invasive cervical cancer worldwide. J Pathol 1999;189:12–9.

2. Schlosser BJ, Howett MK. Human papillomaviruses: molecular aspects of the viral life cycle and pathogenesis. In: Apgar BS, Brotzman GL, Spitzer M, editors. Colposcopy principles and practice: an integrated textbook and atlas. Philadelphia (PA): WB Saunders; 2002. p. 23–39.

3. Schiffman MH, Hildesheim A. Cervical cancer. In: Schottenfeld D, Fraumeni JF, editors. Cancer epidemiology and prevention, 3rd ed. New York (NY): Oxford University Press; 2006.

4. Wright TC Jr, Massad LS, Dunton CJ, Spitzer M, Wilkinson EJ, Solomon D. 2006 consensus guidelines for the management of women with abnormal cervical screening tests. J Low Genit Tract Dis 2007;11:201–22.

5. Wright TC Jr, Massad LS, Dunton CJ, Spitzer M, Wilkinson EJ, Solomon D. 2006 consensus guidelines for the management of women with cervical intraepithelial neoplasia and adenocarcinoma in situ. J Low Genit Tract Dis 2007;11:223–39.

6. Bosch FX, Munoz N, de Sanjose S, Izarzugaza I, Gili M, Viladiu P, et al. Risk factors for cervical cancer in Colombia and Spain. Int J Cancer 1992;52:750–8.

7. Khan MJ, Castle PE, Lorincz AT, Wacholder S, Sherman M, Scott DR, et al. The elevated 10-year risk of cervical precancer and cancer in women with human papillomavirus (HPV) type 16 or 18 and the possible utility of type-specific HPV testing in clinical practice. J Natl Cancer Inst 2005;97:1072–9.

8. Koutsky L, Holmes KK, Critchlow CW, Stevens CE, Paavonen J, Beckman AM, et al. A cohort study of the risk of cervical intraepithelial neoplasia grade 2 or 3 in relation to papillomavirus infection. N Engl J Med 1992;327: 1272–8.

9. Schiffman M, Herrero R, DeSalle R, Hildesheim A, Wacholder S, Rodriguez AC, et al. The carcinogenicity of human papillomavirus types reflects viral evolution. Virology 2005;337:76–84.

10. Ahlbom A, Lichtenstein P, Malmstrom H, Feychting M, Hemminki K, Pedersen NL. Cancer in twins: genetic and nongenetic familial risk factors. J Natl Cancer Inst 1997; 89:287–93.

11. Prokopczyk B, Cox JE, Hoffmann D, Waggoner SE. Identification of tobacco-specific carcinogen in the cervical mucus of smokers and nonsmokers. J Natl Cancer Inst 1997;89:868–73.

12. Turek LP. The structure, function, and regulation of papillomaviral genes in infection and cervical cancer. Adv Virus Res 1994;44:305–56.

13. Slee EA, O'Connor DJ, Lu X. To die or not to die: how does p53 decide? Oncogene 2004;23:2809–18.

14. Kuhne C, Banks L. Cellular targets of the papillomavirus E6 proteins. Papillomavirus Rep 1999;10:139-45.

15. Duensing S, Munger K. Centrosome abnormalities and genomic instability induced by human papillomavirus oncoproteins. Prog Cell Cycle Res 2003;5:383–91.

16. Arroyo M, Bagchi S, Raychaudhuri P. Association of the human papillomavirus type 16 E7 protein with the S-phase-specific E2F-cyclin A complex. Mol Cell Biol 1993;13:6537–46.

17. Munger K, Basile JR, Duensing S, Eichten A, Gonzalez SL, Grace M, et al. Biological activities and molecular targets of the human papillomavirus E7 oncoprotein. Oncogene 2001;20:7888–98.

18. Hopman AH, Smedts F, Dignef W, Ummelen M, Sonke G, Mravunac M, et al. Transition of high-grade cervical intraepithelial neoplasia to micro-invasive carcinoma is characterized by integration of HPV 16/18 and numerical chromosome abnormalities. J Pathol 2004;202:23–33.

19. Lazo PA. The molecular genetics of cervical carcinoma. Br J Cancer 1999;80:2008–18.

20. Toussaint-Smith E, Donner DB, Roman A. Expression of human papillomavirus type 16 E6 and E7 oncoproteins in primary foreskin keratinocytes is sufficient to alter the expression of angiogenic factors. Oncogene 2004;23: 2988–95.

21. Moscicki AB, Shiboski S, Broering J, Powell K, Clayton L, Jay N, et al. The natural history of human papillomavirus infection as measured by repeated DNA testing in adolescent and young women. J Pediatr 1998;132: 277–84.

22. Ho GY, Bierman R, Beardsley L, Chang CJ, Burk RD. Natural history of cervicovaginal papillomavirus infection in young women. N Engl J Med 1998;338:423–8.

23. Ries LA, Melbert D, Krapcho M, Mariotto A, Miller BA, Feuer EJ, et al., editors. SEER cancer statistics review, 1975–2004. Bethesda (MD): National Cancer Institute; 2007. Available at: http://seer.cancer.gov/csr/1975_2004. Retrieved August 17, 2007.

24. Saslow D, Runowicz CD, Solomon D, Moscicki AB, Smith RA, Eyre HJ, et al. American Cancer Society guideline for the early detection of cervical neoplasia and cancer. CA Cancer J Clin 2002;52:342–62.

25. Routine cancer screening. ACOG Committee Opinion No. 356. American College of Obstetricians and Gynecologists. Obstet Gynecol 2006;108:1611–3.

26. Wright TC Jr, Schiffman M, Solomon D, Cox JT, Garcia F, Goldie S, et al. Interim guidance for the use of human papillomavirus DNA testing as an adjunct to cervical cytology for screening. Obstet Gynecol 2004;103:304–9.

27. Wright TC Jr, Cox JT, Massad LS, Twiggs LB, Wilkinson EJ. 2001 Consensus Guidelines for the Management of Women with Cervical Cytological Abnormalities. JAMA 2002;287:2120–9.

28. Schiffman M, Herrero R, Hildesheim A, Sherman ME, Bratti M, Wacholder S, et al. HPV DNA testing in cervi-

cal cancer screening: results from women in a high-risk province of Costa Rica. JAMA 2000;283:87–93.

29. Petry KU, Menton S, Menton M, van Loenen-Frosch F, de Carvalho Gomes H, Holz B, et al. Inclusion of HPV testing in routine cervical cancer screening for women above 29 years in Germany: results for 8466 patients. Br J Cancer 2003;88:1570–7.

30. Sherman ME, Lorincz AT, Scott DR, Wacholder S, Castle PE, Glass AG, et al. Baseline cytology, human papillomavirus testing, and risk for cervical neoplasia: a 10-year cohort analysis. J Natl Cancer Inst 2003;95:46–52.

31. Goldie SJ, Kim JJ, Wright TC. Cost-effectiveness of human papillomavirus DNA testing for cervical cancer screening in women aged 30 years or more. Obstet Gynecol 2004;103:619–31.

32. Sawaya GF, Grady D, Kerlikowske K, Valleur JL, Barnabei VM, Bass K, et al. The positive predictive value of cervical tests in previously screened postmenopausal women: the Heart and Estrogen/progestin Replacement Study (HERS). Ann Intern Med 2000;133:942–50.

33. U.S. Preventive Services Task Force. Screening for cervical cancer. Rockville (MD): Agency for Healthcare Research and Quality; 2003. Available at: http://www.ahrq.gov/clinic/3rduspstf/cervcan/cervcanwh.pdf. Retrieved October 11, 2007.

34. Cervical cytology screening. ACOG Practice Bulletin No. 45. American College of Obstetricians and Gynecologists. Obstet Gynecol 2003;102:417–27.

35. Davey DD, Neal MH, Wilbur DC, Colgan TJ, Styer PE, Mody DR. Bethesda 2001 implementation and reporting rates: 2003 practices of participants in the College of American Pathologists Interlaboratory Comparison Program in Cervicovaginal Cytology. Arch Pathol Lab Med 2004;128:1224–9.

36. Cox JT, Schiffman M, Solomon D. Prospective follow-up suggests similar risk of subsequent cervical intraepithelial neoplasia grade 2 or 3 among women with cervical intraepithelial neoplasia grade 1 or negative colposcopy and directed biopsy. ASCUS-LSIL Triage Study (ALTS) Group. Am J Obstet Gynecol 2003;188:1406–12.

37. Kyrgiou M, Tsoumpou I, Vrekoussis T, Martin-Hirsch P, Arbyn M, Prendiville W, et al. The up-to-date evidence on colposcopy practice and treatment of cervical intraepithelial neoplasia: the Cochrane colposcopy & cervical cytopathology collaborative group (C5 group) approach. Cancer Treat Rev 2006;32:516–23.

38. Sadler L, Saftlas A, Wang W, Exeter M, Whittaker J, McCowan L. Treatment for cervical intraepithelial neoplasia and risk of preterm delivery. JAMA 2004;291:2100–6.

39. Spitzer M, Chernys AE, Shifrin A, Ryskin M. Indications for cone biopsy: pathologic correlations. Am J Obstet Gynecol 1998;178:74–9.

40. Moscicki AB, Schiffman M, Kjaer S, Villa LL. Chapter updating the natural history of HPV and anogenital cancer. Vaccine 2006;24(suppl 3):S42–51.

41. Boardman LA, Stanko C, Weitzen S, Sung CJ. Atypical squamous cells of undetermined significance: human papillomavirus testing in adolescents. Obstet Gynecol 2005;105:741–6.

42. Moscicki AB, Shiboski S, Hills NK, Powell KJ, Jay N, Hanson EN, et al. Regression of low-grade squamous intra-epithelial lesions in young women. Lancet 2004; 364:1678–83.

43. Jain AG, Higgins RV, Boyle MJ. Management of low-grade squamous intraepithelial lesions during pregnancy. Am J Obstet Gynecol 1997;177:298–302.

44. Insinga RP, Glass AG, Rush BB. Diagnoses and outcomes in cervical cancer screening: a population-based study. Am J Obstet Gynecol. 2004;191:105–13.

45. Sherman ME, Schiffman M, Cox JT. Effects of age and human papilloma viral load on colposcopy triage: data from the randomized Atypical Sqaumous Cells of Undeterrmined Significance/Low-Grade Squamous Intraepithelial Lesion Triage Study (ALTS). Atypical Sqaumous Cells of Undeterrmined Significance/Low-Grade Squamous Intraepithelial Lesion Triage Study Group. J Natl Cancer Inst 2002;94:102–7.

46. Kirby TO, Allen ME, Alvarez RD, Hoesley CJ, Huh WK. High-risk human papillomavirus and cervical intraepithelial neoplasia at time of atypical squamous cells of undetermined significance cytologic results in a population with human immunodeficiency virus. J Low Genit Tract Dis 2004;8:298–303.

47. Massad LS, Ahdieh L, Benning L, Minkoff H, Greenblatt RM, Watts H, et al. Evolution of cervical abnormalities among women with HIV-evidence from surveillance cytology in the women's interagency HIV study. J Acquir Immune Defic Syndr 2001;27:432–42.

48. Massad LS, Collins YC, Meyer PM. Biopsy correlates of abnormal cervical cytology classified using the Bethesda system. Gynecol Oncol 2001;82:516–22.

49. Jones BA, Davey DD. Quality management in gynecologic cytology using interlaboratory comparison. Arch Pathol Lab Med 2000;124:672–81.

50. Sharpless KE, Schnatz PF, Mandavilli S, Greene JF, Sorosky JI. Dysplasia associated with atypical glandular cells on cervical cytology [published erratum appears in Obstet Gynecol 2005;105:1495]. Obstet Gynecol 2005; 105:494–500.

51. Desimone CP, Day ME, Tovar MM, Dietrich CS 3rd, Eastham ML, Modesitt SC. Rate of pathology from atypical glandular cell Pap tests classified by the Bethesda 2001 nomenclature. Obstet Gynecol 2006;107:1285–91.

52. Derchain SF, Rabelo-Santos SH, Sarian LO, Zeferino LC, de Oliveira Zambeli ER, do Amaral Westin MC, et al. Human papillomavirus DNA detection and histological findings in women referred for atypical glandular cells or adenocarcinoma in situ in their Pap smears. Gynecol Oncol 2004;95:618–23.

53. Greenspan DL, Cardillo M, Davey DD, Heller DS, Moriarty AT. Endometrial cells in cervical cytology:

review of cytological features and clinical assessment. J Low Genit Tract Dis 2006;10:111–22.

54. Simsir A, Carter W, Elgert P, Cangiarella J. Reporting endometrial cells in women 40 years and older: assessing the clinical usefulness of Bethesda 2001. Am J Clin Pathol 2005;123:571–5.

55. Jakobsson M, Gissler M, Sainio S, Paavonen J, Tapper AM. Preterm delivery after surgical treatment for cervical intraepithelial neoplasia. Obstet Gynecol 2007;109:309–13.

56. El-Bastawissi AY, Becker TM, Daling JR. Effect of cervical carcinoma in situ and its management on pregnancy outcome. Obstet Gynecol 1999;93:207–12.

57. Wang SS, Sherman ME, Hildesheim A, Lacey JV Jr, Devesa S. Cervical adenocarcinoma and squamous cell carcinoma incidence trends among white women and black women in the United States for 1976–2000. Cancer 2004;100:1035–44.

58. Yost NP, Santoso JT, McIntire DD, Iliya FA. Postpartum regression rates of antepartum cervical intraepithelial neoplasia II and III lesions. Obstet Gynecol 1999;93:359–62.

59. Connor JP. Noninvasive cervical cancer complicating pregnancy. Obstet Gynecol Clin North Am 1998;25:331–42.

60. Stoler MH, Schiffman M. Interobserver reproducibility of cervical cytologic and histologic interpretations: realistic estimates from the ASCUS-LSIL Triage Study. Atypical Squamous Cells of Undetermined Significance/Low-Grade Squamous Intraepithelial Lesion Triage Study (ALTS) Group. JAMA 2001;285:1500–5.

61. Soutter WP, Haidopoulos D, Gornall RJ, McIndoe GA, Fox J, Mason WP, et al. Is conservative treatment for adenocarcinoma in situ of the cervix safe? BJOG 2001;108:1184–9.

62. McHale MT, Le TD, Burger RA, Gu M, Rutgers JL, Monk BJ. Fertility sparing treatment for in situ and early invasive adenocarcinoma of the cervix. Obstet Gynecol 2001;98:726–31.

63. American Cancer Society. Cancer facts and figures 2008. Atlanta (GA): ACS; 2008. Available at: http://www.cancer.org/downloads/STT/2008CAFFfinalsecured.pdf. Retrieved February 20, 2008.

64. Franco EL, Schlecht NF, Saslow D. The epidemiology of cervical cancer. Cancer J 2003;9:348–59.

65. Lee KB, Lee JM, Park CY, Lee KB, Cho HY, Ha SY. Lymph node metastasis and lymph vascular space invasion in microinvasive squamous cell carcinoma of the uterine cervix. Int J Gynecol Cancer 2006;16:1184–7.

66. Hricak H, Gatsonis C, Chi DS, Amendola MA, Brandt K, Schwartz LH, et al. Role of imaging in pretreatment evaluation of early invasive cervical cancer: results of the intergroup study American College of Radiology Imaging Network 6651-Gynecologic Oncology Group 183. American College of Radiology Imaging Network 6651; Gynecologic Oncology Group 183. J Clin Oncol 2005;23:9329–37.

67. Mitchell DG, Snyder B, Coakley F, Reinhold C, Thomas G, Amendola M, et al. Early invasive cervical cancer: tumor delineation by magnetic resonance imaging, computed tomography, and clinical examination, verified by pathologic results, in the ACRIN 6651/GOG 183 Intergroup Study. J Clin Oncol 2006;24:5687–94.

68. Grigsby PW, Siegel BA, Dehdashti F. Lymph node staging by positron emission tomography in patients with carcinoma of the cervix. J Clin Oncol 2001;19:3745–9.

69. Yen TC, Ng KK, Ma SY, Chou HH, Tsai CS, Hsueh S, et al. Value of dual-phase 2-fluoro-2-deoxy-d-glucose positron emission tomography in cervical cancer [published erratum appears in J Clin Oncol 2004;22:209]. J Clin Oncol 2003;21:3651–8.

70. Kesic V. Management of cervical cancer. Eur J Surg Oncol 2006;32:832–7.

71. Mota F. Microinvasive squamous carcinoma of the cervix: treatment modalities. Acta Obstet Gynecol Scand 2003;82:505–9.

72. Gadducci A, Sartori E, Maggino T, Landoni F, Zola P, Cosio S, et al. The clinical outcome of patients with stage Ia1 and Ia2 squamous cell carcinoma of the uterine cervix: a Cooperation Task Force (CTF) study. Eur J Gynaecol Oncol 2003;24:513–6.

73. Marana HR, de Andrade JM, Matthes AC, Spina LA, Carrara HH, Bighetti S. Microinvasive carcinoma of the cervix: analysis of prognostic factors. Eur J Gynaecol Oncol 2001;22:64–6.

74. Kodama J, Mizutani Y, Hongo A, Yoshinouchi M, Kudo T, Okuda H. Optimal surgery and diagnostic approach of stage IA2 squamous cell carcinoma of the cervix. Eur J Obstet Gynecol Reprod Biol 2002;101:192–5.

75. Ceballos KM, Shaw D, Daya D. Microinvasive cervical adenocarcinoma (FIGO stage 1A tumors): results of surgical staging and outcome analysis. Am J Surg Pathol 2006;30:370–4.

76. Balega J, Michael H, Hurteau J, Moore DH, Santiesteban J, Sutton GP, et al. The risk of nodal metastasis in early adenocarcinoma of the uterine cervix. Int J Gynecol Cancer 2004;14:104–9.

77. Webb JC, Key CR, Qualls CR, Smith HO. Population-based study of microinvasive adenocarcinoma of the uterine cervix. Obstet Gynecol 2001;97:701–6.

78. Smith HO, Qualls CR, Romero AA, Webb JC, Dorin MH, Padilla LA, et al. Is there a difference in survival for IA1 and IA2 adenocarcinoma of the uterine cervix? Gynecol Oncol 2002;85:229–41.

79. Yamashita H, Nakagawa K, Tago M, Shiraishi K, Nakamura N, Ohtomo K, et al. Comparison between conventional surgery and radiotherapy for FIGO stage I-II cervical carcinoma: a retrospective Japanese study. Gynecol Oncol 2005;97:834–9.

80. Ayhan A, Al RA, Baykal C, Demirtas E, Yuce K, Ayhan A. A comparison of prognoses of FIGO stage IB adenocarcinoma and squamous cell carcinoma. Int J Gynecol Cancer 2004;14:279–85.

81. Rotman M, Sedlis A, Piedmonte MR, Bundy B, Lentz SS, Muderspach LI, et al. A phase III randomized trial of postoperative pelvic irradiation in stage IB cervical carcinoma with poor prognostic features: follow-up of a Gynecologic Oncology Group study. Int J Radiat Oncol Biol Phys 2006;65:169–76.

82. Rutledge TL, Kamelle SA, Tillmanns TD, Gould NS, Wright JD, Cohn DE, et al. A comparison of stages IB1 and IB2 cervical cancers treated with radical hysterectomy: is size the real difference? Gynecol Oncol 2004; 95:70–6.

83. Rocconi RP, Estes JM, Leath CA 3rd, Kilgore LC, Huh WK, Straughn JM Jr. Management strategies for stage IB2 cervical cancer: a cost-effectiveness analysis. Gynecol Oncol 2005;97:387–94.

84. National Institutes of Health Consensus Development Conference statement on cervical cancer. April 1–3, 1996. Gynecol Oncol 1997;66:351–61.

85. Moore DH. Treatment of stage IB2 (bulky) cervical carcinoma. Cancer Treat Rev 2003;29:401–6.

86. Monk BJ, Wang J, Im S, Stock RJ, Peters WA 3rd, Liu PY, et al. Rethinking the use of radiation and chemotherapy after radical hysterectomy: a clinical-pathologic analysis of a Gynecologic Oncology Group/Southwest Oncology Group/Radiation Therapy Oncology Group trial. Gynecologic Oncology Group; Southwest Oncology Group; Radiation Therapy Oncology Group. Gynecol Oncol 2005;96:721–8.

87. Benedetti-Panici P, Greggi S, Colombo A, Amoroso M, Smaniotto D, Giannarelli D, et al. Neoadjuvant chemotherapy and radical surgery versus exclusive radiotherapy in locally advanced squamous cell cervical cancer: results from the Italian multicenter randomized study. J Clin Oncol 2002;20:179–88.

88. Behtash N, Nazari Z, Ayatollahi H, Modarres M, Ghaemmaghami F, Mousavi A. Neoadjuvant chemotherapy and radical surgery compared to radical surgery alone in bulky stage IB-IIA cervical cancer. Eur J Surg Oncol 2006;32:1226–30.

89. Cai HB, Chen HZ, Yin HH. Randomized study of preoperative chemotherapy versus primary surgery for stage IB cervical cancer. J Obstet Gynaecol Res 2006;32:315–23.

90. Tierney JF, Stewart LA, Parmar MK. Can the published data tell us about the effectiveness of neoadjuvant chemotherapy for locally advanced cancer of the uterine cervix? Eur J Cancer 1999;35:406–9.

91. Neoadjuvant chemotherapy for locally advanced cervical cancer: a systematic review and meta-analysis of individual patient data from 21 randomised trials. Neoadjuvant Chemotherapy for Locally Advanced Cervical Cancer Meta-analysis Collaboration. Eur J Cancer 2003;39:2470–86.

92. Modarress M, Maghami FQ, Golnavaz M, Behtash N, Mousavi A, Khalili GR. Comparative study of chemoradiation and neoadjuvant chemotherapy effects before radical hysterectomy in stage IB-IIB bulky cervical cancer and with tumor diameter greater than 4 cm. Int J Gynecol Cancer 2005;15:483–8.

93. Panici PB, Plotti F, Zullo MA, Muzii L, Manci N, Palaia I, et al. Pelvic lymphadenectomy for cervical carcinoma: laparotomy extraperitoneal, transperitoneal or laparoscopic approach? A randomized study. Gynecol Oncol 2006;103:859–64.

94. Sharma R, Bailey J, Anderson R, Murdoch J. Laparoscopically assisted radical vaginal hysterectomy (Coelio-Schauta): comparison with open Wertheim/Meigs hysterectomy. Int J Gynecol Cancer 2006;16:1927–32.

95. Steed H, Rosen B, Murphy J, Laframboise S, De Petrillo D, Covens A. A comparison of laparoscopic-assisted radical vaginal hysterectomy and radical abdominal hysterectomy in the treatment of cervical cancer. Gynecol Oncol 2004;93:588–93.

96. Bernardini M, Barrett J, Seaward G, Covens A. Pregnancy outcomes in patients with radical trachelectomy. Am J Obstet Gynecol 2003;189:1378–82.

97. Plante M, Renaud MC, Francois H, Roy M. Vaginal radical trachelectomy: an oncologically safe fertility-preserving surgery. An updated series of 72 cases and review of the literature. Gynecol Oncol 2004;94:614–23.

98. Smith JR, Boyle DC, Corless DJ, Ungar LE, Lawson AD, Del Piore G, et al. Abdominal radical trachelectomy: a new surgical technique for the conservative management of cervical carcinoma. Br J Obstet Gynaecol 1997;104: 1196–200.

99. Kuzuya K. Chemoradiotherapy for uterine cancer: current status and perspectives. Int J Clin Oncol 2004;9:458–70.

100. Berek JS, Howe C, Lagasse LD, Hacker NF. Pelvic exenteration for recurrent gynecologic malignancy: survival and morbidity analysis of the 45-year experience at UCLA. Gynecol Oncol 2005;99:153–9.

101. Lambrou NC, Pearson JM, Averette HE. Pelvic exenteration of gynecologic malignancy: indications and technical reconstructive considerations. Surg Oncol Clin N Am 2005;14:289–300.

102. Moore DH, Blessing JA, McQuellon RP, Thaler HT, Cella D, Benda J, et al. Phase III study of cisplatin with or without paclitaxel in stage IVB, recurrent, or persistent squamous cell carcinoma of the cervix: a gynecologic oncology group study. J Clin Oncol 2004;22:3113–9.

103. Long HJ, Bundy BN, Grendys EC Jr, Benda JA, McMeekin DS, Sorosky J, et al. Randomized phase III trial of cisplatin with or without topotecan in carcinoma of the uterine cervix: a Gynecologic Oncology Group study. J Clin Oncol 2005;23:4626–33.

Cancer of the Uterine Corpus

Peter G. Rose, MD

Uterine cancer is the most common malignancy of the female genital tract, accounting for more than one half of all gynecologic cancers in the United States. Approximately 41,200 new cases are diagnosed annually, resulting in more than 7,350 deaths—more than double the number of deaths a decade ago. Uterine cancer is the fourth most common cancer in women, ranking behind breast, lung, and colon cancer, and it is the eighth leading cause of female death from malignancy. Overall, approximately 2–3% of women will develop uterine cancer during their lifetime. Ninety-seven percent of all cases of uterine cancer arise from the glands of the endometrium and are known as *endometrial carcinomas*. The remaining 3% of cases of uterine cancer arise from mesenchymal uterine components and are classified as *sarcomas*.

EPIDEMIOLOGY AND RISK FACTORS

Endometrial carcinoma most often occurs in women older than 50 years, with a median age 60 years. Two different pathogenetic types of endometrial carcinoma exist (Table 17). Type I tumors, the most common type of endometrial carcinoma, occur more often in younger or perimenopausal women and tend to be better differentiated than type II tumors. Most are estrogen dependent, and many have positive estrogen and progesterone receptors. Type II endometrial carcinomas are poorly differentiated or of papillary serous or clear cell histology and tend to occur in older, thin, postmenopausal women with no source of excess estrogen, arising in a background of atrophic endometrium. Type II tumors are associated with a poorer prognosis than are estrogen-dependent tumors.

Type I endometrial cancer cases are associated with genetic mutations of *K-ras*, *PTEN*, and *MLH1*, whereas aneuploidy, allelic imbalance, mutations in *p53*, and *erb-B2* overexpression are seen in type II cancer cases. African-American women with endometrial carcinoma have a poorer prognosis because of the disproportionately higher percentage of type II carcinomas. A population-based study indicated that the high-risk type II carcinomas occur in equal frequency in the African-American and white population but that the frequency of type I endometrial cancer was threefold greater in the white population. This situation may contribute to most of the decreased mortality rate for white patients who have endometrial cancer.

Most risk factors for the development of type I endometrial cancer are related to prolonged, unopposed estrogen stimulation of the endometrium (Table 18). Women who are 50 lb overweight are at the greatest risk for developing endometrial cancer (relative risk, 10.8). Obesity increases the risk of endometrial carcinoma as a result of peripheral conversion of adrenally derived androstenedione by aromatization to excessive levels of estrone by fat tissue. A history of oligomenorrhea as a result of anovulatory cycles results in prolonged exposure to estrogen without sufficient progesterone, thus increasing the risk. Other factors leading to long-term estrogen exposure, such as polycystic ovary syndrome and estrogen-producing ovarian tumors, are associated with an increased risk of endometrial cancer. Postmenopausal estrogen therapy without progestin increases the risk of endometrial cancer four to eight times. The addition of progestin significantly reduces this risk. Tamoxifen, although an estrogen antagonist in the breast, has an estrogen-agonist effect on the endometrium and increases the risk of endometrial carcinoma (relative risk, 2.2). In addition, diabetes and other medical conditions, such as hypertension and hypothyroidism, have been associated with endometrial cancer. However, a causal relationship has not been confirmed.

A hereditary disposition to endometrial carcinoma has been described in two hereditary syndromes. The Lynch II syndrome (hereditary nonpolyposis colorectal cancer syndrome) is caused by inherited germline mutations in DNA-mismatch repair genes. A second rare hereditary syndrome, site-specific uterine cancer syndrome, also has been identified and is associated with a defect in DNA mismatch repair.

DIAGNOSIS

There are no cost-effective screening techniques for early detection of endometrial cancer in asymptomatic women. Pap tests or routine endometrial biopsies, even in women with risk factors, are not adequate for screening. The diagnosis is based on evaluation of signs and symptoms.

Most patients who have endometrial cancer present with abnormal uterine bleeding early in the development of the disease. Appropriate testing in this situation usually results in early diagnosis, timely treatment, and a high

TABLE 17. Two Pathogenic Types of Endometrial Carcinoma

Association With	Type I	Type II
Estrogen Use	Associated	Not associated
Obesity	Associated	Not associated
Tumor		
Grade	Grades 1, 2	Grade 3, serous, clear cell
Depth of invasion	Superficial	Deep
Nodal metastasis	Infrequent	Frequent
Estrogen and progesterone receptor positivity	Frequent	Infrequent
Stage	Low	High
Prognosis	Excellent	Poor

TABLE 18. Risk Ratio Estimated for Certain Factors Correlated With Endometrial Cancer

Factor	Risk Ratio
Overweight (age 50–59 years) 20–50 lb	3
Overweight (age 50–59 years) more than 50 lb	10
Nulliparity vs one child	2
Nulliparity vs five children	5
Late menopause (women aged 52 years or older compared with women younger than 49 years)	2.4
Diabetes by personal history	2.8
Irradiation to the pelvis	8
Exogenous unopposed estrogen use	6
Tamoxifen	2.2
Sequential oral contraceptive use	7
Combination oral contraceptive use	0.5

cure rate. Only approximately 10% of patients with postmenopausal bleeding have endometrial cancer. However, the likelihood of endometrial cancer with postmenopausal bleeding is variable and age dependent, occurring in 9.3%, 16.3%, 27.9%, and 60% of patients in their 50s, 60s, 70s, and 80s, respectively. Abnormal bleeding, especially in perimenopausal women, and any bleeding in postmenopausal women should always be investigated. Nongenital tract sites should be considered, and testing for blood in the urine and stool should be considered. Bleeding may not occur in some patients with endometrial cancer because of cervical stenosis and associated hematometra. This finding often is associated with a poor prognosis. Less than 5% of women with diagnosed endometrial cancer are asymptomatic. In the absence of symptoms, endometrial cancer usually is detected as the result of investigation of abnormal Pap test results, removal of the uterus for some other reason, or evaluation of an abnormal finding on pelvic ultrasonography or computed tomography performed for an unrelated reason.

Premenopausal women with endometrial cancer usually have abnormal uterine bleeding, which often is characterized as menorrhagia or menometrorrhagia. The diagnosis of endometrial cancer must be considered in premenopausal women with abnormal bleeding, especially if the patient is obese or has a history of chronic anovulation.

The use of endometrial ablation for the treatment of patients with abnormal uterine bleeding is becoming more common, and cases of subsequent diagnosis of endometrial carcinoma have been reported. A pretreatment biopsy is essential before ablative procedures are undertaken to identify endometrial pathologic conditions that will not be managed well with ablation.

Physical examination seldom reveals any evidence of endometrial carcinoma. Abdominal examination usually is unremarkable except in advanced cases, in which ascites or hepatic or omental metastases may be palpable. On gynecologic examination, the vaginal introitus and suburethral area, as well as the entire vagina and cervix, should be carefully inspected and palpated. Bimanual rectovaginal examination should be done to specifically evaluate the uterus for size and mobility, the adnexa for masses, the parametrium for induration, and the cul-de-sac for nodularity.

To evaluate patients with abnormal vaginal bleeding, a Pap test and office endometrial biopsy should be performed. A normal Pap test result does not exclude endometrial cancer, because only 30–50% of patients with endometrial cancer have abnormal Pap test results. Outpatient endometrial biopsy generally is well tolerated and has a diagnostic accuracy of 93–98% when compared with subsequent findings of hysterectomy or dilation and curettage (D&C). In the absence of a diagnosis of endometrial cancer based on endometrial biopsy, a transvaginal ultrasound examination may be useful in determining the need for additional testing. Findings of an endometrial thickness greater than 5 mm, a polypoid endometrial mass, or a fluid collection within the uterus require further evaluation. However, the ultrasound finding of an endometrial thickness less than 5 mm does not eliminate the need for endometrial sampling in a symptomatic postmenopausal woman. Performance of a D&C should be reserved for situations in which cervical stenosis or patient tolerance does not permit adequate evaluation by an endometrial biopsy. Additionally, a D&C should be performed if bleeding recurs after a negative endometrial biopsy, or if the specimen obtained is inadequate to explain the abnormal bleeding. Hysteroscopy is more accurate than endometrial biopsy or D&C alone in identifying polyps and submucous myomata.

ENDOMETRIAL HYPERPLASIA

Endometrial hyperplasia is an overabundance of nonsecretory endometrium that makes up more than 50% of the tissue specimen. Endometrial hyperplasia usually evolves within a background of proliferative endometrium that is a result of protracted estrogen stimulation in the absence of progestin. It may precede or occur simultaneously with endometrial cancer. The risk of endometrial hyperplasia's progressing to carcinoma is related to the type of hyperplasia and the presence and severity of cytologic atypia. Progression to carcinoma occurs in approximately 1% of patients with simple hyperplasia, 3% of patients with complex hyperplasia without atypia, 8% of patients with simple hyperplasia with atypia, and approximately 30–40 % of patients with complex hyperplasia with atypia. The premalignant potential of hyperplasia is influenced by underlying ovarian disease, endocrinopathy, obesity, and exogenous hormone exposure.

Progestin therapy is very effective in reversing endometrial hyperplasia without atypia, but it is less effective in the management of endometrial hyperplasia with atypia. For women with endometrial hyperplasia, cyclical progestin therapy (for example, 10–20 mg of medroxyprogesterone acetate per day for 14 days per month) or continuous progestin therapy (for example, megestrol acetate, 20–40 mg per day) seems to be effective.

Hysterectomy usually is advised for patients with complex hyperplasia with atypia because endometrial carcinoma will subsequently develop or is concurrently present in many patients. In a recent study of 289 evaluable patients with complex hyperplasia with atypia, 123 (42.6%) had endometrial cancer (1). Although almost 70% of cases were limited to the endometrium, 38 (30.9%) had myometrial invasion, and 13 (10.6%) had outer-half myometrial invasion. Therefore, atypical complex hyperplasia should be managed as a potential low-grade endometrial cancer. At the time of hysterectomy, peritoneal cytologic sampling and an intraoperative frozen section should be obtained. The patient should be counseled about the potential need for pelvic and paraaortic selective lymphadenectomy if more than minimally invasive carcinoma is found.

In patients who are poor surgical candidates, high-dose hormone therapy with the progestin megestrol acetate (160 mg per day in divided doses) probably is the most reliable management for reversing atypical hyperplasia. Therapy should be continued for 3 months, after which an endometrial biopsy should be performed to assess response. For patients in whom systemic progesterone is contraindicated or complicates preexisting medical problems such as diabetes, a progesterone-eluting intrauterine device may be considered. Hormone therapy in this circumstance produces a standard response in as many as 50–75% of patients. For patients who respond, lifelong therapy usually is required.

ENDOMETRIAL CARCINOMA

From a practical viewpoint, most endometrial carcinomas can be classified into three major types: endometrioid carcinoma and its variants, papillary serous carcinoma, and clear cell carcinoma. The latter two are considered poorly differentiated tumors.

The histologic classification of carcinoma arising in the endometrium is shown in Box 10. Endometrioid carcinomas account for approximately 80% of endometrial carcinomas. These tumors are composed of glands that resemble normal endometrial glands with varying amounts of solid tumor. The differentiation, expressed as its grade, is determined by architectural growth pattern and nuclear features (Box 11).

Less differentiated tumors contain more solid areas, less glandular formation, and more cytologic atypia. The well-differentiated endometrial cancers may be difficult to separate from atypical hyperplasia. Approximately 15–25% of endometrioid carcinomas have areas of squa-

Classification of Endometrial Carcinomas

Endometrioid adenocarcinoma

    Variants

    Villoglandular or papillary

    Secretory

    With squamous differentiation

Mucinous carcinoma

Papillary serous carcinoma

Clear cell carcinoma

Squamous carcinoma

Undifferentiated carcinoma

Mixed carcinoma

Lurain JR. Uterine cancer. In: Berek JS, editor. Berek and Novak's gynecology. 14th ed. Philadelphia (PA): Lippincott Williams and Wilkins; 2007. p. 1351.

International Federation of Gynecology and Obstetrics Definition for Grading of Endometrial Carcinoma

Histopathologic degree of differentiation:

    Grade 1: less than 5% nonsquamous or nonmorular growth pattern

    Grade 2: 6–50% nonsquamous or nonmorular growth pattern

    Grade 3: greater than 50% nonsquamous or nonmorular growth pattern

Notes on pathologic grading:

1. Notable nuclear atypia, inappropriate for the architectural grade, raises the grade of a grade 1 or grade 2 tumor by one grade.

2. In serous adenocarcinoma, clear cell adenocarcinoma, and squamous cell carcinoma, nuclear grading takes precedence.

3. Adenocarcinomas with squamous differentiation are graded according to the nuclear grade of the glandular component.

Lurain JR. Uterine cancer. In: Berek JS, editor. Berek and Novak's gynecology. 14th ed. Philadelphia (PA): Lippincott Williams and Wilkins; 2007. p. 1352.

mous differentiation. Previously called *adenosquamous carcinoma*, they are now referred to as *adenocarcinoma with squamous differentiation*. The behavior of these adenosquamous tumors depends largely on the grade of the glandular component rather than the benign or malignant appearance of the squamous component.

A villoglandular configuration is present in approximately 2% of endometrioid carcinomas. These lesions are always well differentiated and behave like endometrioid carcinomas; however, they should be distinguished from papillary serous carcinomas that have a more aggressive behavior. Secretory carcinomas are rare variants of endometrioid carcinomas that account for approximately 1% of cases. They occur mostly in early postmenopausal women and generally have an excellent prognosis; they must be distinguished from clear cell carcinomas, which also have predominantly clear cells.

Approximately 5% of endometrial carcinomas have a predominant mucinous pattern with a well-differentiated glandular architecture. Their clinical behavior is similar to that of common well-differentiated endometrioid carcinomas.

Approximately 5–7% of endometrial carcinomas resemble papillary serous carcinoma of the ovary and fallopian tube and have an aggressive behavior. These tumors are composed of fibrovascular stalks lined by highly atypical cells with tufted stratification. Psammoma bodies frequently are observed. They are commonly admixed with other histologic patterns, but mixed tumors containing 25% or more of the papillary serous carcinoma behave as aggressively as pure papillary serous carcinomas. Of patients with clinical stage I disease, more than one half are found to have deep myometrial invasion, three fourths manifest lymph–vascular space invasion, and approximately 50% have extrauterine disease detected at surgery. Initial studies suggested that these tumors, even when confined to the endometrium or endometrial polyps without myometrial or vascular invasion, behave more aggressively than endometrioid carcinomas and have a propensity for intraabdominal spread. However, after careful staging with peritoneal cytology, pelvic and paraaortic lymphadenectomy, and partial omentectomy, these tumors, when confined to the endometrium or endometrial polyps without myometrial or vascular invasion, have a better prognosis.

Clear cell carcinomas account for approximately 3% of all endometrial carcinomas. Although they once were considered to behave as aggressively as serous carcinomas, more recent studies suggest a behavior similar to poorly differentiated endometrioid carcinoma when limited to the uterus.

Squamous carcinomas of the endometrium are extremely rare. Some tumors are pure, but most have a few glands. To establish primary origin within the endometrium, there must be no connection with, or spread from, cervical squamous epithelium. Squamous carcinomas often are associated with cervical stenosis, chronic inflammation, and pyometra at the time of diagnosis. These tumors have a poor prognosis, with an estimated 36% survival rate for women with clinical stage I disease.

Synchronous endometrial and ovarian cancers are the most common simultaneously occurring gynecologic malignancies, with a reported incidence of 1.4–3.8%. Both the ovarian and endometrial tumors usually are well-differentiated endometrioid adenocarcinomas of low stage, with an excellent prognosis. Because of the symptomatic endometrial tumor, the ovarian cancer usually is discovered as an incidental finding and is diagnosed at an earlier stage, resulting in a more favorable outcome. Approximately 30% of patients with endometrioid ovarian adenocarcinomas will have an associated endometrial cancer. Granulosa cell tumors, which can produce estrogen, have an associated endometrial carcinoma in 15–20% of cases.

Pretreatment Evaluation

After the diagnosis of endometrial carcinoma (or atypical complex hyperplasia) has been established, obtaining a complete history and performing a thorough physical examination are important to determine the best and safest approach to management of the disease. Patients with endometrial carcinomas often are elderly or obese and have a variety of medical problems, such as diabetes mellitus and hypertension, that affect surgical management. Any abnormal symptoms should be evaluated. Physical examination should be directed to the supraclavicular and inguinal lymph nodes (to ensure they are not enlarged and do not feel abnormal), abdominal masses, and possible areas of cancer spread within the pelvis. Stool should be tested for occult blood.

Chest radiography should be performed to rule out pulmonary metastasis and to evaluate the cardiorespiratory status of the patient. Complete blood count and renal and liver function tests are recommended as part of a preoperative evaluation and clinical staging. Although preoperative CA 125 values often are elevated in patients with advanced or metastatic disease, elevated CA 125 baseline levels may be helpful in the subsequent follow-up. No other preoperative or staging studies are required or necessary for most patients with endometrial cancer. Studies such as cystoscopy, colonoscopy, mammography, intravenous pyelography, barium enema, and computed tomography scanning of the abdomen and pelvis are not indicated unless dictated by patient symptoms, physical findings, or other laboratory tests. Ultrasonography and magnetic resonance imaging obtained preoperatively do not reproducibly assess myometrial invasion accurately. Ideally, patients should be referred to a gynecologic oncologist to perform a complete pelvic and paraaortic lymphadenectomy as part of surgical staging.

Treatment

Surgery is the cornerstone of staging and therapy for most patients with endometrial cancer. Depending on the stage of the disease, surgery may be followed by adjuvant therapy. Other forms of primary therapy—primary radiation therapy and hormone therapy—may be considered in patients who are not candidates for surgery.

PRIMARY RADIATION THERAPY

Primary surgery followed by individualized radiation therapy has become the most widely accepted treatment for patients with early-stage endometrial cancers. However, approximately 3–5% of patients with endometrial cancer have severe medical conditions that render them unsuitable for surgery. These patients tend to be elderly and obese and to have multiple chronic or acute medical illnesses, such as hypertension, cardiac disease, and diabetes mellitus, as well as pulmonary, renal, and neurologic diseases.

Several studies have demonstrated that radiotherapy is effective treatment for patients with inoperable endometrial cancer. Because of the high incidence of death caused by intercurrent illness in this group of patients, the 5- and 10-year overall survival rates are only 55% and 28%, respectively, compared with disease-specific survival rates of 87% and 85%, respectively.

The decision to treat a patient who has endometrial cancer with radiation therapy alone must involve a careful analysis of the relative risks and benefits of surgery. Although radiation therapy alone can produce excellent survival and local control, it should be considered for definitive treatment only if the operative risk is estimated to exceed the 10–15% risk of uterine recurrence expected with radiation treatment alone.

HORMONE THERAPY

It is reasonable to consider hormone therapy (progestins) as primary management for a grade 1 endometrial carcinoma in a young patient who desires fertility preservation. In a literature review of 81 patients, 62 patients (76%) responded to therapy, but 15 patients (24%) had subsequent recurrence at a median of 19 months, with 10 patients requiring hysterectomy (2). Twenty patients were able to become pregnant, and there were no disease-related patient deaths.

SURGERY

Hysterectomy and bilateral salpingo-oophorectomy are the primary operative procedures in the management of carcinoma of the endometrium. The adnexa should be removed because they may be the site of microscopic metastasis; also, patients with endometrial carcinoma are at increased risk for ovarian cancer, which may develop simultaneously or later. Although the type of hysterectomy has not been shown to affect survival, total abdominal hysterectomy and bilateral salpingo-oophorectomy have been most commonly employed. A laparotomy through an adequate abdominal incision, which allows a thorough intraabdominal exploration and retroperitoneal lymphadenectomy, should be performed. After the abdomen has been opened, pelvic peritoneal washings are obtained and sent for cytopathology evaluation.

Most patients with endometrial cancer should undergo surgical staging based on the 1988 International Federation of Gynecology and Obstetrics (FIGO) system (Table 19) (3). The minimum surgical procedure should include sampling of peritoneal fluid for cytologic evaluation, extrafascial hysterectomy, bilateral salpingo-oophorectomy, and pelvic and paraaortic lymphadenectomy. Because fewer than 10% of patients with lymphatic metastasis have grossly enlarged nodes, palpation is not an acceptable alternative to lymphadenectomy. A standard lymphadenectomy should be performed. An omental biopsy or partial omentectomy also should be performed for patients with nonendometrioid carcinomas (papillary serous or clear cell types). Extended surgical staging, including selective pelvic and paraaortic lymphadenectomy, in patients with endometrial cancer prolongs anesthesia time, increases blood loss, and extends the duration of the hospital stay, but it does not add significantly to the morbidity from hysterectomy. Morbidity is related primarily to other factors, such as patient weight, age, and race; operating time; and surgical technique (4).

TABLE 19. International Federation of Gynecology and Obstetrics Surgical Staging of Endometrial Carcinoma

Stage	Description
IA	Tumor limited to endometrium
IB	Invasion to less than one half of myometrium
IC	Invasion to greater than one half of myometrium
IIA	Endocervical glandular involvement only
IIB	Cervical stromal invasion
IIIA	Tumor invades serosa or adnexa or both or positive peritoneal cytologic findings or both
IIIB	Vaginal metastasis
IIIC	Metastasis to pelvic or paraaortic lymph nodes or both
IVA	Tumor invasion of bladder or bowel mucosa or both
IVB	Distant metastasis including intraabdominal nodes or inguinal lymph nodes or both

This table was published in International Journal of Gynecology and Obstetrics, volume 95, supplement, Creasman WT, Odicino F, Maisonneuve MA, Quinn P, Beller U, Benedet JL, et al. Carcinoma of the corpus uteri. International Federation of Gynecology and Obstetrics. FIGO annual report on the results of treatment in gynecological cancer, s105–43, copyright Elsevier 2006.

The incidence of lymph node metastasis in clinical stage I endometrial cancer is approximately 3% in grade 1 tumors, 9% in grade 2 tumors, and 18% in grade 3 tumors. Fewer than 5% of patients with no myometrial invasion or with superficial (less than one half) myometrial invasion have lymph node metastasis, compared with approximately 20% of patients with deep (greater than one half) myometrial invasion. Pelvic lymph node metastases are present in fewer than 5% of grade 1 and grade 2 tumors with superficial myometrial invasion, in approximately 15% of grade 1 and grade 2 tumors with deep myometrial invasion or grade 3 tumors with superficial invasion, and in more than 40% of grade 3 tumors with deep myometrial invasion. Approximately one half to two thirds of patients with positive pelvic lymph nodes also will have paraaortic lymph node metastases. However, in one study among patients with positive pelvic nodes, the paraaortic nodes were the only nodes involved in 14% of the patients. Cervical involvement is associated with an approximately 15% risk of pelvic or paraaortic node metastasis. The incidence of lymph node metastasis also correlates with tumor size (smaller than 2 cm, 4%; larger than 2 cm, 15%; entire cavity, 35%). Extrauterine spread of disease also increases the risk of pelvic and paraaortic nodal metastasis to 32% and 20%, respectively.

Evidence of the efficacy of routine lymphadenectomy is limited. Although some researchers have reported a survival benefit from lymphadenectomy, the indications for adjuvant radiation therapy are not clearly specified. Data from the National Cancer Institute's Surveillance, Epidemiology, and End Results program representing 9,185 women with stage I or II endometrial cancer showed that the 5-year relative survival for 6,363 women with stage I endometrial cancer who did not undergo lymph node sampling was not statistically different from that of the 2,831 women who did undergo lymph node sampling (0.98 and 0.96, respectively) (1). Among those women with stage I, grade 3 disease, lymph node sampling was associated with increased survival (relative 5-year survival of 0.89, compared with 0.81, $P=.0110$). In a recent updated analysis of this study of 12,333 patients, a significant benefit could be seen in the intermediate IB grade 3, IC, and II–IV stages because more nodes were removed (1, 2–5, 6–10, 11–20, and greater than 20) (5). More extensive nodal resection remained a significant prognostic factor for improved survival ($P<.001$) in intermediate- and high-risk patients after correcting for other factors including age, stage, grade, adjuvant radiation therapy, and nodal metastasis. Improved survival rates have been found when more than 11 pelvic nodes were removed at lymphadenectomy for poorly differentiated tumors but not for moderately differentiated or well-differentiated tumors (4).

In a trial in which 1,408 patients were randomized between hysterectomy and bilateral salpingo-oophorectomy, with or without pelvic lymphadenectomy (6), baseline characteristics were well balanced between the groups.

A similar percentage of patients, 39% in both arms, received postoperative pelvic radiation therapy. No difference in overall survival was seen, and progression-free survival slightly improved in the patients who did not undergo pelvic lymphadenectomy.

Vaginal hysterectomy with bilateral salpingo-oophorectomy is an alternative to abdominal hysterectomy. In the past this route was typically reserved for selected patients who were extremely obese and had a poor medical status or for patients with extensive uterovaginal prolapse. The disadvantages to this approach are that bilateral salpingo-oophorectomy often is technically difficult, and abdominal exploration and lymph node sampling cannot be performed. However, laparoscopically assisted vaginal hysterectomy is now in wider use and can facilitate this modality. A prospective study of laparoscopic lymphadenectomy followed by immediate laparotomy and lymphadenectomy reviewed a mean of 31 pelvic and 12 paraaortic lymph nodes obtained by laparoscopy, and only 3 of 40 patients were found to have had an inadequate lymphadenectomy (7).

The Gynecologic Oncology Group recently has completed accrual to a randomized trial of laparoscopy compared with laparotomy with hysterectomy, bilateral salpingo-oophorectomy, and pelvic and paraaortic lymphadenectomy for endometrial cancer (8). In all, 2,616 patients were enrolled in the study and randomized to receive laparotomy (n=920) or laparoscopy (n=1696). Approximately 23% of the patients randomized to laparoscopy required laparotomy to complete the staging. Length of stay was shorter with laparoscopy (median, 3 days; range, 0–95 days) than with laparotomy (median, 4 days; range, 1–49), and operative times were longer with laparoscopy (median, 3.3 hours; range, 0.7–10.1) than with laparotomy (median, 2.2 hours; range, 0.7–6.3). Perioperative deaths due to treatment were caused chiefly by pulmonary emboli, which occurred rarely in both arms, and wound complications resulted in readmission and reoperation in a small number of cases. The current data suggest that laparoscopic surgical staging is feasible for most patients with clinical stage I or IIA uterine cancer. The long-term results of the progression-free and overall survival of this study are awaited.

The outcome of radical hysterectomy, with removal of the parametria and upper vagina, compared with that of extrafascial hysterectomy and bilateral salpingo-oophorectomy alone, depends on the stage of disease. In clinical stage I disease, radical hysterectomy does not improve survival and increases intraoperative and postoperative morbidity. In stage II disease, however, radical hysterectomy results in improved survival with or without the use of adjuvant radiation therapy.

Prognostic Factors

A number of individual prognostic factors for disease recurrence or survival have been identified. Most, but not all, of these factors have been incorporated into the current staging system. As a result, stage of disease is the most significant variable affecting survival. Based on the most recent FIGO data, the 5-year survival for surgically staged patients is 89.6%, 78.3%, 61.9%, and 21.1% for stage I, II, III, and IV disease stages, respectively (Table 20).

TABLE 20. Carcinoma of the Endometrium: Stage Distribution and Actuarial Survival by Stage (Surgical and Clinical)

Stage	Patients Treated		Survival (%)	
	Number	%	3-Year	5-Year
Surgical Stage				
I	5,313	67	93.4	89.6
II	973	12	84.2	78.3
III	1,048	13	69.6	61.9
IV	255	3	30.0	21.1
Clinical Stage				
I	161	2	65.1	53.5
II	46	0.5	72.5	67.7
III	79	0.9	48.2	37.7
IV	45	0.6	19.6	15.3

This table was adapted from International Journal of Gynecology and Obstetrics, volume 95, supplement, Creasman WT, Odicino F, Maisonneuve MA, Quinn P, Beller U, Benedet JL, et al. Carcinoma of the corpus uteri. International Federation of Gynecology and Obstetrics. FIGO annual report on the results of treatment in gynecological cancer, s105–43, copyright Elsevier 2006.

Extrauterine metastasis, excluding peritoneal cytology and lymph node metastasis, occurs in approximately 4–6% of patients with clinical stage I endometrial cancer. Tumor recurrence is almost five times more likely in patients with extrauterine disease spread.

Lymph node metastasis is probably the most important prognostic factor in apparent early-stage endometrial cancer. Of patients with clinical stage I disease, approximately 10% will have pelvic metastases, and 6% will have paraaortic lymph node metastases. Patients with lymph node metastases have almost a sixfold higher likelihood of developing recurrent cancer than patients without lymph node metastases. The 5-year disease-free survival rate for patients with lymph node metastases is approximately 50% compared with 90% for patients without lymph node metastases.

Most patients with adnexal spread have other poor prognostic factors that place them at high risk for recurrence. However, for patients with well-differentiated tumors with adnexal spread as their only high-risk factor, a survival rate has been reported to be as high as 85%.

The significance of malignant peritoneal cytologic findings in patients with endometrial cancer is controversial. Increased recurrence rates and decreased survival rates have been noted, and on this basis, treatment has been recommended when cytologic findings are positive. Others have found no significant relationship between malignant peritoneal cytologic findings and an increased incidence of disease recurrence in patients with early endometrial cancer. In the absence of other evidence of extrauterine disease or other poor prognostic factors, malignant peritoneal cytologic findings probably have no significant effect on recurrence and survival. When associated with other poor prognostic factors or extrauterine disease, malignant peritoneal cytologic findings increase the likelihood of distant and intraabdominal disease recurrence and have a significant adverse effect on survival. The use of several different therapeutic modalities in patients with malignant peritoneal cytologic findings has not resulted in any proven benefit.

Involvement of the uterine isthmus, or cervix, or both is associated with an increased risk of extrauterine disease and lymph node metastasis. Patients with cervical involvement also tend to have higher-grade, larger, and more deeply invasive tumors, undoubtedly contributing to the increased risk of recurrence (relative risk, 1.6).

Increasing depth of invasion is associated with increasing likelihood of extrauterine spread, recurrence, and death. In general, patients with noninvasive or superficially invasive tumors have an 80–90% 5-year survival rate, whereas patients with deeply invasive tumors have a 60% 5-year survival rate.

The histologic grade of the endometrial tumor is strongly associated with prognosis. Patients with grade 3 tumors are more than five times more likely to have a recurrence than are patients with grade 1 and grade 2 tumors. The 5-year disease-free survival rate for patients with grade 1 and grade 2 tumors is approximately 90%, compared with approximately 65% for patients with grade 3 tumors. Increasing tumor grade is associated with deep myometrial invasion, cervical extension, lymph node metastasis, and local recurrence and distant metastasis.

Nonendometrioid histologic subtypes account for approximately 10% of endometrial cancers and carry an increased risk of recurrence and distant spread. In contrast to the approximately 90% survival rate among patients with endometrioid tumors, the overall survival rate for patients with one of the more aggressive subtypes, such as papillary serous or clear cell tumors, is only 30–50%. At the time of surgical staging, more than one half of the patients with an unfavorable histologic subtype have extrauterine spread of disease.

Lymph–vascular space invasion appears to be an independent risk factor for recurrence and death in patients with all types of endometrial cancer. The overall incidence of lymph–vascular space invasion in early endometrial cancer is approximately 15%, although it increases with increasing tumor grade and depth of myometrial invasion. The 5-year survival rate for patients without demonstrable lymph–vascular space invasion is approximately 85%, compared with a 65% survival rate for individuals in whom lymph–vascular space invasion is present.

Tumor size is a significant prognostic factor for survival in patients with endometrial cancer. Five-year survival rates are higher than 95% for patients with tumors 2 cm or smaller, approximately 85% for patients with tumors larger than 2 cm, and approximately 65% for patients with tumors involving the whole uterine cavity.

Estrogen receptor and progesterone receptor levels have been shown to be prognostic indicators for endometrial cancer independent of grade in several studies. Patients whose tumors are positive for one or both receptors have longer survival times than patients whose carcinomas lack the corresponding receptors.

Approximately two thirds of endometrial adenocarcinomas have a diploid DNA content as determined by flow cytometric analysis. The proportion of nondiploid tumors increases with stage, lack of tumor differentiation, and depth of myometrial invasion. In several studies, DNA content has been related to the clinical course of the disease, with death rates generally reported to be higher in women whose tumors contained aneuploid populations of cells. The proliferative index also is related to prognosis.

Death from endometrial carcinoma increases with increasing age. Although type II tumors are more common in older patients, older age remains a significant risk factor for recurrence even when corrected for pathologic variables. Five-year disease-specific survival rates are higher than 95% for patients aged 50 years or younger, 75% for patients aged 51–75 years, and 50% for patients older than 75 years.

Postoperative Adjuvant Therapy

Options for postoperative care of patients with endometrial cancer include observation, vaginal vault irradiation, external pelvic irradiation, extended-field (pelvic and paraaortic) irradiation, whole-abdomen irradiation, administration of progestins, or systemic chemotherapy. The decision to use adjuvant therapy after surgery should be based on the risk of recurrence determined by surgical–pathologic risk factors. Patients with grade 1 or grade 2 lesions with minimal or no myometrial invasion (stage IA, grades 1 and 2) have an excellent prognosis and require no postoperative therapy.

The role of adjuvant pelvic radiation therapy for patients treated for endometrial carcinoma has been studied. One trial evaluated 540 patients with surgical stage I endometrial cancer who received whole-pelvic radiation therapy (45 Gy) compared with observation after total abdominal hysterectomy and bilateral salpingo-oophorectomy and vaginal brachytherapy (9). Patients who received pelvic radiation therapy had a statistically lower frequency of pelvic recurrences but no improvement in survival. The only exception to this finding was among patients with stage IC, grade 3 tumors; these patients had survival rates of 73% with observation compared with 82% with pelvic radiation therapy.

In another study of patients who did not undergo staging lymphadenectomy, 715 patients with intermediate-risk endometrial carcinoma (stage IC, grades 1 and 2, and stage IB, grades 2 and 3) had an increased rate of localized recurrence but no survival difference with observation (10). In still another study, 448 patients who underwent negative staging surgery that included a pelvic and paraaortic lymphadenectomy were randomized to receiving no further therapy or pelvic radiation therapy (11). Those patients who were irradiated (50.4 Gy) had a 3% recurrence rate, compared with a 12% recurrence in those patients who underwent observation ($P=.007$). The researchers found no difference in survival with a median follow-up of 69 months. A subgroup of patients was defined as "high risk" based on patient age and the presence of risk factors (grade 2 or 3 tumors, outer one third myometrial invasion, vascular lymphatic invasion, or both). Patients younger than 50 years were required to have three risk factors; patients aged 50–70 years, two risk factors; and patients older than 70 years, one risk factor. Among the high-risk patients, the risk of recurrence was 26% with observation and 6% with pelvic radiation therapy, which was significant (relative risk, 0.42).

In a study of 21,249 patients from the Surveillance, Epidemiology, and End Results database, the frequency of lymphadenectomy increased with increasing tumor grade and depth of myometrial invasion (12). Women with stage IA, grade 1 disease underwent nodal sampling in 25% of cases compared with 67% for stage IC, grade 3 disease. Similarly, adjuvant radiation therapy was used more frequently with increasing tumor grade and depth of myometrial invasion, ranging from 2% of patients with stage IA, grade 1 tumors up to 63% of patients with stage IC, grade 3 tumors. For patients with stage IC, grade 3 tumors, radiation therapy decreased the risk of recurrence (relative risk, 0.72; $P=.009$). Pelvic radiation therapy is most commonly associated with gastrointestinal adverse effects, usually abdominal cramps and diarrhea; however, more serious complications, such as bleeding, proctitis, bowel obstruction, and fistula formation, may occur and require surgical correction in approximately 5–8% of patients.

Lymphadenectomy is helpful in selecting patients who might benefit from adjuvant radiation therapy. Many authors have demonstrated that surgically staged patients with negative nodes but intermediate disease in the uterus can be treated with vaginal irradiation with excellent outcomes and be spared the morbidity of whole-pelvis radiation therapy. Most of these studies have reported high numbers of lymph nodes removed, which is important in determining whether the lymphadenectomy was adequately thorough. Although no randomized trials of vaginal radiation therapy have been performed, large institutional experiences suggest that vaginal irradiation can reduce the incidence of local recurrence in stage I patients from 15% to 1–2%. Morbidity is low, although vaginal dryness, stenosis, and dyspareunia may be a problem for sexually active patients. Pelvic irradiation commonly is used for patients with stage IC or grade 3 disease who did not have lymphadenectomy, although based on the Postoperative Radiation Therapy for Endometrial Carcinoma trial, observation and treatment at recurrence would be a reasonable alternative. Observation or vaginal irradiation are treatment options for patients who have surgical stage I, grade 1 and grade 2 tumors with less than one half of myometrial invasion.

A large randomized trial was performed to evaluate the effectiveness of external beam radiotherapy in the treatment of patients with uterine cancer (13). Of 906 patients with stage I endometrial cancer, 452 patients received external beam radiotherapy (40–46 Gy in 20–25 fractions to the pelvis) immediately after the surgery, and 454 patients received no external beam radiotherapy until clinically indicated. Brachytherapy was used regardless of external beam radiotherapy allocation. The preliminary results showed no benefit in overall survival or progression-free survival. Furthermore, morbidity was higher in the patients who received external beam radiotherapy. These studies demonstrated that external beam radiotherapy does not improve survival in women with intermediate risk, stage I endometrial cancer.

Approximately 15% of patients with endometrial carcinoma have stage II disease, which conveys an increased risk of mortality (relative risk, 2.2). The clinical staging of endometrial carcinoma by fractional D&C overcalls cervical involvement; only approximately 40% of patients are found to have cervical involvement at hysterectomy.

Because of this fact and the high incidence of extrapelvic disease when the cervix is involved, the preferred method for management is an initial surgical approach, provided the tumor is felt to be resectable. Adjuvant therapy then can be determined based on the extent of cervical disease and the results of surgical staging. Although pelvic and vaginal irradiation are most commonly employed, vaginal irradiation alone or observation are the National Comprehensive Cancer Network guideline options for patients with stage IIA disease and limited uterine disease (14). Vaginal radiation therapy alone has been used for patients with minimal stage IIB disease.

For patients with endometrial carcinoma of a more advanced stage, individualized treatment plans must be developed that are directed toward both the local and systemic disease. In patients who are medically fit, surgery could be considered to determine the extent of disease and, if possible, to remove the bulk of the disease.

Patients with pelvic lymph node metastasis and negative paraaortic nodes have a relatively high (65–70%) survival after treatment with pelvic radiation therapy alone. When paraaortic node metastases are present but there is no other evidence of disease, pelvic and extended-field irradiation results in 5-year survival rates ranging from 15% to 20% for macroscopic nodal metastasis and from 42% to 59% for microscopic nodal metastasis. Whole-abdomen radiation therapy has been reported to be effective for patients with adnexal or upper abdominal disease that has been optimally resected with residual disease less than 2 cm. However, in a randomized trial comparing whole-abdomen irradiation versus chemotherapy with doxorubicin and cisplatin, chemotherapy was found to be superior to radiation therapy, as well as to statistically reduce the risk of progression by 29% and decrease the risk of death at 5 years by 32%.

The use of pelvic radiation therapy with or without adjuvant chemotherapy is being evaluated. The researchers reported a randomized study comparing adjuvant pelvic radiation therapy versus chemotherapy plus pelvic radiation therapy in patients with early-stage, high-risk endometrial cancer (15). "High risk" was categorized as having one or more risk factors, including grade 3 disease, deep myometrial invasion, and DNA nondiploidy, or having serous, clear cell, or anaplastic carcinomas. The study showed that the progression-free survival in the platinum-based combination chemotherapy plus radiation therapy group was higher than in the group that received only radiation therapy. Ongoing studies are comparing adjuvant platinum-based combination chemotherapy versus pelvic radiation therapy in patients with high-risk, low-stage endometrial cancer.

As demonstrated in patients with adnexal metastasis and low-grade tumors, hormonal therapy may be effective and well tolerated for managing estrogen receptor (ER)- or progesterone receptor (PR)-expressing tumors. Stage IVA endometrial carcinoma, in which tumor invades the bladder or rectum, is rare, and treatment must be individualized.

Patients with papillary serous or clear cell carcinomas are at high risk for recurrence, and a variety of adjuvant therapy regimens have been used. Comprehensive surgical staging is the most important first step in the treatment of patients with these tumors. When tumors have been comprehensively staged, the risk of recurrence for stage I tumors is appreciably lower than previously reported. More recent pathology studies have demonstrated that when comprehensively staged, clear cell carcinoma behaves more like poorly differentiated endometrioid carcinoma than papillary serous carcinoma, which has a higher risk of recurrence. The best form of treatment has not been determined. For more extensive disease, adjuvant chemotherapy with a taxane and a platinum compound with or without tumor-directed radiation therapy is used most often. However, prospective studies to evaluate such an approach are lacking.

Recurrent Disease

Approximately one fourth of patients undergoing treatment for early endometrial cancer develop recurrent disease. More than one half of the recurrences will develop within 2 years, and approximately three fourths of recurrences will occur within 3 years of initial treatment. The distribution of recurrences depends on the type of primary therapy (surgery alone compared with surgery plus local or regional radiotherapy). In patients with surgical stage I disease, vaginal and pelvic recurrences make up approximately 50% of all recurrences in patients treated with surgery alone, whereas only 30% of recurrences are vaginal or pelvic in patients treated with combined surgery and radiotherapy. The most common sites of extra-pelvic metastases are the lung, abdomen, lymph nodes (aortic, supraclavicular, and inguinal), liver, brain, and bone. In general, patients with isolated vaginal recurrences fare better than patients with pelvic recurrences, who in turn have a better chance of cure than patients with distant metastases. Overall 5-year disease-free survival is 5–10%. However, patients who initially have well-differentiated tumors or who develop recurrent cancer more than 3 years after the primary therapy also tend to have an improved outlook.

The choice of systemic therapy is best determined based on the ER/PR status of the tumor. In patients with tumors expressing ER or PR, systemic hormonal therapy is an acceptable alternative to cytotoxic chemotherapy, and it has significantly less toxicity. The most active chemotherapeutic agents are taxanes (paclitaxel and docetaxel), the platinum compounds (cisplatin and carboplatin), and anthracyclines (doxorubicin or epirubicin). The three-drug combination of paclitaxel, doxorubin, and cisplatin is superior to doxorubin and cisplatin, with improvements in response rate (57% versus 34%), progression-free intervals (8.3 months versus 5.3 months) and overall survival (15.3 months versus 12.3 months) (16).

Follow-up After Treatment

Patients should be examined every 3–4 months during the first 2 years after treatment and every 6 months thereafter. Approximately one half of patients discovered to have recurrent cancer will be symptomatic, and 75–80% of recurrences will be detected initially on physical examination. Particular attention should be given to peripheral lymph nodes, the abdomen, and the pelvis. Vaginal cytologic testing should be performed at each visit. Although vaginal cytologic testing detects very few asymptomatic recurrences, these early recurrences often are amenable to successful therapy. If the CA 125 level was elevated at the time of treatment or initial recurrence, serum CA 125 measurements may be useful.

Estrogen therapy after treatment for patients with endometrial cancer has long been considered contraindicated because of the concern that estrogen might activate occult metastatic disease. The position of the American College of Obstetricians and Gynecologists for women with a history of endometrial cancer is that hormone therapy could be used in the presence of the same indications as for any other woman, except that the selection of appropriate candidates for estrogen treatment should be based on prognostic indicators and the patient must be willing to assume the risk. The Gynecologic Oncology Group conducted a randomized trial evaluating hormone therapy in patients with endometrial carcinoma. This trial was closed prematurely; however, after a 3-year follow-up there was no difference in recurrence (17).

UTERINE SARCOMA

Uterine sarcomas make up only 3% of uterine cancers. However, they are virulent and account for 15% of the deaths from uterine cancer.

Classification

A large variety of histologic types of uterine sarcoma have been identified, and many systems of classification have been proposed. One classification divides these tumors, based on their histology, into pure or mixed and further divides the mixed tumors as having either homologous or heterologous components (18). Other classification systems that are more or less specific have been suggested. The two most common histologic variants of uterine sarcoma are carcinosarcoma (homologous and heterologous types) and leiomyosarcoma, which make up 2% and 1% of uterine cancer cases, respectively. Endometrial stromal sarcoma and other sarcomas make up less than 1% of uterine cancer cases.

CARCINOSARCOMA

The term *carcinosarcoma*, originally used to specify a tumor with a malignant epithelial element and a malignant homologous sarcomatous element, is now considered to include malignant müllerian mixed tumor, malignant mesodermal mixed tumor, and metaplastic carcinoma. Histologically, these tumors appear to be composed of a mixture of sarcoma and carcinoma.

Almost all uterine sarcomas occur after menopause, at a median age of 62 years. As with endometrial carcinoma, obesity, hypertension, and diabetes are frequently associated diseases, occurring in 18%, 11%, and 8% of patients with uterine sarcoma, respectively. Additionally, tamoxifen has been associated with a high risk of carcinosarcoma. Carcinosarcoma has a 2.5-fold higher incidence in African-American women (4.3 per 100,000 women) compared with Caucasian women (1.7 per 100,000 women) (19). A history of previous pelvic irradiation is found in 7–37% of patients.

The metastatic pattern of these neoplasms is similar to that of endometrial adenocarcinoma, based on local extension and regional lymph node metastasis. At the time of diagnosis the tumor has spread outside the uterus in 40–60% of cases. Patients with tumor apparently confined to the uterine corpus (stage I) have approximately a 50% 2-year survival, whereas survival decreases to less than 10% when disease extends to the cervix or outside the uterus. In a large study, factors significantly related to progression-free interval by multivariate analysis were adnexal spread, lymph node metastases, histologic cell type (homologous compared with heterologous), and grade of sarcoma. In another study, women who were postmenopausal or had a history of pelvic radiation therapy, pain at presentation, clinical stage II–III disease, uterine enlargement (identical to a gestational age of 12 weeks or greater), or an abnormal Pap test result had a significantly poorer prognosis than the other patients in the series (20).

Adenosarcoma is an uncommon variant of sarcoma in which the glandular component is benign and admixed with a malignant stromal sarcoma. The prognosis for patients with this type of sarcoma is better than that seen in patients with carcinosarcoma. Treatment consists of a hysterectomy and bilateral salpingo-oophorectomy with or without adjuvant radiotherapy. Recurrences, mostly local pelvic or vaginal, have been reported in 40–50% of cases, leading some authors to recommend adjuvant postoperative intravaginal or pelvic irradiation. However, a subset of patients with adenosarcoma with sarcomatous overgrowth experiences an aggressive course similar to that of carcinosarcomas.

LEIOMYOSARCOMA

The diagnosis of leiomyosarcoma is dependent on three histopathologic findings: mitotic count, cellular atypia, and the presence of coagulative necrosis. Patients who have tumors with mitotic counts of less than 5 mitoses per 10 high-power fields (HPF) have a much better prognosis than patients with tumors of intermediate mitotic counts (5–10 mitoses per 10 HPF). Patients who have tumors with mitotic counts greater than 10 mitoses per 10 HPF have the poorest prognosis. Uterine smooth muscle tumors with any two of these three features are associated with a poor prognosis. The median age of women with leiomyosarcoma (52 years) is somewhat lower than the age for other uterine sarcomas, and premenopausal patients have a better chance for survival. This malignancy has no relationship with parity, and the incidence of associated diseases is not as high in carcinosarcoma as it is in endometrial adenocarcinoma. African Americans have a 1.65-fold higher incidence (1.61 per 100,000 women) compared with Caucasians (0.91 per 100,000 women) (19). The incidence of sarcomatous change in benign uterine leiomyomata is reported to be between 0.13% and 0.81%.

Survival rates of patients with uterine leiomyosarcoma range from 20% to 63% (mean, 47%). The pattern of tumor spread is to the myometrium, pelvic blood vessels and lymphatics, contiguous pelvic structures, and abdomen, and then distantly, most often to the lungs.

ENDOMETRIAL STROMAL TUMORS

Endometrial stromal tumors are divided into two types based on mitotic activity, vascular invasion, and observed differences in prognosis. These types are low-grade stromal sarcoma and undifferentiated stromal sarcoma.

Low-grade endometrial stromal sarcoma, previously referred to as *endolymphatic stromal myosis*, is characterized microscopically by a mitotic rate of less than 10 mitoses per 10 HPF. Clinically these tumors occur in younger patients than do undifferentiated endometrial stromal sarcomas, have a protracted course, and recur late and locally. Low-grade stromal sarcoma extends beyond the uterus in 24% of cases at the time of diagnosis, but the extrauterine spread is confined to the pelvis in two thirds of the cases. Recurrence occurs in almost 50% of cases at an average interval of 5 years after initial therapy. Prolonged survival may be achieved with progestin therapy.

Undifferentiated endometrial stromal sarcoma histologically exhibits more than 10 mitoses per 10 HPF and often completely lacks recognizable stromal differentiation. This tumor has a much more aggressive clinical course and poorer prognosis than does low-grade stromal sarcoma. The 5-year disease-free survival is approximately 25%. There is no relationship to parity, associated diseases, or prior pelvic radiotherapy. The occurrence rates of these tumors are not increased in African Americans.

Clinical Presentation

The most frequent symptom of carcinosarcomas is abnormal uterine bleeding, which occurs in 80–90% of cases. Other, less common symptoms are vaginal discharge, abdominal–pelvic pain, weight loss, and passage of tissue from the vagina. The duration of symptoms usually is only a few months. On physical examination, uterine enlargement is present in 50–95% of patients, and a polypoid

mass may be seen within or protruding from the endocervical canal in as many as 50% of patients with carcinosarcoma. Diagnosis usually can be determined by biopsy of an endocervical mass or endometrial curettage.

In patients with endometrial stromal sarcomas, abnormal uterine bleeding is the most common symptom; abdominal pain and pressure due to an enlarging pelvic mass occur less often, and some patients may be asymptomatic. Pelvic examination usually reveals regular or irregular uterine enlargement, sometimes associated with rubbery parametrial induration. The diagnosis may be established with endometrial biopsy, but the usual preoperative diagnosis is uterine leiomyoma. At surgery, the presence of an enlarged uterus filled with soft, grayish white to yellow necrotic and hemorrhagic tumors with bulging surfaces associated with wormlike elastic extensions into the pelvic veins indicates the possibility of uterine sarcoma.

Patients with leiomyosarcoma present with uterine enlargement and abnormal bleeding. Although the classic presentation of leiomyosarcoma is a rapidly growing uterus, leiomyosarcoma is uncommon, occurring in only 0.23% of patients with this finding.

Treatment

Because uterine sarcomas are aggressive tumors, appropriate management plans are best designed after computed tomographic imaging of the chest, abdomen, and pelvis. Most patients with apparent localized disease are treated with surgery initially.

SURGERY

Management of most stage I and stage II uterine sarcomas should include hysterectomy and bilateral salpingo-oophorectomy. At the time of surgery, the peritoneal cavity should be carefully explored and peritoneal washings obtained. A pelvic and paraaortic lymphadenectomy should be performed in all patients with uterine sarcomas with the exception of patients with leiomyosarcoma, which rarely involves lymph nodes. The standard practice has been the removal of the adnexa because of the potential for tumor extension, as well as the stimulating effect that estrogen from retained ovaries might have on residual tumor cells. Some authors have noted a similar risk of recurrence with ovarian preservation and bilateral salpingo-oophorectomy in premenopausal women with low-grade endometrial stromal sarcoma and leiomyosarcoma and have advocated this treatment option (21, 22).

RADIATION THERAPY

Adjuvant pelvic radiation therapy decreases pelvic recurrences for patients with localized endometrial stromal sarcoma and malignant mixed müllerian tumor. In one study, patients with carcinosarcoma treated with pelvic radiation therapy had a lower rate of pelvic recurrence than patients treated with surgery alone (28% versus 48%, $P=.0002$), but the overall survival rates (36% versus 27%, $P=.1$) and distant metastasis rates (57% versus 54%, $P=.96$) were not significantly different (20). However, patients treated with pelvic radiation therapy had a longer mean time to any distant relapse (17.3 months versus 7 months, $P=.001$) than did patients treated with surgery alone. For leiomyosarcoma, the use of pelvic radiation therapy has not affected the progression-free interval, 2-year survival rate, or site of first recurrence. Radiation therapy may be beneficial for inadequately excised or locally recurrent pelvic disease.

CHEMOTHERAPY

Recurrences develop in more than one half of cases of uterine sarcoma treated by surgery or surgery and radiation therapy, even when disease is apparently localized at the time of initial treatment. Furthermore, because isolated pelvic failures account for fewer than 10% of recurrences, there is an obvious need for effective systemic therapy. Among uterine sarcomas, only low-grade endometrial stromal sarcoma is consistently hormone receptor positive and responsive to progestin therapy. Because progesterone therapy is considered the treatment of choice for recurrent low-grade endometrial stromal sarcoma, adjuvant progesterone therapy has been advocated.

Based on limited data, it had been determined that carcinosarcomas rarely respond to doxorubicin. The combined use of localized radiation therapy and systemic chemotherapy for patients with uterine carcinosarcoma of clinical stages I or II followed by platinum–anthracycline chemotherapy has resulted in improved survival rates for those patients who completed treatment. Adjuvant chemotherapy with cisplatin, ifosfamide, and doxorubicin for three cycles followed by radiotherapy in 18 patients with localized uterine sarcomas resulted in a 3-year recurrence-free survival rate of 76% for those patients treated with both modalities compared with a 43% rate for historical controls treated with radiation therapy alone (23). A comparison of patients with stages I through IV carcinosarcoma who underwent whole-abdomen radiation therapy compared with those who underwent three cycles of therapy with cisplatin and ifosfamide found that chemotherapy reduced the risk of recurrence by 28.5% (hazard ratio, 0.71) and the risk of death by 32.8% (hazard ratio, 0.67) (24).

Recurrent disease usually is managed with chemotherapy; although isolated, late (more than 2 years) pulmonary lesions may be amenable to surgical excision. In patients with recurrent disease not amenable to surgery or with stage IV disease, chemotherapy is an option. Paclitaxel, platinum compounds, and ifosfamide are active in carcinosarcomas, whereas doxorubicin, ifosfamide, docetaxel, and gemcitabine are active in leiomyosarcoma. The combination of paclitaxel and ifosfamide has demonstrated superiority over single-agent ifosfamide, with improve-

ments in response rate and survival (25). The combination of gemcitabine and docetaxel has the highest response rate reported for leiomyosarcoma (26).

References

1. Trimble CL, Kauderer J, Zaino R, Silverberg S, Lim PC, Burke JJ 2nd, et al. Concurrent endometrial carcinoma in women with a biopsy diagnosis of atypical endometrial hyperplasia: a Gynecologic Oncology Group study. Cancer 2006;106:812–9.

2. Ramirez PT, Fromovitz M, Bodurka DC, Sun CC, Levenback C. Hormonal therapy for the management of grade 1 endometrial adenocarcinoma: a literature review. Gynecol Oncol 2004;95:133–8.

3. Management of endometrial cancer. ACOG Practice Bulletin No. 65. American College of Obstetricians and Gynecologists. Obstet Gynecol 2005;106:413–25.

4. Cragun JM, Havrilesky LJ, Calingaert B, Synan I, Secord AA, Soper JT, et al. Retrospective analysis of selective lymphanedectomy in apparent early-stage endometrial cancer. J Clin Oncol 2005;23:3668–75.

5. Chan JK, Cheung MK, Huh WK, Osann K, Husain A, Teng NN, et al. Therapeutic role of lymph node resection in endometrioid corpus cancer: a study of 12,333 patients. Cancer 2006;107:1823–30.

6. Kitchener H, Redman CW, Swart AM. ASTEC: a study in treatment of endometrial cancer: a randomised trial of lymphadenectomy in treatment of endometrial cancer [abstract]. Gynecol Oncol 2006;101(suppl):s21–s22.

7. Schlaer JB, Spirtos NM, Carson LF, Boike G, Adamec T, Stonebraker B. Laparoscopic retroperitoneal lymphadenectomy followed by immediate laparotomy in women with cervical cancer: a Gynecologic Oncology Group study. Gynecol Oncol 2002;85:81–8.

8. Walker JL, Mannel RS, Piedmonte M, Schlaerth J, Spirtos N, Eisenkop S, Spiegel G. Phase III trial of laparoscopy versus laparotomy for surgical resection and comprehensive surgical staging of uterine cancer: a Gynecologic Oncology Group study (GOG): preliminary results [abstract]. Gynecol Oncol 2006;101(suppl):s11–12.

9. Aalders J, Abeler V, Kolstad P, Onsrud M. Postoperative external irradiation and prognostic parameters in stage I endometrial carcinoma: clinical and histopathologic study of 540 patients. Obstet Gynecol 1980;56:419–27.

10. Creutzberg CL, van Putten WL, Warlam-Rodenhuis CC, van den Bergh AC, de Winter KA, Koper PC, et al. Outcome of high-risk stage IC, grade 3, compared with stage I endometrial carcinoma patients: the Postoperative Radiation Therapy in Endometrial Carcinoma Trial. J Clin Oncol 2004;22:1234–41.

11. Keys HM, Roberts JA, Brunetto VL, Zaino RJ, Spirtos NM, Bloss JD, et al. A phase III trial of surgery with or without adjunctive external pelvic radiation therapy in intermediate risk endometrial adenocarcinoma: a Gynecologic Oncology Group study. Gynecologic Oncology Group [published

erratum appears in Gynecol Oncol 2004;94:241–2]. Gynecol Oncol 2004;92:744–51.

12. Lee CM, Szabo A, Shrieve DC, Macdonald OK, Gaffney DK. Frequency and effect of adjuvant radiation therapy among women with stage I endometrial adenocarcinoma [published erratum appears in JAMA 2006;295:2482]. JAMA 2006;295:389–97.

13. Orton J, Blake P. Adjuvant external beam radiotherapy (EBRT) in the treatment of endometrial cancer: results of the randomized MRC ASTEC and NCIC CTG EN.5 trial [abstract]. J Clin Oncol 2007;25(suppl):275s.

14. National Comprehensive Cancer Network. Practice guidelines in oncology: uterine neoplasms. Available at: http://www.nccn.org/professionals/physician_gls/PDF/uterine.pdf. Retrieved August 10, 2007.

15. Hogberg T, Rosenberg P, Kristensen G, de Oliveira CF, de Pont Christensen R, Sorbe B, et al. A randomized phase-III study on adjuvant treatment with radiation (RT) +-chemotherapy (CT) in early-stage high-risk endometrial cancer (NSGO-EC-9501/EORTC 55991). Nordic Society of Gynecologic Oncology and European Organization for Research and Treatment of Cancer [abstract]. J Clin Oncol 2007;25(suppl):274s.

16. Fleming GF, Brunetto VL, Cella D, Look KY, Reid GC, Munkarah AR, et al. Phase III trial of doxorubicin plus cisplatin with or without paclitaxel plus filgrastim in advanced endometrial carcinoma: a Gynecologic Oncology Group study. J Clin Oncol 2004;22:2159–66.

17. Barakat RR, Bundy BN, Spirtos NM, Bell J, Mannel RS. Randomized double-blind trial of estrogen replacement therapy versus placebo in stage I or II endometrial cancer: a Gynecologic Oncology Group study. Gynecologic Oncology Group. J Clin Oncol 2006;24:587–92.

18. Ober WB, Towell HM. Mesenchymal sarcomas of the uterus. Am J Obstet Gynecol 1959;77:246–68.

19. Brooks SE, Zhan M, Cote T, Baquet CR. Surveillance, epidemiology and end results analysis of 2677 cases of uterine sarcoma 1989–1999. Gynecol Oncol 2004;93:204–8.

20. Callister M, Ramondetta LM, Jhingran A, Burke TW, Eifel PJ. Malignant mixed Mullerian tumors of the uterus: analysis of patterns of failure, prognostic factors, and treatment outcome. Int J Radiat Oncol Biol Phys 2004;58:786–96.

21. Giuntoli RL 2nd, Metzinger DS, DiMarco CS, Cha SS, Sloan JA, Keeney GL, et al. Retrospective review of 208 patients with leiomyosarcoma of the uterus: prognostic indicators, surgical management, and adjuvant therapy. Gynecol Oncol 2003;89:460–9.

22. Li AJ, Giuntoli RL 2nd, Drake R, Byun SY, Rojas F, Barbuto D, et al. Ovarian preservation in stage I low-grade endometrial stromal sarcomas. Obstet Gynecol 2005;106:1304–8.

23. Pautier P, Rey A, Haie-Meder C, Kirbrat P, Dutel JL, Getsa P, et al. Adjuvant chemotherapy with cisplatin, ifosfamide, and doxorubicin followed by radiotherapy in localized uterine sarcomas: results of a case-control study with radiotherapy alone. Int J Gynecol Cancer 2004;14:1112–7.

24. Wolfson AH, Brady MF, Rocereto T, Mannel RS, Lee YC, Futoran RJ, et al. A gynecologic oncology group randomized phase trial III of whole abdominal irradiation (WAI) vs. cisplatin-isfomide and mesna (CIM) as post-surgical therapy in stage I-IV carcinosarcoma (CS) of the uterus. Gynecol Oncol 2007;107:177–85.

25. Homesley HD, Filiaci VL, Markman M, Bitterman P, Eaton L, Kilgore LC, et al. Phase III trial of ifosfamide with or without paclitaxel in advanced uterine carcinosarcoma: a Gynecologic Oncology Group study. Gynecologic Oncology Group. J Clin Oncol 2007;25:526–31.

26. Hensley ML, Maki R, Venkatraman E, Geller G, Lovegren M, Aghajanian C, et al. Gemcitabine and docetaxel in patients with unresectable leiomyosarcoma: results of a phase II trial. J Clin Oncol 2002;20:2824–31.

Cancer of the Ovary, Peritoneum, and Fallopian Tube

Dennis S. Chi, MD, and Noah D. Kauff, MD

EPIDEMIOLOGY AND DIAGNOSIS

In 2008, approximately 21,650 American women are expected to receive the diagnosis of ovarian cancer and an estimated 15,520 are expected to die of the disease, making it the fifth most common cancer in women and the most common cause of gynecologic cancer mortality (1). Approximately 1 in 70 women will develop ovarian cancer in her lifetime. Ovarian cancer is more common in northern European countries and North America than in Asia, developing countries, or southern continents.

The etiology of ovarian cancer is not known, but risk factors have been identified. Recognized risk factors for the disease include advancing age, with an annual incidence of 1 in 11,000 at age 40 years, 1 in 4,500 at age 50 years, 1 in 2,600 at age 60 years, and 1 in 2,000 at age 70 years (2). Other factors associated with an increased risk include infertility, endometriosis, and application of talcum powder to the perineum (3). The incremental risk of developing ovarian cancer associated with any of these age-independent risk factors is relatively small, with relative risks of no more than 2–3 compared with the general population. Smoking, alcohol use, coffee consumption, and viral infections (such as mumps) have not been associated with increased risk. Approximately 8–13% of cases of ovarian cancer are caused by inherited mutations in the cancer-susceptibility genes *BRCA1* and *BRCA2* (see "Genetics and Gynecologic Cancer") (4, 5).

In the absence of genetic testing information, a family history of ovarian cancer or early-onset breast cancer has been associated with an increased risk of ovarian cancer, with a relative risk of approximately 3–5 compared with the general population (6). It is not clear, however, how much of this increased risk is accounted for by mutations in the known ovarian cancer-susceptibility genes.

In regard to protective factors, multiple studies have demonstrated that oral contraceptive use and parity are associated with a decreased risk of ovarian cancer (7). Use of oral contraceptives is protective for ovarian cancer, with an average relative risk of approximately 0.7 for women who have used oral contraceptives for 2 years and 0.5 for women who have used oral contraceptives for 5 years or longer. The protective effect of oral contraceptive use appears to be long term, with some studies indicating a lifetime risk reduction. A woman's risk of ovarian cancer also may be reduced if she has had tubal sterilization, undergone a hysterectomy, or given birth to at least one child whom she has breast-fed (8).

The 5-year survival rate for ovarian cancer by stage is not significantly different from the 5-year survival rate for other gynecologic cancers. However, two thirds of patients with ovarian cancer have advanced-stage disease at the time of diagnosis, unlike patients with cancer of the uterine corpus or cervix, in whom the disease is likely to be found at an early stage. It is clear from these data that the single most important factor in the large number of deaths from ovarian cancer is the failure to establish the diagnosis while the disease is at an early stage. The reasons for this failure correspond with the growth and spread patterns of this type of cancer. Because the ovary floats freely in the pelvic cavity, a tumor may grow for some time while producing only vague symptoms associated with involvement of, or pressure on, other organs. These vague symptoms frequently either are ignored by the patient or are not recognized as potential signs and symptoms of ovarian cancer by her physician.

SCREENING

One of the best ways to improve survival for patients with ovarian cancer would be to find a way to screen women for ovarian cancer and detect the disease before it spreads beyond the ovary. Recommendations for ovarian cancer screening traditionally have been stratified according to level of risk, with different recommendations put forth for women at average risk compared with women at increased risk. With the identification of autosomal dominant ovarian cancer susceptibility syndromes, the increased-risk group has been further stratified into two groups: 1) a group with a clear inherited risk and 2) a group with increased risk by virtue of family history but in the absence of a known inherited cancer predisposition.

A great deal of the incremental risk of ovarian cancer for women with a family history of ovarian or early-onset breast cancer is likely the result of mutations in the known ovarian cancer-susceptibility genes. Preliminary evidence has suggested that individuals with a strong family history of breast cancer but no demonstrable mutation in *BRCA1* or *BRCA2* may not be at significantly increased risk of ovarian cancer (9). For this reason and because of the limitations of the currently available ovarian cancer screening tests described in the following section, women at increased risk should be encouraged to consider genetic counseling and testing before initiating ovarian cancer screening or other ovarian cancer risk reduction strategies.

Tests for Early Detection

A number of tests have been evaluated as potential methods for early detection of ovarian cancer. To date, there is no evidence that routine pelvic examination is effective in the early diagnosis of ovarian cancer. Tests that have been investigated most include serum CA 125 measurement and transvaginal ultrasonography. Less information is available regarding a number of other serum markers, used alone or in combination. A newer technology, proteomics, is being investigated; this method involves simultaneous evaluation of dozens to hundreds of low-molecular-weight proteins.

The high-molecular-weight protein CA 125, which is excreted by more than 90% of advanced epithelial ovarian cancers, has been the most evaluated serum marker for early detection of ovarian cancer. In the largest study to date, 22,000 postmenopausal women at average risk of ovarian cancer were randomized to receive either annual serum CA 125 measurement or usual gynecologic care. Ultrasonography was performed in women in the early detection arm if the CA 125 level was greater than 30 units/mL. In this study, women with ovarian cancer that was detected early by the test had improved survival rates compared with women with ovarian cancer who were randomized to usual care. Although these results were promising, there was no difference between the two groups in the number of deaths caused by ovarian cancer. Additionally, despite having 8,732 women undergo early testing, only six cases of ovarian cancer were detected by testing, with three of these cases being in the advanced stage.

Other studies have suggested that CA 125 level also is elevated in 2–3% of healthy postmenopausal women. Given this fact and the relatively low annual incidence of ovarian cancer, detection of one additional ovarian cancer using annual CA 125 measurement as primary screening requires recalling 100–150 women for further evaluation and approximately 30 diagnostic surgeries.

To improve the utility of CA 125 measurements for early detection of ovarian cancer, a method has been proposed that focuses on the change in CA 125 concentration over time as opposed to the absolute value. This approach

is being used in the ongoing United Kingdom Collaborative Trial of Ovarian Cancer Screening study in Great Britain in which 200,000 women will be randomized to either testing with serial CA 125 measurement, transvaginal ultrasound testing, or usual care. Results from this study are expected in 2012.

A number of imaging modalities have been evaluated for possible use in ovarian cancer screening. Because of the position of the ovaries deep in the pelvis and the fact that they are mobile organs with solid and cystic components, however, transvaginal ultrasonography consistently has been the most promising imaging modality for routine screening for ovarian cancer. In the largest study to date evaluating ultrasonography as a screening method for ovarian cancer, 14,469 women predominantly at average risk of ovarian cancer were monitored with annual transvaginal ultrasonography (10). In this study, ultrasonography was associated with an 81% sensitivity and a 98.9% specificity, resulting in a positive predictive value of 9.4%. The authors also suggested that transvaginal ultrasonography was associated with an early detection of ovarian cancer. Of the 17 cases of ovarian cancer detected by this screening, 11 were stage I. Critics, however, have pointed out that only two of the 11 cases of stage I cancer detected by the screen were high grade, compared with all six cases of advanced-stage ovarian cancer detected by the screen. However, this result may in fact have been reflective of the rarity of ovarian cancer in the population, as opposed to necessarily being the result of the ability of ultrasonography to rule out disease.

Several studies have evaluated the simultaneous use of transvaginal ultrasonography and CA 125 measurement. These studies have suggested that the combination of these tests results in a higher sensitivity for ovarian cancer detection, but at the cost of an increased rate of false-positive results. In the ongoing Prostate, Lung, Colorectal, and Ovarian Cancer Screening Trial, 28,816 women were randomized to receive annual transvaginal ultrasound examination and CA 125 measurement. At baseline, 1,338 ultrasound results (4.7%) and 402 CA 125 levels (1.4%) were abnormal. Workup of these abnormalities led to the diagnosis of 20 cases of invasive ovarian cancer. The positive predictive values for an abnormal test were 1.0% for transvaginal ultrasonography and 3.7% for CA 125 measurement. This value, however, did increase to 23.5% when both results were abnormal (11). Final results comparing this screened cohort with a control group of 39,000 women randomized to usual care are expected in 2015.

Many other serum markers, including osteopontin, YKL-40, prostasin, and lysophosphatidic acid, have been evaluated alone and in combination for primary screening of ovarian cancer. Although several preliminary studies have suggested that some of these approaches may have better sensitivity and specificity profiles than CA 125 measurement alone, none of these approaches has been demonstrated in prospective screening trials to detect ovarian cancer at earlier stages than the CA 125 test in women at any level of risk.

In 2002, a report from researchers at the National Cancer Institute suggested that by evaluating the low-molecular-weight protein spectrum in peripheral serum, one could identify a characteristic "proteomic" pattern that was highly sensitive (100%) and specific (95%) for early ovarian cancer (12). Although this initial report was promising, this approach has not been validated.

Screening Guidelines

Many national organizations, such as the American Cancer Society, the American College of Obstetricians and Gynecologists (ACOG), the Society of Gynecologic Oncologists (SGO), and the National Comprehensive Cancer Network, have issued ovarian cancer screening guidelines. These organizations do not recommend ovarian cancer screening. An annual gynecologic examination with pelvic examination is recommended for preventive health care.

HISTOLOGY

Ovarian tumors usually are categorized by their tissue of origin: epithelial (from the coelomic epithelial cells that line the ovary), germ cell (from the germinal epithelium), and sex cord–stromal (from the mesenchymal tissue of the ovary). Epithelial tumors account for approximately 85% of all cases of ovarian cancer, germ cell cancers account for approximately 10% of tumors, and the remaining 5% of tumors are sex cord–stromal.

Of the malignant epithelial ovarian cancers, 40–50% are serous tumors, 15–25% are endometrioid tumors, 6–16% are mucinous tumors, and 5–11% are clear cell tumors (Box 12). Transitional cell (Brenner), mixed epithelial, and undifferentiated carcinomas are encountered less frequently. Epithelial tumors may be benign, have low malignant potential, or be frankly malignant. The vast majority of borderline tumors (or tumors of low malignant potential), especially those of the serous type, have a benign course, but a small proportion have a more malignant behavior. Malignant tumors are further subdivided by histologic grade into either three grades based on architecture (classification of the International Federation of Gynecology and Obstetrics [FIGO]) or four grades based on nuclear atypia (Broders' index).

DIAGNOSIS

Most patients receive the diagnosis of ovarian cancer after the disease has spread beyond the ovary. In these patients, symptoms may be abdominal pain or a bloated feeling, gastrointestinal or urinary tract disturbances, or in many cases, the onset of clinically detectable ascites. Some patients with advanced disease have menstrual irregularity or postmenopausal bleeding. Occasionally, a patient may

have a palpable inguinal lymph node, tumor in a hernia sac, or a pleural effusion. For patients with advanced disease, diagnosis is established by analysis of tissue obtained at exploratory laparotomy. In rare instances when a patient cannot undergo surgery because of medical problems, the histologic or cytologic diagnosis is established by needle biopsy.

Studies have shown that women with ovarian cancer, even women with early-stage disease, often experience symptoms several months before the diagnosis. In a survey of 1,725 women with ovarian cancer, 70% recalled having had symptoms for 3 months or longer before the diagnosis, and 35% recalled having had symptoms for at least 6 months (13). Approximately three fourths of these women had abdominal symptoms, and one half had pain or constitutional symptoms. It appears that the best way to detect early ovarian cancer is for both the patient and her clinician to have a high index of suspicion regarding the diagnosis (14). Persistent symptoms such as an increase in abdominal size, abdominal bloating, fatigue, abdominal pain, indigestion, inability to eat normally, urinary frequency, pelvic pain, constipation, back pain, urinary incontinence of recent onset, or unexplained weight loss should be evaluated, with the inclusion of ovarian cancer in the differential diagnosis.

Early ovarian cancer is diagnosed by surgical evaluation of an adnexal mass. The decision to subject a patient to surgical exploration is difficult to make, however. Ultrasound evaluation of adnexal masses has improved the ability to distinguish patients who should have surgical exploration from patients who can be evaluated further through observation, but it also has resulted in an increasing number of patients who are found to have an asymptomatic ovarian cyst. This result is of particular concern in postmenopausal women.

The use of tumor markers to assist in the evaluation of a patient with an adnexal mass is appropriate, but misinformation may result. Serum CA 125 is the only serum marker available with the potential accuracy to be beneficial, but even this marker is less than optimal. Approximately one half of patients with early-stage ovarian cancer and other types of cancer do not have elevated serum CA 125 levels. Also, a variety of nonmalignant and nonovarian malignant conditions can result in elevated serum CA 125 levels. These conditions are listed in Box 13. A serum CA 125 elevation above 35 units may be helpful in deciding whether to recommend surgery in a postmenopausal patient with an ovarian mass, but a normal value is not helpful. Likewise, a serum CA 125 elevation in women of reproductive age with both an ovarian mass and leiomyomata or endometriosis may not be helpful.

Figure 19 shows an algorithm for the management of a patient with an adnexal mass. As with any diagnostic or therapeutic schema, the criteria for surgery cannot be absolute. For example, a patient with known endometriosis may meet the criteria for surgical exploration when it

Histologic Classification of Common Epithelial Tumors of the Ovary

Serous Tumors

Cellular type: endosalpingeal

- Benign

  Cystadenoma and papillary cystadenoma

  Surface papilloma

  Adenofibroma and cystadenofibroma

- Of borderline malignancy (carcinoma of low malignant potential)

  Cystadenoma and papillary cystadenoma

  Surface papilloma

  Adenofibroma and cystadenofibroma

- Malignant

  Adenocarcinoma

  Surface papillary carcinoma

  Malignant adenofibroma and cystadenofibroma

Mucinous Tumors

Cellular type: endocervical

- Benign

  Cystadenoma

  Adenofibroma and cystadenofibroma

- Of borderline malignancy (carcinoma of low malignant potential)

  Cystadenoma

  Adenofibroma and cystadenofibroma

- Malignant

  Adenocarcinoma and cystadenofibroma

  Malignant adenofibroma and cystadenofibroma

Endometrioid Tumors

Cellular type: endometrial

- Benign

  Adenoma and cystadenoma

  Adenofibroma and cystadenofibroma

- Of borderline malignancy (carcinoma of low malignant potential)

  Adenoma and cystadenoma

  Adenofibroma and cystadenofibroma

- Malignant

  Adenocarcinoma

  Adenocanthoma

  Adenosquamous carcinoma

  Malignant adenofibroma and cystadenofibroma

- Epithelial: stroma and stromal

  Adenosarcoma

  Stromal sarcoma

  Carcinosarcoma: homologous and heterologous

Clear Cell Tumors

Cellular type: müllerian

- Benign

- Of borderline malignancy (carcinoma of low malignant potential)

- Malignant

  Adenocarcinoma

Cellular type: transitional

  Brenner tumor

  Brenner tumor of borderline malignancy (proliferating)

  Malignant Brenner tumor

  Transitional cell carcinoma (non-Brenner type)

Squamous Cell Carcinoma

Mixed Epithelial Tumors (specify types)

Cellular type: mixed

- Benign

- Of borderline malignancy

- Malignant

Undifferentiated Carcinoma

Cellular type: anaplastic

Unclassified

Cellular type: mesothelioma

Modified from Ozols RF, Rubin SC, Thomas GM, Robboy SJ. Epithelial ovarian cancer. In: Hoskins WJ, Perez CA, Young RC, Barakat R, Markman M, Randall M, editors. Principles and practice of gynecologic oncology. 4th ed. Philadelphia (PA): Lippincott Williams and Wilkins; 2005. p. 895–987.

actually is not the best treatment option. In postmenopausal women with unilocular cysts measuring 8–10 cm or less, no family history of breast or ovarian cancer, and normal serial CA 125 levels, expectant management instead of surgical evaluation is a reasonable option (15, 16). In some circumstances (for example, germ cell tumors and stromal tumors), conservative evaluative surgery may be warranted.

Conditions That May Cause Elevated Serum CA 125 Levels

Malignant Conditions

Gynecologic cancer

Epithelial ovarian cancer

Some germ cell tumors

Some stromal tumors

Fallopian tube cancer

Endometrial cancer

Endocervical cancer

Nongynecologic cancer

Pancreatic cancer

Lung cancer

Breast cancer

Colon cancer

Benign Conditions

Gynecologic conditions

Endometriosis

Adenomyosis

Leiomyomata uteri

Ectopic pregnancy

Normal pregnancy

Pelvic inflammatory disease

Menses

Nongynecologic conditions

Pancreatitis

Cholecystitis

Cirrhosis

Passive liver congestion

Peritonitis

Peritoneal tuberculosis

Peritoneal sarcoidosis

Recent laparotomy

Laparoscopic evaluation of an adnexal mass is possible under some circumstances. Masses too large to be removed intact by way of the cul-de-sac, a laparoscopy bag, or a small incision require surgical exploration. It is not appropriate to aspirate a mass or open a mass in the abdominal cavity because of the danger of seeding the abdomen with clonogenic cancer cells and because there are no data to show that the cytologic diagnosis of aspirated cyst fluid is accurate. A frozen section diagnosis of

ovarian cancer in a mass removed by laparoscopy may necessitate surgical exploration for appropriate surgical staging and therapy, although a well-trained gynecologic oncologist may perform appropriate surgical staging with laparoscopy (17).

In an attempt to promote a consensus that would improve referral patterns for women at risk of malignancy, ACOG in conjunction with the SGO issued a 2002 Joint Committee Opinion regarding the role of the generalist obstetrician–gynecologist in the early detection of ovarian cancer (14). The ACOG and SGO Joint Opinion advises clinicians to recommend patient referral to a gynecologic oncologist under the following circumstances:

- Postmenopausal women who have a pelvic mass that raises suspicion for a malignant ovarian neoplasm as suggested by at least one of the following indicators: an elevated CA 125 level, ascites, a nodular or fixed pelvic mass, evidence of abdominal or distant metastasis, and a family history of one or more first-degree relatives with ovarian or breast cancer

- Premenopausal women who have a pelvic mass that raises suspicion for a malignant neoplasm, as suggested by at least one of the following indicators: a very elevated CA 125 level (for example, greater than 200 units/mL), ascites, evidence of abdominal or distant metastasis, and a family history of one or more first-degree relatives with ovarian or breast cancer

Despite a persistent effort to educate the public and medical professionals, the referral of patients with malignant pelvic masses to gynecologic oncologists lags far behind the standards set forth in the guidelines. A recent multicenter study analyzed the performance of the ACOG and SGO referral guidelines with regard to the preoperative identification of malignant pelvic masses (18). The study involved seven large academic medical centers and 1,035 women with a diagnosis of a pelvic mass. Of this group, 318 women had ovarian cancer diagnosed at surgery. Referral would have identified 70% of the premenopausal women and 94% of the postmenopausal women with cancer. Approximately 30–40% of women with benign masses would have been referred to a gynecologic oncologist if the guidelines had been applied. However, given the extremely poor prognosis for women with ovarian cancer who undergo surgery with a nongynecologic oncologist, excessive referral appears to be preferable to insufficient referral.

STAGING

Staging classification is based on surgical evaluation, and removal of as much tumor as possible is the cornerstone of treatment. Despite the importance of surgery, some type of adjuvant treatment almost always is required. The proper

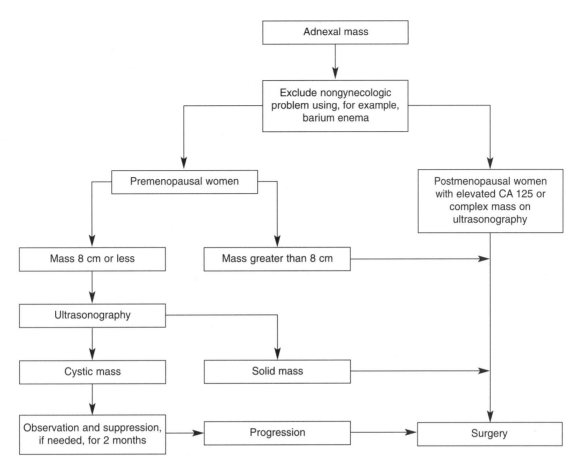

■ FIG. 19. Preoperative evaluation of the patient with an adnexal mass. Berek JS. Epithelial ovarian cancer. In: Berek JS, Hacker NF, editors. Practical gynecologic oncology. 4th ed. Philadelphia (PA): Lippincott Williams and Wilkins; 2005. p. 443–509.

surgical procedure and the appropriate choice of adjuvant therapy depend on the findings at initial exploration, the histologic type of the tumor, and the age and reproductive desires of the patient.

The FIGO staging classification scheme for ovarian cancer is outlined in Table 21. The staging of advanced disease (disease spread throughout the abdomen) may be obvious to most physicians, but a surgeon must be meticulous in the staging of early ovarian cancer. One study found that one third of patients referred with stage I or stage II disease were found to actually have stage III disease when the appropriate staging procedure was performed. Other researchers have reported similar results.

Box 14 outlines the recommended surgical staging procedures for ovarian carcinoma that appears to be confined to the pelvis. The appropriate performance of a staging operation requires an understanding of the spread patterns of the cancer. The cancer can spread by direct infiltration of pelvic structures, such as the pelvic peritoneum, bladder surface, rectal surface, fallopian tube, broad ligament, or uterus. Lymphatic spread occurs early in ovarian cancer, with nodal metastases occurring in 10–12% of patients with stage I cancer and 20–25% of patients with stage II disease. In stage III and stage IV, the

incidence of positive lymph nodes is 50–70%. By far the most significant spread of ovarian cancer, however, is due to exfoliation of clonogenic cells into the peritoneal cavity. These cells are swept up the right abdominal gutter to the diaphragm and omentum by the clockwise flow of peritoneal fluid in the abdomen. The cells implant, form tumor nodules, and, in turn, exfoliate more cells. The normal daily activities of the patient and normal peristalsis of the intestine can result in spread of the disease throughout the abdominal cavity. Proper staging requires a generous lower and upper midline incision and meticulous exploration with multiple peritoneal and nodal biopsies.

MANAGEMENT OF EPITHELIAL OVARIAN CANCER

The management of epithelial ovarian cancer usually involves several types of therapy. Surgical therapy is the initial form of intervention, but it is curative in only a small percentage of cases. Usually, adjuvant chemotherapy is necessary. In a large percentage of patients, some type of salvage therapy is important. Table 22 and Box 15 outline current therapeutic recommendations for patients with epithelial ovarian cancer.

TABLE 21. International Federation of Gynecology and Obstetrics Staging of Carcinoma of the Ovary

Stage	Description
I	Growth limited to the ovaries
IA	Growth limited to one ovary; no ascites containing malignant cells present; no tumor on the external surface; capsule intact
IB	Growth limited to both ovaries; no ascites containing malignant cells present; no tumor on the external surfaces; capsules intact
IC*	Tumor either stage IA or IB, but with tumor on the surface of one or both ovaries, or with capsule ruptured, or with ascites containing malignant cells present, or with positive peritoneal washings
II	Growth involving one or both ovaries with pelvic extension
IIA	Extension or metastases or both to the uterus or fallopian tubes or both
IIB	Extension to other pelvic tissues
IIC*	Tumor either stage IIA or IIB, but with tumor on the surface of one or both ovaries, or with capsule(s) ruptured, or with ascites present containing malignant cells, or with positive peritoneal washings
III	Tumor involving one or both ovaries with histologically confirmed peritoneal implants outside the pelvis or positive retroperitoneal or inguinal nodes or both; superficial liver metastasis equals stage III; tumor is limited to the true pelvis but with histologically proven malignant extension to small bowel or omentum
IIIA	Tumor grossly limited to the true pelvis with negative nodes, but with histologically confirmed microscopic seeding of abdominal peritoneal surfaces, or histologically proven extension to small bowel or mesentery
IIIB	Tumor of one or both ovaries with histologically confirmed implants, peritoneal metastasis of abdominal peritoneal surfaces, none exceeding 2 cm in diameter; nodes are negative
IIC	Peritoneal metastasis beyond the pelvis larger than 2 cm in diameter or positive retroperitoneal or inguinal nodes or all
IV	Growth involving one or both ovaries with distant metastases; if pleural effusion is present, there must be positive cytologic findings to allot a case to stage IV; parenchymal liver metastasis equals stage IV

*To evaluate the effect on prognosis of the different criteria for allotting cases to stage IC or IIC, it would be of value to know if rupture of the capsule was spontaneous or caused by the surgeon, and if the source of malignant cells detected was peritoneal washings or ascites.

This table was published in International Journal of Gynecology and Obstetrics, volume 95, supplement, Heintz AP, Odicino F, Maisonneuve P, Quinn MA, Benedet JL, Creasman WT, et al. Carcinoma of the ovary. International Federation of Gynecology and Obstetrics. FIGO annual report on the results of treatment in gynecological cancer. s161–92, copyright Elsevier 2006.

Surgery

Surgical removal of epithelial cancer that is confined to the ovary, followed by a full surgical staging procedure, may be adequate therapy for selected patients. Generally, a patient with a fully staged IA, grade 1 epithelial cancer will not benefit from adjuvant therapy. There is debate among gynecologic oncologists as to whether a stage IA, grade 2 cancer requires adjuvant chemotherapy. In other early-stage disease, some type of adjuvant treatment usually is required. Epithelial ovarian cancer is categorized as early disease (stages I and IIA with no residual cancer) or advanced disease (stage IIB with residual cancer and stages III and IV).

Table 22 and Box 15 provide a classification system for patients within broad categories. Early ovarian cancer can be divided into low-risk and high-risk disease. For properly staged low-risk epithelial ovarian cancer, the survival rate is approximately 95%. No therapy has been shown to be more effective than surgical removal of the cancer. For patients who wish to retain childbearing capabilities, unilateral salpingo-oophorectomy is acceptable, providing

that a full surgical staging procedure was performed. Some, but not all, authorities would recommend removal of the retained ovary when childbearing is complete.

High-risk cancer, however, requires adjuvant treatment with chemotherapy. Survival rates for patients with high-risk cancer who have adjuvant chemotherapy are 75–95%. In these patients, the role of conservative surgery is more controversial, although some oncologists will preserve childbearing capability in these women despite the requirement for adjuvant chemotherapy.

PRIMARY CYTOREDUCTIVE SURGERY

Decades of studies comparing patients with "optimal" compared with "suboptimal" residual disease have demonstrated that patients who undergo optimal cytoreduction have improved response rates to chemotherapy, prolonged disease-free survival, and improved overall survival. However, if cytoreduction is suboptimal, there is no survival benefit to debulking, no matter how much of the tumor is removed. With current postoperative chemotherapeutic regimens, overall survival for patients with advanced ovarian cancer who undergo optimal cytoreduction is 47–66 months compared with 33–36 months for patients who are suboptimally debulked.

BOX 14

Recommended Primary Surgical Staging Procedure for Patients With Apparently Early Ovarian Carcinoma

- Vertical incision
- Multiple peritoneal washings
- Total abdominal hysterectomy and bilateral salpingo-oophorectomy (unilateral salpingo-oophorectomy may be appropriate for selected patients with stage IA disease who desire to defer definitive surgery until completion of childbearing)
- Infracolic omentectomy
- Pelvic and paraaortic lymph node sampling
- Peritoneal biopsies of the following:

   Cul-de-sac

   Rectal and bladder serosas

   Right and left pelvic side walls

   Right and left paracolic gutters

   Right and left diaphragm

   Any adhesions

Chi DS, Hoskins WJ. Primary surgical management of ovarian cancer. In: Bartlett JM, editor. Ovarian cancer: methods and protocols. Totowa (NJ): Humana Press; 2000. p. 75–87.

In a meta-analysis of studies of the effects of cytoreductive surgery for patients with stage III or stage IV ovarian carcinoma, investigators found that survival rates improved among patients referred to expert centers for primary surgery (19). Expert centers were described as those that attained optimal cytoreduction in 75% or more of advanced-stage cases. To achieve this goal, upper abdominal surgical procedures such as liver mobilization, diaphragm peritonectomy, and splenectomy may be required (20). In expert centers, the performance of these procedures if necessary to attain optimal cytoreduction can lead to significantly improved survival rates (21). Although different authors have used various cutoffs to define optimal cytoreduction, the cutoff used by the Gynecologic Oncology Group (GOG) and the one most commonly reported is tumor measuring 1 cm or less. This amount of residual disease is associated with a survival advantage; however, the best survival rates are achieved in cases where all of the grossly visible tumor is removed.

INTERVAL CYTOREDUCTIVE SURGERY

Even in expert centers, a significant percentage of patients with advanced ovarian cancer will not be able to have optimal cytoreduction. Thus, a significant number of patients begin initial adjuvant therapy with large-volume disease. To address this issue, a European cooperative group trial analyzed the benefit of a second cytoreductive procedure during the primary chemotherapy. This second surgery was referred to as *interval cytoreduction*. In this trial, patients with suboptimal residual disease were randomized to receive six courses of cisplatin and cyclophosphamide compared with three courses of the same regimen, interval cytoreduction, and then another three

---

TABLE 22. Recommended Therapy for Epithelial Ovarian Cancer

Category of Ovarian Cancer Based on Surgical Staging	Recommended (Standard) Therapy
Early ovarian cancer	
Low risk (stages IA and IB, grade 1)	TAH, BSO
High risk (stages IA and IB, grades 2 and 3; stages IC, IIA, IIB, and IIC, no residual)	TAH, BSO Adjuvant therapy with combination carboplatin or paclitaxel chemotherapy
Advanced ovarian cancer	
Stage III with optimal residual disease	Maximal surgical cytoreduction Combination chemotherapy with systemic carboplatin and paclitaxel or systemic pacitaxel plus intraperitoneal cisplatin and paclitaxel
Stage IV, or suboptimal disease, or both	Maximal surgical cytoreduction Combination chemotherapy with carboplatin and paclitaxel

Abbreviations: BSO indicates bilateral salpingo-oophorectomy; TAH, total abdominal hysterectomy.

Additional Notes on Recommended Therapy for Epithelial Ovarian Cancer

- Some investigators include grade 2 in the low-risk category.
- Unilateral salpingo-oophorectomy is permissible in patients who desire further childbearing.
- Optimal disease occurs when the residual tumor is 1 cm or smaller.
- Suboptimal disease occurs with stage III or stage IV and a residual tumor larger than 1 cm.

courses of the same chemotherapy. The investigators reported a statistically significant improvement in progression-free survival rates and overall survival rates for the patients undergoing interval cytoreduction (22).

The GOG subsequently performed another randomized trial of interval debulking, which was similar to the European trial except that, in the U.S. trial, the chemotherapeutic agents were cisplatin and paclitaxel (23). The researchers concluded that interval debulking did not improve progression-free survival or overall survival. The most accepted reason why these two trials yielded conflicting results is that in the U.S. trial the initial surgeries were generally performed by gynecologic oncologists, and, therefore, an aggressive attempt at cytoreduction was attempted, whereas in the European trial this was not the case. Therefore, one can conclude that these randomized trials have demonstrated that there is a survival benefit to cytoreductive surgery (the European trial), but if a valid attempt has been made by a trained gynecologic oncologist at primary surgery, there is no benefit to performing a second, interval cytoreductive procedure during the primary chemotherapy (the U.S. trial).

Second-Look Operation

At present, no randomized trials have definitively proved the benefits of second-look surgical reevaluation. Approximately one half of patients who undergo negative second-look operations harbor occult cancer that eventually will lead to a recurrence. Based on the current literature, second-look operations should be used in the context of experimental trials (24).

A recently published randomized trial of the GOG demonstrated an improvement in progression-free survival with the administration of 1 year (versus 3 months) of monthly paclitaxel without any second-look operation as a consolidation treatment for patients in a complete clinical remission (25). This trial met early stopping rules based on the disease-free survival difference, so the impli-

cations of this strategy with regard to overall survival are unknown. Therefore, the benefits of this approach are still controversial.

Secondary Cytoreductive Surgery

Primary cytoreductive surgery is well accepted as the cornerstone of the initial management of ovarian cancer, but the use of cytoreductive surgery in the setting of recurrent disease is less clearly defined. A recent study suggested that until randomized data become available, the selection of patients who undergo secondary cytoreduction should be based on the disease-free interval from the completion of primary therapy, the number of sites of recurrence, and the probability that cytoreduction to minimal residual disease can be achieved (26).

Chemotherapy

Although surgery is important in the management of epithelial ovarian cancer, surgery alone is rarely curative and provides only brief palliation of advanced disease. Most patients with ovarian cancer require adjuvant chemotherapy; 75–80% of patients will respond to chemotherapy. However, many patients develop resistance to chemotherapy before eradication of the cancer is complete. For these patients, secondary or salvage chemotherapy is an important part of treatment.

Primary Chemotherapy

The standard primary chemotherapy agents for patients with advanced ovarian cancer are carboplatin and paclitaxel. However, the GOG recently published the results of a randomized phase 3 trial that compared intravenous (IV) paclitaxel plus cisplatin to IV paclitaxel plus intraperitoneal (IP) cisplatin and paclitaxel in patients with optimally cytoreduced stage III ovarian cancer (27). The study arm receiving the IV/IP regimen had a 16-month improvement from 50 months to 66 months in median overall survival compared with the IV-only control arm. This trial, along with others that have demonstrated improved survival for the IV/IP approach, led the National Cancer Institute to issue a clinical announcement in January 2006 that recommended that women with optimally debulked stage III ovarian cancer be counseled about the potential clinical benefit associated with combined IV and IP administration of chemotherapy. However, because of concerns regarding increased toxicity, studies are ongoing to determine the best drug dosing and the most safe and effective combined IV/IP regimen.

Chemotherapy for Persistent Disease

Approximately 20–25% of patients with advanced epithelial ovarian cancer will be "cured" by initial surgery and primary chemotherapy. Most patients (75–80%) either will have residual disease at the conclusion of initial therapy or will develop recurrent disease. For these patients, second-line therapies may be required. The most important issues to consider in this setting are the size and location of the persistent disease and whether the patient responded to primary chemotherapy. Patients are considered to be platinum or paclitaxel sensitive if they had an initial response to chemotherapy drugs and did not develop regrowth of disease within 6 months.

For patients with small-volume persistent or recurrent disease confined to the peritoneal cavity who are felt to have platinum-sensitive disease, IP chemotherapy may be a reasonable regimen if they have not already received it (24). Systemic chemotherapy should be considered for patients with large tumors (larger than 1 cm) or patients with disease outside the peritoneal cavity. Patients who respond to platinum therapy often can be repeatedly treated with one of the platinum compounds alone or in combination with other agents. The longer the disease-free interval from primary chemotherapy, the better the chances of response; patients who have a disease-free interval of 2 years or more respond at a rate similar to that of patients with newly diagnosed cancer.

Patients who have platinum- or paclitaxel-resistant disease are candidates for experimental trials. In the absence of an experimental trial, modest response rates have been reported with topotecan, liposomally encapsulated doxorubicin, gemcitabine plus carboplatin, etoposide, and bevacizumab. Low-dose etoposide administered orally, however, has been associated with an increased risk of leukemia, so its use has not been recommended for patients who have a long life expectancy (rarely a consideration for patients with platinum-resistant disease).

Follow-up Care

Early-stage ovarian cancer usually has a low recurrence rate, providing patients had full surgical staging and received appropriate therapy. Exceptions include patients with clear cell cancers of the ovary. Because of the low recurrence rate, patients should be monitored with a gynecologic examination and a serum CA 125 test every 3–4 months for the first 2 years and every 6 months for the next 3 years. After 5 years, annual examinations are recommended. Annual Pap tests also are recommended. There is no proven benefit of diagnostic radiography or computed tomography in asymptomatic patients with normal serum CA 125 levels.

Advanced ovarian cancer has a high recurrence rate, approaching 75%. For these patients, follow-up care should be more intensive. They should have a gynecologic examination and a serum CA 125 test every 3 months for the first 3 years. Follow-up examinations at 6-month intervals are recommended for the next 2 years. The use of routine computed tomographic scanning is debatable, although many experts recommend it. The optimal frequency for such tests has not been established.

The value of the serum CA 125 test in the follow-up care of patients depends in large part on whether the patient had an elevated serum level before therapy, even though CA 125 levels do not always correlate with tumor volume. The serum test, however, does appear to be the best follow-up test available. One of the problems in CA 125 follow-up testing of patients in complete clinical remission is care of the patient with an increasing CA 125 level and normal results in clinical and radiologic evaluation. No data indicate whether such a patient should be treated or be monitored closely until clinical recurrence is detected.

Primary peritoneal carcinoma is a serous carcinoma arising in the peritoneal lining that is histologically indistinguishable from serous epithelial ovarian cancer. The diagnosis is inexact and usually established when there is widespread abdominal disease with only surface ovarian involvement. This entity responds to therapy in a similar fashion to epithelial ovarian cancer and is managed in an identical manner.

OVARIAN GERM CELL TUMORS

Malignant germ cell tumors of the ovary occur primarily in the second and third decades of life, although they are occasionally found in young girls and older women. The tumors usually are accompanied by abdominal pain, and almost 10% of patients will contact a physician because of an acute episode of torsion, hemorrhage, or rupture of the tumor.

Germ cell tumors may be associated with elevated serum levels of β-hCG, alpha-fetoprotein, or lactic dehydrogenase. Measurement of these markers may aid in the diagnosis of germ cell tumors and may be useful in management and follow-up care. Markers vary considerably, although most endodermal sinus tumors produce alpha-fetoprotein, and most choriocarcinomas and dysgerminomas produce β-hCG and lactic dehydrogenase.

Prognosis is good for most patients treated with platinum-based multidrug chemotherapy. Of 85 patients given adjuvant therapy of either a bleomycin–etoposide–platinum regimen or a platinum–vinblastine–bleomycin regimen, 83 patients (98%) were progression-free (28). In comparison, patients who had residual disease, had persistent disease, or developed recurrences had a progression-free survival rate of only 59% (71 of 120 patients) when treated with similar regimens.

Survival is enhanced by complete cytoreduction of malignant germ cell tumors. The surgeon should make every effort to resect the disease completely, but there is no need to remove reproductive organs not involved with the cancer. These tumors are seldom bilateral. Thus, even patients with advanced disease who do not have involvement of the other ovary and the uterus should have those organs conserved. Because high cure rates are achieved with the use of multidrug chemotherapy, many patients are able to retain reproductive capability.

Patients with malignant germ cell tumors of the ovary should undergo surgical staging similar to staging for epithelial ovarian cancer. However, because most patients will require chemotherapy, reexploration for staging is not indicated unless the goal is to resect residual cancer completely. It is best to begin chemotherapy as soon as possible, because tumors can recur and grow rapidly. The benefit of second-look laparotomy in patients with germ cell tumors has not been clearly demonstrated, although it has been recommended in selected patients, such as those with marker-negative incompletely resected immature teratomas.

STROMAL TUMORS

Sex cord–stromal tumors or sex cord–mesenchymal tumors include those of the female type (granulosa cell tumors and granulosa–theca cell tumors), the male type (Sertoli–Leydig cell tumors), and rare types, such as lipid cell tumors and gynandroblastoma. In general, the therapy is total abdominal hysterectomy and bilateral salpingo-oophorectomy, with full surgical staging for patients who do not desire childbearing capabilities. For younger patients, unilateral salpingo-oophorectomy and full surgical staging are indicated.

The granulosa cell tumor is the most common malignant tumor of this group of neoplasms. These tumors occur throughout a woman's lifetime but are more common in the first four decades. They are bilateral in only approximately 5% of cases. All granulosa cell tumors should be considered potentially malignant, and late recurrences are common. There are two major histologic types: the adult variety and the juvenile form. The juvenile form is much more likely to result in a malignancy.

The therapy for granulosa cell tumors involves surgical removal; there is no proven benefit of adjuvant therapy. Inhibin is secreted by granulosa tumors, and it is a good marker. In younger patients who desire to retain their childbearing capability, unilateral salpingo-oophorectomy and full surgical staging are the treatments of choice. In granulosa cell tumors, as in germ cell tumors, the traditional choice of chemotherapy for metastatic disease is bleomycin, etoposide, and platinum; however, recent studies have shown that taxanes demonstrate activity against sex cord–stromal tumors, and the combination of taxanes and platinum may be less toxic than the bleomycin, etoposide, and platinum regimen. There are too few reported series on granulosa cell tumors managed with chemotherapy to provide accurate figures on response rates to chemotherapy.

Young patients with granulosa cell tumors may show precocious puberty, because these tumors may produce estrogen. In older women, menstrual irregularity or postmenopausal bleeding due to estrogen production may be the presenting symptom. Sertoli–Leydig cell tumors occur less frequently than granulosa cell tumors and are rarely bilateral. These tumors may produce androgens and have clinical symptoms of defeminization or masculinization. The malignant potential of these tumors is related directly to the degree of differentiation, and they usually are classified as well differentiated, moderately differentiated, or poorly differentiated. A fourth classification is Sertoli–Leydig cell tumors with heterologous elements.

CANCER OF THE FALLOPIAN TUBE

Histologically, cancer of the fallopian tube resembles papillary serous carcinoma of the ovary in more than 90% of cases. The staging system used is modified from the staging system for ovarian cancer (Table 23).

Fallopian tube cancer and ovarian cancer spread in a similar manner. The classic triad of colicky pain, abnormal bleeding, and leukorrhea is rarely seen in its entirety; the most common symptom is abnormal vaginal bleeding. Pain is reported frequently as an early symptom, however.

The therapy for fallopian tube cancer is similar to the therapy for ovarian cancer; the most important initial therapy is effective cytoreductive surgery. As in ovarian cancer, the amount of residual disease is a good predictor of survival rates. The adjuvant therapy is determined in a similar fashion to that for ovarian cancer and is based on the stage, grade, and residual disease.

The risk of fallopian tube cancer is increased in patients with *BRCA1* or *BRCA2* genes. This risk is decreased with prophylactic removal of the tube and the ovary (29).

References

1. American Cancer Society. Cancer facts and figures 2008. Atlanta (GA): ACS; 2008. Available at: http://www.cancer.org/downloads/STT/2008CAFFfinalsecured.pdf. Retrieved February 20, 2008.

2. Ries LA, Melbert D, Krapcho M, Mariotto A, Miller BA, Feuer EJ, et al, editors. SEER cancer statistics review, 1975–2004. Bethesda (MD): National Cancer Institute; 2007. Available at: http://seer.cancer.gov/csr/1975_2004. Retrieved August 17, 2007.

3. Ness RB, Cramer DW, Goodman MT, Kjaer SK, Mallin K, Mosgaard BJ, et al. Infertility, fertility drugs, and ovarian cancer: a pooled analysis of case-control studies. Am J Epidemiol 2002;155:217–24.

4. Risch HA, McLaughlin JR, Cole DE, Rosen B, Bradley L, Kwan E, et al. Prevalence and penetrance of germline BRCA1 and BRCA2 mutations in a population series of 649 women with ovarian cancer. Am J Hum Genet 2001; 68:700–10.

5. Pal T, Permuth-Wey J, Betts JA, Krischer JP, Fiorica J, Arango H, et al. BRCA1 and BRCA2 mutations account for a large proportion of ovarian carcinoma cases. Cancer 2005; 104:2807–16.

TABLE 23. International Federation of Gynecology and Obstetrics Staging of Carcinoma of the Fallopian Tube

Stage	Description
0	Carcinoma in situ (limited to tubal mucosa)
I	Growth limited to the fallopian tubes
IA	Growth limited to one tube, with extension into the submucosa, or muscularis, or both, but not penetrating the serosal surface; no ascites
IB	Growth limited to both tubes, with extension into the submucosa, or muscularis, or both, but not penetrating the serosal surface; no ascites
IC	Tumor either stage IA or IB, but with tumor extension through or onto tubal serosa, or with ascites present containing malignant cells, or with positive peritoneal washings
II	Growth involving one or both fallopian tubes with pelvic extension
IIA	Extension, or metastasis, or both to the uterus, or ovaries, or both
IIB	Extension to other pelvic tissues
IIC	Tumor either stage IIA or IIB and with ascites present containing malignant cells or with positive peritoneal washings
III	Tumor involves one or both fallopian tubes, with peritoneal implants outside the pelvis, or positive retroperitoneal nodes, or inguinal nodes, or all; superficial liver metastasis equals stage III; tumor appears limited to the true pelvis, but with histologically proven malignant extension to the small bowel or omentum
IIIA	Tumor grossly limited to the true pelvis, with negative nodes, but with histologically confirmed microscopic seeding of abdominal peritoneal surfaces
IIIB	Tumor involving one or both tubes, with histologically confirmed implants of abdominal peritoneal surfaces, none exceeding 2 cm in diameter; lymph nodes are negative
IIIC	Abdominal implants greater than 2 cm in diameter, or positive retroperitoneal nodes, or inguinal nodes, or all
IV	Growth involving one or both fallopian tubes with distant metastases; if pleural effusion is present, there must be positive cytologic findings to be stage IV; parenchymal liver metastases equals stage IV

This table was published in the International Journal of Gynecology and Obstetrics, volume 95, supplement, Heintz AP, Odicino F, Maisonneuve P, Quinn MA, Benedet JL, Creasman WT, et al. Carcinoma of the fallopian tube. International Federation of Gynecology and Obstetrics. FIGO annual report on the results of treatment in gynecological cancer, s145–60, copyright Elsevier 2006.

6. Bergfeldt K, Rydh B, Granath F, Gronberg H, Thalib L, Adami HO, et al. Risk of ovarian cancer in breast-cancer patients with a family history of breast or ovarian cancer: a population-based cohort study. Lancet 2002;360:891–4.

7. Edmondson RJ, Monaghan JM. The epidemiology of ovarian cancer. Int J Gynecol Cancer 2001;11:423–9.

8. Kjaer SK, Mellemkjaer L, Brinton LA, Johansen C, Gridley G, Olsen JH. Tubal sterilization and risk of ovarian, endometrial and cervical cancer. A Danish population-based follow-up study of more than 65 000 sterilized women. Int J Epidemiol 2004;33:596–602.

9. Kauff ND, Mitra M, Robson ME, Hurley KE, Chuai S, Godlfrank D, et al. Risk of ovarian cancer in BRCA1 and BRCA2 mutation-negative hereditary breast cancer families. J Natl Cancer Inst 2005;97:1382–4.

10. van Nagell JR Jr, DePriest PD, Reedy MB, Gallion HH, Ueland FR, Pavlik EJ, et al. The efficacy of transvaginal sonographic screening in asymptomatic women at risk for ovarian cancer. Gynecol Oncol 2000;77:350–6.

11. Buys SS, Partridge E, Greene MH, Prorok PC, Reding D, Riley TL, et al. Ovarian cancer screening in the Prostate, Lung, Colorectal and Ovarian (PLCO) cancer screening trial: findings from the initial screen of a randomized trial [published erratum appears in Am J Obstet Gynecol 2005; 193:2183–4]. Am J Obstet Gynecol 2005;193:1630–9.

12. Petricoin EF, Ardekani AM, Hitt BA, Levine PJ, Fusaro VA, Steinberg SM, et al. Use of proteomic patterns in serum to identify ovarian cancer. Lancet 2002;359:572–7.

13. Goff BA, Mandel L, Muntz HG, Melancon CH. Ovarian carcinoma diagnosis. Cancer 2000;89:2068–75.

14. The role of the generalist obstetrician–gynecologist in the early detection of ovarian cancer. ACOG Committee Opinion No. 280. American College of Obstetricians and Gynecologists. Obstet Gynecol 2002;100:1413–6.

15. Nardo LG, Kroon ND, Reginald PW. Persistent unilocular ovarian cysts in a general population of postmenopausal women: is there a place for expectant management? Gynecol Oncol 2003;102:589–93.

16. Modesitt SC, Pavlik EJ, Ueland R, DePriest PD, Kryscio RJ, van Nagell JR. Risk of malignancy in unilocular ovarian cystic tumors less than 10 centimeters in diameter. Obstet Gynecol 2003;102:594–9.

17. Chi DS, Abu-Rustum NR, Sonoda Y, Ivy J, Rhee E, Moore K, et al. The safety and efficacy of laparoscopic surgical staging of apparent stage I ovarian and fallopian tube cancers. Am J Obstet Gynecol 2005;192:1614–9.

18. Gostout BS, Brewer MA. Guidelines for referral of the patient with an adnexal mass. Clin Obstet Gynecol 2006; 49:448–58.

19. Bristow RE, Tomacruz RS, Armstrong DK, Trimble EL, Montz FJ. Survival effect of maximal cytoreductive surgery for advanced ovarian carcinoma during the platinum era: a meta-analysis. J Clin Oncol 2002;20:1248–59.

20. Chi DS, Franklin CC, Levine DA, Akselrod F, Sabbatini P, Jarnagin WR, et al. Improved optimal cytoreduction rates for stages IIIC and IV epithelial ovarian, fallopian tube, and primary peritoneal cancer: a change in surgical approach. Gynecol Oncol 2004;94:650–4.

21. Eisenhauer EL, Abu-Rustum NR, Sonoda Y, Levine DA, Poynor EA, Aghajanian CA, et al. The addition of extensive upper abdominal surgery to achieve optimal cytoreduction improves survival in patients with stage IIIC-IV epithelial ovarian cancer. Gynecol Oncol 2006;103:1083–90.

22. van der Burg ME, van Lent M, Buyse M, Kobierska A, Colombo N, Favalli G, et al. The effect of debulking surgery after induction chemotherapy on the prognosis in advanced epithelial ovarian cancer: Gynecological Cancer Cooperative Group of the European Organization for Research and Treatment of Cancer. N Engl J Med 1995; 332:629–34.

23. Rose PG, Nerenstone S, Brady M, Clarke-Pearson D, Olt G, Rubin SC, et al. Secondary surgical cytoreduction for advanced ovarian carcinoma. N Engl J Med 2004;351: 2489–97.

24. Barakat RR, Sabatini P, Bhaskaran D, Revzin M, Smith A, Venkatraman E, et al. Intraperitoneal chemotherapy for ovarian carcinoma: results of long-term follow-up. J Clin Oncol 2002;20:694–8.

25. Markman M, Liu PY, Wilczynski S, Monk B, Copeland LJ, Alvarez RD, et al. Phase III randomized trial of 12 versus 3 months of maintenance paclitaxel in patients with advanced ovarian cancer after complete response to platinum and paclitaxel-based chemotherapy: a Southwest Oncology Group and Gynecologic Oncology Group trial. J Clin Oncol 2003;21:2460–5.

26. Chi DS, McCaughty K, Diaz J, Huh J, Schwabenbauer S, Hummer AJ, et al. Guidelines and selection criteria for secondary cytoreductive surgery in patients with recurrent, platinum-sensitive epithelial ovarian carcinoma. Cancer 2006;106:1933–9.

27. Armstrong DK, Bundy B, Wenzel L, Huang HQ, Baergen R, Lele S, et al. Intraperitoneal cisplatin and paclitaxel in ovarian cancer. N Engl J Med 2006;354:34–43.

28. Williams SD, Gershenson DM. Management of germ cell tumors of the ovary. In: Markman M, Hoskins WJ, editors. Cancer of the ovary. New York (NY): Raven Press; 1993. p. 375–84.

29. Kauff ND, Satagopan JM, Robson ME, Scheuer L, Hensley M, Hudis CA, et al. Risk-reducing salpingo-oophorectomy in women with a BRCA1 or BRCA2 mutation. N Engl J Med 2002;346:1609–15.

Gestational Trophoblastic Disease

John R. Lurain, MD

Gestational trophoblastic disease encompasses four clinicopathologic forms of growth disturbances of the human placenta: hydatidiform mole (complete and partial), invasive mole, choriocarcinoma, and placental-site trophoblastic tumor. The term *gestational trophoblastic neoplasia* has been applied collectively to the latter three conditions (Table 24).

If untreated, these tumors can progress, invade, metastasize, and lead to death. The overall cure rate in the treatment of patients with gestational trophoblastic neoplasia now exceeds 90% (1). This high rate is the result of the chemotherapy-sensitive nature of trophoblastic tumors; the ability to establish a diagnosis and monitor therapy effectively by using hCG as a tumor marker; the referral of patients to specialized treatment centers; the identification of prognostic factors to enhance individualization of therapy; and the aggressive use of combination chemotherapy, irradiation, and surgery in high-risk patients.

HYDATIDIFORM MOLE

Hydatidiform mole refers to a pregnancy characterized by vesicular swelling of placental villi and, usually, the absence of an intact fetus. There is microscopic proliferation of the trophoblast (the cytotrophoblast and the syncytiotrophoblast), with varying degrees of hyperplasia and anaplasia. The chorionic villi are filled with fluid and distended, and blood vessels are scant. Two syndromes of hydatidiform mole have been described based on morphologic and cytogenetic criteria (Table 24).

Complete hydatidiform mole undergoes early and total hydatidiform enlargement of villi in the absence of an ascertainable fetus or embryo (Fig. 20), and the trophoblast is consistently hyperplastic, with varying degrees of atypia. It usually has a 46,XX karyotype derived from fertilization by a haploid (23,X) sperm that totally replaces the maternal contribution and reaches the 46,XX status by its own duplication. The nucleus of the ovum may be either absent or inactivated after fertilization. Occasionally, a 46,XY karyotype occurs as a result of dispermic fertilization of an empty egg. Although the chromosomes of complete hydatidiform moles are entirely paternal, mitochondrial DNA is of maternal origin.

Partial hydatidiform mole is characterized by slowly progressive hydatidiform change in the presence of functioning villous capillaries. This change affects only some of the villi. The result is chorionic villi that vary in size and shape and have scalloping and prominent stromal trophoblastic inclusions. Trophoblastic immaturity is constant, and there is only focal hyperplasia with mild atypia. Partial hydatidiform mole is associated with an identifiable abnormal fetus or embryo (alive or dead) or fetal membranes or erythrocytes. Most partial hydatidiform moles have a triploid karyotype, usually 69,XXY, with the extra haploid set of chromosomes derived from the father. It may be difficult to distinguish partial hydatidiform moles from fetuses with hydropic degeneration.

Trophoblastic neoplasia (invasive mole or choriocarcinoma) follows complete hydatidiform mole in 15–20% of cases. Of patients who have trophoblastic persistence, 75–85% have nonmetastatic disease, and 15–25% have evidence of metastasis. The reported incidence of trophoblastic neoplasia after partial hydatidiform mole is less than 5%, with metastasis occurring rarely. Several case reports of choriocarcinoma after partial hydatidiform mole have been published (2).

Incidence

The incidence of hydatidiform mole varies greatly throughout the world. In the United States and Europe, the incidence is approximately 0.6–1.1 per 1,000 pregnancies. In other areas, especially Asia, the incidence has been reported to be more than three times higher: 2–10 per 1,000 pregnancies (3). Much of this geographic variation may result from reporting differences rather than true incidence differences, although the high incidence of molar pregnancy in some populations has been attributed to low dietary intake of carotene and animal fat, resulting in vitamin A deficiency. There is an increased risk of molar pregnancy for women older than 40 years and women at the lower end of the reproductive range, although there does not appear to be any significant association with gravidity. The risk of complete and partial hydatidiform mole is increased in women who had a previous spontaneous abortion, although there is no association between maternal age or dietary factors and the risk of partial hydatidiform mole. Hydatidiform moles recur in 0.5–2.6% of patients, with a greater risk of developing invasive mole or choriocarcinoma after repeated molar pregnancies.

TABLE 24. Clinicopathologic Features of Gestational Trophoblastic Disease

Clinicopathologic Form	Pathologic Features	Clinical Features
Hydatidiform mole		
Complete	Diploid (46,XX; 46,XY)	15–20% trophoblastic sequelae
	Absent fetus or embryo	Human chorionic gonadotropin level often higher than 100,000 milli-International Units/mL
	Diffuse swelling of villi	Medical complications, such as preeclampsia, hyperthyroidism, or trophoblastic embolization
	Diffuse trophoblastic hyperplasia	
Partial	Triploid (69,XXY; 69,XXX)	Less than 5% trophoblastic sequelae
	Abnormal fetus or embryo	Human chorionic gonadotropin level usually lower than 100,000 milli-International Units/mL
	Focal swelling of villi	Medical complications rare
	Focal trophoblastic hyperplasia	
Invasive mole	Myometrial invasion	15% metastatic to lung or vagina
	Swollen villi	Most often diagnosed clinically rather than pathologically
	Hyperplastic trophoblast	
Choriocarcinoma	Abnormal trophoblastic hyperplasia and anaplasia	Vascular spread to distant sites, such as lung, brain, or liver
	Absent villi	Malignant disease
	Hemorrhage, necrosis	
Placental-site trophoblastic tumor	Tumor cells infiltrate myometrium with vascular or lymphatic invasion	Extremely rare
	Intermediate cells and absent villi	Human chorionic gonadotropin level less reliable indicator
	Less hemorrhage, necrosis	Relatively chemoresistant
	Human placental lactogen in tumor cells	Chiefly surgical treatment

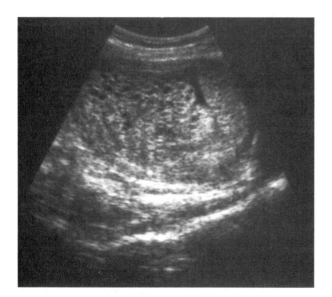

■ **FIG. 20.** Ultrasound image of a complete molar pregnancy with the characteristic vesicular ultrasound pattern secondary to diffuse hydropic swelling that demonstrates multiple echoes, holes within the placental mass, and usually no fetus.

Diagnosis

The clinical presentation of complete hydatidiform mole has changed considerably over the past several years. Widespread use of ultrasonography and the administration of accurate tests for hCG have resulted in earlier diagnosis. Vaginal bleeding continues to be the most common presenting symptom, occurring at 6–16 weeks of gestation in 80–90% of patients. The other classic clinical signs and symptoms, such as uterine enlargement greater than expected for gestational dates (28%), hyperemesis (8%), and pregnancy-induced hypertension in the first or second trimester (1%), now occur less frequently. Clinical hyperthyroidism and trophoblastic embolization with symptoms and signs of congestive heart failure and pulmonary edema are rare. Bilateral theca-lutein cyst enlargement of the ovaries occurs in approximately 15% of cases. Fetal heart tones usually are absent.

Human chorionic gonadotropin levels in patients with complete hydatidiform mole usually, but not always, are elevated above levels of normal pregnancy, often exceeding 100,000 milli-International Units per mL. A single hCG level determination, however, is seldom helpful in differentiating complete hydatidiform mole from a normal intrauterine pregnancy, an intrauterine pregnancy complicated by multiple gestation or diseases associated with an enlarged placenta (for example, erythroblastosis fetalis or intrauterine infections), or an enlarged uterus caused by uterine leiomyomata during a normal intrauterine pregnancy.

Ultrasonography is a reliable and sensitive test for the diagnosis of complete hydatidiform mole, and it has virtually replaced all other means of preoperative diagnosis. Because the chorionic villi of complete hydatidiform moles exhibit diffuse hydropic swelling, a characteristic vesicular ultrasonographic pattern can be observed. It consists of multiple echoes, holes within the placental mass, and usually no fetus (see Fig. 20). Correlating the ultrasonographic findings with the hCG level may aid in differentiating an early complete hydatidiform mole from abortion.

Patients with partial hydatidiform moles usually do not exhibit the classic clinical features of complete hydatidiform moles previously described. More than 90% of patients have symptoms of incomplete or missed abortion, and the diagnosis of partial hydatidiform mole usually is established after histologic review of specimens. The main presenting symptom is vaginal bleeding, which occurs in approximately 75% of patients. Excessive uterine enlargement, pregnancy-induced hypertension, hyperemesis, hyperthyroidism, and theca-lutein ovarian cysts develop infrequently. Preevacuation hCG levels usually are not as high as they are for complete hydatidiform moles, exceeding 100,000 milli-International Units per mL in fewer than 10% of patients with partial hydatidiform moles. Ultrasonography may facilitate the early diagnosis of a partial hydatidiform mole by demonstrating focal cystic spaces within the placenta and an increase in the transverse diameter of the gestational sac (see Table 24).

FALSE-POSITIVE (PHANTOM) HUMAN CHORIONIC GONADOTROPIN LEVELS

Although hCG levels are invaluable in diagnosing and monitoring gestational trophoblastic disease, laboratory assays for hCG may yield false-positive results. Such false-positive hCG results, as high as 800 milli-International Units per mL, have led to treatment of healthy patients with surgery and chemotherapy in what has been termed *phantom hCG syndrome or phantom choriocarcinoma syndrome* (4). The causes of these false-positive test results are proteolytic enzymes that produce nonspecific protein interference and heterophilic antibodies (human antimouse antibodies); these antibodies are found in 3–4% of healthy individuals and can mimic hCG immunoreactivity by linking and capturing tracer mouse immunoglobulin G.

When the clinical findings suggest phantom hCG syndrome, three methods can be used to determine whether serum hCG assay results are false positive:

- Determination of the urine hCG level—urinary hCG assay results should be negative, because the interfering substances are not excreted in the urine

- Serial dilution of the serum, which should not show a parallel decrease with dilution

- Testing the patient's serum at a national hCG reference laboratory

COEXISTING TWIN PREGNANCY AND MOLE

Since the introduction of ovulation-inducing agents in the 1970s, a number of multiple pregnancies consisting of a normal fetus or fetuses and a molar gestation have been reported (Fig. 21). This phenomenon most commonly occurs as a twin pregnancy with a complete hydatidiform mole and a normal fetus, with an estimated incidence of 1 in 22,000–100,000 pregnancies. A twin pregnancy consisting of a complete hydatidiform mole and a normal fetus is distinguished from a partial molar pregnancy (a single, usually triploid conceptus with an anomalous fetus) by the fact that the normal fetoplacental unit and the molar placenta are two different conceptuses, analogous to dizygotic twins. The diagnosis of this rare entity often is based on ultrasound findings—though with less reliability than in complete or partial hydatidiform moles—and on symptomatology similar to molar pregnancies. Definitive diagnosis is based on a diploid fetal karyotype and normal fetal development.

Compared with complete or partial hydatidiform moles, these pregnancies are at increased risk for hemorrhage, preeclampsia, thyroid storm, and hyperemesis, as well as at markedly increased risk (40–57%) for persistent gestational trophoblastic neoplasia requiring chemotherapy after delivery or evacuation (5). The rate of survival of the coexisting fetus is approximately 25–30% when the pregnancy can continue to viability in the absence of hemorrhage or severe medical complications. Patients require extensive counseling while deciding whether to continue or to terminate the pregnancy. Although it has not been proved that ovulation induction can increase the rate of molar pregnancy per se, the number of multiple pregnancies has increased appreciably, likely resulting in the emergence of this rare entity. In any case, ovulation induction leads to the release of relatively immature ova and an increased rate of nuclear "empty" ova, which theoretically increases the risk of complete molar gestation.

Treatment

The patient with hydatidiform mole should be evaluated carefully for the presence of associated medical complications and be stabilized. Next, the most appropriate method of molar evacuation should be determined (Fig. 22). The

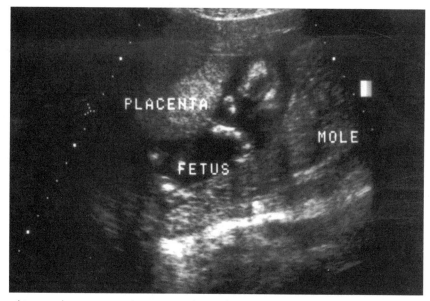

■ **FIG. 21.** Ultrasound image demonstrating the rare condition of a twin pregnancy consisting of a complete molar pregnancy and a normal fetus.

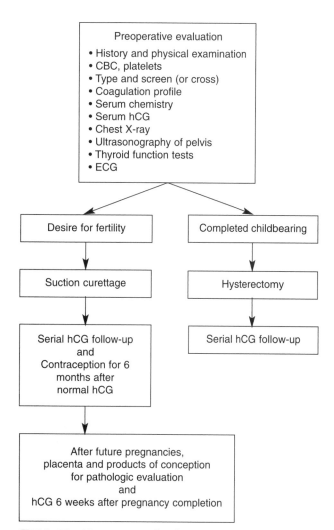

■ **FIG. 22.** Management of molar pregnancy. Abbreviations: CBC indicates complete blood count; ECG, electrocardiography; hCG, human chorionic gonadotropin

preoperative evaluation should include gathering information on the patient's history; a physical examination; tests for complete blood and platelet counts, coagulation profile, serum chemistry, thyroid function, blood type and crossmatch, and serum hCG level; urinalysis; chest radiography; electrocardiography; and pelvic ultrasonography.

Suction curettage is the preferred method of evacuation of a hydatidiform mole, independent of uterine size, in patients who wish to maintain their fertility. Suction evacuation should be followed by gentle sharp curettage. An oxytocic agent should be infused intravenously near the end of evacuation and be continued for several hours to enhance uterine contractility. Attention to blood and crystalloid replacement decreases pulmonary complications. Because trophoblastic cells express the CDE (Rh) factor, patients whose blood type is D negative should receive anti-D immune globulin at the time of evacuation.

Hysterectomy is an alternative to suction curettage if childbearing has been completed (Fig. 22). The adnexa may be preserved even in the presence of theca-lutein cysts. Although hysterectomy reduces the risk of postmolar gestational trophoblastic tumor to approximately 3–5%, continued hCG follow-up is still required. Hysterotomy and medical induction of labor with oxytocin or prostaglandins are not recommended, because these methods increase morbidity and the subsequent development of postmolar gestational trophoblastic neoplasia.

Follow-up Care

Follow-up of patients after evacuation of a hydatidiform mole indicates that this therapy cures more than 80% of patients (6). Incomplete involution of the uterus and vaginal bleeding may be signs of persistent trophoblastic disease. Another curettage may be performed if there is significant bleeding and ultrasound evidence of retained molar tissue within the cavity of the uterus; however, repeated curettage rarely is curative without chemotherapy, it has associated risks such as uterine perforation, and tissue obtained for histologic examination rarely changes management (7).

Clinical findings such as prompt uterine involution, ovarian cyst regression, and cessation of bleeding are reassuring signs. Definitive follow-up, however, requires serial hCG testing with an assay of sufficient sensitivity. Testing should include the following:

- Determination of serum hCG levels every 2 weeks until three consecutive test results show normal levels

- Determination of serum hCG levels every month for 6–12 months

- Avoidance of pregnancy for 6 months after the first normal hCG test results

- Sending the placenta and other products of conception for pathologic evaluation after any future pregnancy

- Determination of serum hCG level 6 weeks after the completion of future pregnancies

Contraception should be prescribed for 6 months after evacuation of the molar pregnancy. The use of oral contraceptives is acceptable and has the advantage of suppressing endogenous luteinizing hormone, which may interfere with the measurement of hCG at low levels.

For patients at highest risk of postmolar trophoblastic tumors (Box 16), prophylactic chemotherapy at the time of, or immediately after, molar evacuation may be considered. The need for treatment in patients with postmolar trophoblastic neoplasia is determined primarily by monitoring hCG levels (Box 17).

GESTATIONAL TROPHOBLASTIC NEOPLASIA

Invasive mole arises from myometrial invasion by a hydatidiform mole by way of direct extension through tissue or venous channels (Table 24). Invasive mole tends to undergo spontaneous regression. The overall incidence of invasive mole has been estimated to be 1 in 15,000 pregnancies. Approximately 10–17% of hydatidiform moles will result in invasive mole. The diagnosis most often is established clinically, on the basis of increasing or persistently elevated hCG levels after evacuation of a hydatidiform mole. Hysterectomy or biopsy of metastatic lesions to obtain pathologic confirmation usually are not performed because of the excellent success in managing the disease with chemotherapy.

Choriocarcinoma is characterized by abnormal trophoblastic hyperplasia and anaplasia; absence of chorion-

---

BOX 16

Risk Factors of Postmolar Gestational Trophoblastic Neoplasia

- Preevacuation uterine size greater than gestational age or larger than 20 weeks of gestation
- Theca-lutein cysts larger than 6 cm
- Age older than 40 years
- Serum human chorionic gonadotropin levels higher than 100,000 milli-International Units/mL
- Medical complications of molar pregnancy
- Previous hydatidiform mole

BOX 17

Indications for Treatment of Postmolar Gestational Trophoblastic Neoplasia

- Plateau in hCG level for 3 consecutive weeks
- Increase in hCG level for 2 consecutive weeks
- Persistently elevated hCG levels 6 months after molar evacuation
- Presence of metastatic disease
- Histopathologic diagnosis of choriocarcinoma

Abbreviation: hCG indicates human chorionic gonadotropin.

---

ic villi; hemorrhage and necrosis; direct invasion of the myometrium; and vascular spread to the myometrium and distant sites, the most common being the lungs, brain, liver, pelvis and vagina, spleen, intestines, and kidney (Table 24). Gestational choriocarcinoma may arise in association with any type of pregnancy. Approximately 25% of cases of gestational choriocarcinoma follow abortion or tubal pregnancy, and 25% are associated with term gestation; the remaining cases arise from hydatidiform moles. Overall, only 2–3% of hydatidiform moles progress to choriocarcinoma. The incidence of choriocarcinoma, therefore, is approximately 1 per 40,000 pregnancies.

Placental-site trophoblastic tumor, an extremely rare disease, arises from the placental implantation site and consists predominantly of intermediate trophoblasts that secrete human placental lactogen. This tumor is associated with less vascular invasion, necrosis, and hemorrhage than typical choriocarcinoma, and it has a propensity for lymphatic spread (Table 24). The most common symptom is irregular vaginal bleeding, often distant from a preceding nonmolar gestation. Placental-site tumors tend to remain within the uterus, disseminate late, and produce low levels of hCG relative to their tumor mass. The clinical classification schemes and scoring systems used for other gestational trophoblastic neoplasms do not apply to placental-site trophoblastic tumor. These tumors are relatively resistant to chemotherapy, and surgery has been the mainstay of treatment.

Diagnosis

The diagnosis of gestational trophoblastic neoplasia can be established based on an increase or plateau in hCG levels after the evacuation of a molar pregnancy. Occasionally, the diagnosis is established based on a persistent elevation in hCG levels, frequently in conjunction with the demonstration of metastases, after other pregnancy events. Pathologic diagnosis sometimes can be established by curettage, biopsy of metastatic lesions, or occasionally, examination of hysterectomy specimens or placenta. Biopsy of any cervical or vaginal lesion suggestive of gestational trophoblastic tumor is dangerous because of the massive, uncontrolled bleeding that may occur. When the diagnosis of gestational trophoblastic neoplasia is suspected, the patient should undergo a metastatic workup that includes computed tomography of the abdomen and pelvis, as well as chest radiography or computed tomography of the chest. Computed tomography or magnetic resonance imaging of the brain should be considered, especially in the presence of pulmonary metastases, neurologic symptoms, or both.

Symptoms and Signs

The symptom most suggestive of persistent trophoblastic tumor is continued uterine bleeding after evacuation of a hydatidiform mole or after any pregnancy event. Bleeding as a result of uterine perforation or metastatic lesions may result in abdominal pain; hemoptysis; melena; or evidence of increased intracranial pressure from intracerebral hemorrhage leading to headaches, seizures, or hemiplegia. Patients also may exhibit pulmonary symptoms, such as dyspnea, cough, and chest pain, caused by extensive lung metastases.

Signs suggestive of postmolar trophoblastic neoplasia are an enlarged, irregular uterus and persistent bilateral ovarian enlargement. Occasionally, a metastatic lesion is noted on examination, most commonly in the vagina. Choriocarcinoma associated with a nonmolar gestation has no characteristic physical signs, but it may produce symptoms as a result of metastatic disease. In patients with uterine bleeding and subinvolution after delivery, gestational trophoblastic neoplasia should be considered along with other possible causes (retained products of conception or endometritis, primary or metastatic tumors of other organ systems, and another pregnancy that occurred shortly after the first).

Classification and Staging

When a gestational trophoblastic neoplasm has been confirmed, it is necessary to determine the extent of disease (see the previous discussion). If the physical examination and chest radiography yield normal findings, other sites of metastasis are uncommon. Pelvic ultrasonography also may be useful in detecting extensive uterine disease for which hysterectomy may be of benefit. After these initial studies, patients are categorized on the basis of anatomic extent of disease and likelihood of response to various chemotherapeutic protocols, and treatment is carried out accordingly.

The currently used classification system adopted by the International Federation of Gynecology and Obstetrics (FIGO) in 2000 designates the FIGO stage with a Roman numeral followed by the modified World Health Organization score designated by an Arabic numeral separated by a colon (Tables 25 and 26). Placental-site trophoblastic tumors are classified separately (8).

The FIGO system also outlines the necessary components needed to determine the diagnosis of postmolar gestational trophoblastic neoplasia (Box 17). These components include at least one of the following: 1) an hCG plateau for four values or more for 3 weeks or longer, 2) an hCG increase of 10% or greater for three or more values for 2 weeks or longer, 3) hCG persistence 6 months after molar evacuation, 4) histopathologic diagnosis of choriocarcinoma, or 5) the presence of metastatic disease.

Treatment is based on classification into risk groups defined by the scoring system: low-risk group score, 6 or lower and high-risk group score, 7 or higher. Patients with nonmetastatic (stage I) and low-risk metastatic (stages II and III; score lower than 7) gestational trophoblastic neoplasia can be treated with single-agent chemotherapy with resulting survival rates approaching 100%. Patients classified as having high-risk metastatic disease (stage IV or score of 7 or higher) should be treated in a more aggressive manner with combination chemotherapy and adjuvant radiation therapy or surgery to achieve cure rates of 80–90%. Use of this classification system is essential for determining initial therapy for patients with gestational trophoblastic neoplasia to ensure the best possible outcomes with the least morbidity.

Therapy

NONMETASTATIC DISEASE

Single-agent chemotherapy with either methotrexate or dactinomycin is the treatment of choice for patients with nonmetastatic gestational trophoblastic neoplasia (1). This treatment is markedly different from the regimen used in patients with ectopic pregnancy. Several outpatient chemotherapeutic protocols have been used, all yielding excellent and fairly comparable remission rates. Hysterectomy may be used as part of primary therapy in patients who no longer desire to preserve fertility.

Regardless of the treatment protocol used, chemotherapy is continued until hCG values have returned to normal and one or two courses have been administered after the

TABLE 25. Modified World Health Organization Prognostic Scoring System as Adapted by the International Federation of Gynecology and Obstetrics

Characteristic	Score			
	0	1	2	4
Age	Younger than 40 years	40 years or older	—	—
Antecedent pregnancy	Mole	Abortion	Term	
Interval from index pregnancy	Less than 4 months	4–6 months	7–12 months	More than 12 months
Pretreatment serum human chorionic gonadotropin (International Units per liter)	Less than 10^3	$10^3–10^4$	$10^4–10^5$	Greater than 10^5
Largest tumor size (including uterus)	Less than 3 cm	3–4 cm	Greater than or equal to 5 cm	—
Site of metastases	Lung	Spleen, kidney	Gastrointestinal tract	Liver, brain
Number of metastases	—	1–4	5–8	More than 8
Previous failed chemotherapy	—	—	Single drug	Two or more drugs

This table was published in International Journal of Gynecology and Obstetrics, volume 95, supplement, Ngan HY, Odicino F, Maisonneuve P, Creasman WT, Beller U, Quinn MA. Gestational trophoblastic neoplasia. International Federation of Gynecology and Obstetrics. FIGO annual report on the results of treatment in gynecological cancer, s193–203, copyright Elsevier 2006.

TABLE 26. Gestational Trophoblastic Neoplasia: International Federation of Gynecology and Obstetrics Staging and Classification

Stage	Description
I	Disease is confined to the uterus.
II	Disease extends outside the uterus but is limited to genital structures (adnexa, vagina, and broad ligament).
III	Disease extends to the lungs, with or without genital tract involvement.
IV	Disease involves all other metastatic sites.

This table was published in International Journal of Gynecology and Obstetrics, volume 83, supplement, Ngan HY, Bender H, Benedet JL, Jones H, Montruccoli GC, Pecorelli. Gestational trophoblastic neoplasia, FIGO 2000 staging and classification. FIGO Committee on Gynecologic Oncology, s175–7, copyright Elsevier 2003.

first normal hCG level. Chemotherapy is changed to the alternative single agent if the hCG level plateaus above normal or if toxicity precludes an adequate dose or frequency of treatment. If there is a significant elevation in the hCG level, development of metastases, or resistance to sequential single-agent chemotherapy, multiagent chemotherapy should be initiated. Hysterectomy can be considered for disease remaining in the uterus that is refractory to chemotherapy.

Cure is anticipated in essentially all patients with nonmetastatic disease. Approximately 85–90% of patients will be cured by the initial chemotherapeutic regimen. Most of the remaining patients will go into permanent remission with additional single-agent chemotherapy; multiagent chemotherapy rarely is needed. Fewer than 5% of patients will require hysterectomy for cure, resulting in the preservation of reproductive function in more than 95% of patients.

METASTATIC DISEASE

Therapy differs for low- and high-risk patients. This discussion will cover protocols for the management of low-risk disease, high-risk disease, and placental-site trophoblastic tumors.

Single-agent chemotherapy with 5-day regimens of methotrexate or dactinomycin is the treatment for patients with low-risk metastatic gestational trophoblastic neoplasia. The weekly methotrexate or biweekly dactinomycin single-dose protocols that are in use for the management of nonmetastatic postmolar disease should not be employed for the management of metastatic disease. When resistance to sequential single-agent chemotherapy develops, combination chemotherapy, as for high-risk disease, is used. Hysterectomy may be necessary to eradicate persistent, chemotherapy-resistant disease in the uterus, or it may be performed as adjuvant treatment coincident with the institution of chemotherapy to shorten the duration of therapy.

Cure rates should approach 100% in this group of patients when treatment is administered properly. Approximately 30–50% of patients in this category will develop resistance to the first chemotherapeutic agent and require alternative treatment. Thus, it is important to carefully monitor patients undergoing treatment for evidence of drug resistance so that a change to a second agent can be made at the earliest possible time. Approximately 5–15% of patients treated for low-risk metastatic disease with sequential single-agent chemotherapy will require combination chemotherapy with or without surgery to achieve remission.

Patients with high-risk metastatic gestational trophoblastic neoplasia should be treated more aggressively with initial combination chemotherapy including etoposide, methotrexate, and dactinomycin with or without adjuvant radiation therapy or surgery (9). For recurrent or resistant gestational trophoblastic disease, other chemotherapeutic agents with proven activity in trophoblastic tumors, such as cisplatin, bleomycin, and ifosfamide, should be used in combination with etoposide (10–13). Adjuvant surgical procedures, especially hysterectomy and thoracotomy, may be useful in combination with other procedures to remove known foci of chemotherapy-resistant disease, control hemorrhage, relieve bowel or urinary obstruction, manage infection, or deal with other life-threatening complications (14).

Chemotherapy is continued for at least two or three courses after the first normal hCG level measurement. Intensive therapy with combination chemotherapy and, when indicated, adjuvant radiotherapy and surgery has resulted in cure rates of 80–90% in patients with high-risk metastatic gestational trophoblastic neoplasia. The factors most important in determining treatment response in these patients are clinicopathologic diagnosis of choriocarcinoma, metastases to sites other than the lung and vagina, number of metastases, and failure of previous chemotherapy. Most treatment failures can be attributed to the presence of extensive choriocarcinoma at the time of diagnosis or to lack of appropriate initial treatment (9).

Hysterectomy with lymphadenectomy is the recommended management for a placental-site trophoblastic tumor because of the relative resistance of these tumors to chemotherapy and their propensity to spread through the lymphatic system. Chemotherapy should be used in patients with metastatic placental-site trophoblastic tumor and in patients with nonmetastatic disease who have adverse prognostic factors for survival other than metastatic disease, such as interval from last known pregnancy to diagnosis greater than 2 years, deep myometrial invasion, tumor necrosis, and mitotic count greater than 6 mitoses per 10 high-power fields (15). Although optimal chemotherapy for patients with placental-site trophoblastic tumor remains to be defined, the current clinical impression is that a platinum-containing regimen, such as etoposide/methotrexate/actinomycin–etoposide/cisplatin or a paclitaxel/cisplatin–paclitaxel/etoposide doublet, is the treatment of choice (16). The survival rate is approximately 100% for patients with nonmetastatic disease and 50–60% for patients with metastatic disease.

Consultation and Referral Guidelines

Because most deaths in patients with gestational trophoblastic disease occur because of delayed treatment or inadequate treatment in the setting of advanced disease, appropriate consultation and referral are critical in the management of this disease. Gynecologic oncologists are trained specifically in establishing the diagnosis, evaluation, medical and surgical management, and surveillance of gestational trophoblastic disease. Routine consultation or evaluation by a gynecologic oncologist may benefit women who receive a diagnosis of molar pregnancy confirmed by ultrasonography; a diagnosis of molar pregnancy confirmed histologically; or a diagnosis of persistent postmolar trophoblastic disease, choriocarcinoma, or placental-site trophoblastic tumor. Specialized trophoblastic disease centers may offer patients with high-risk metastatic disease special expertise in multimodal therapy and management of toxicity, as well as new investigational treatments (17).

Follow-up Care

TROPHOBLASTIC DISEASE SURVEILLANCE

After a patient has completed chemotherapy, quantitative serum hCG levels should be determined at 2-week intervals for the first 3 months of remission and then at 1-month intervals until monitoring has shown 1 year of normal hCG levels (17). The risk of recurrence is low after 1 year. Physical examinations are performed at intervals of 6–12 months, and other examinations, such as chest radiography, are performed as indicated. Reliable contraception should be maintained during treatment and for 1 year after the completion of chemotherapy. Because these patients are at increased risk for another gestational trophoblastic disease event, pelvic ultrasonography is recommended in the first trimester of a subsequent pregnancy to confirm a normal gestation. The products of conception or placentas from future pregnancies should undergo careful histopathologic examination, and a serum quantitative hCG level should be determined 6 weeks after any pregnancy.

REPRODUCTIVE PERFORMANCE

The successful management of gestational trophoblastic neoplasia with chemotherapy has resulted in the retention of reproductive potential in a large number of women despite their exposure to drugs that have ovarian toxicity and teratogenic potential. Most women resume normal ovarian function after chemotherapy and exhibit no increase in infertility. Many successful pregnancies have been reported. Generally, these women experience no increase in incidences of abortions, stillbirths, congenital anomalies, prematurity, or major obstetric complications (18). There has been no evidence of reactivation of disease because of a subsequent pregnancy, although patients who have had one trophoblastic disease episode are at greater risk of the development of a second episode in a subsequent pregnancy, unrelated to whether they had previously received chemotherapy. Patients are advised to delay conception for 1 year after cessation of chemotherapy.

This schedule allows for uninterrupted hCG follow-up evaluation to ensure cure. It also may permit the elimination of mature ova damaged by exposure to cytotoxic drugs, thus allowing more immature oocytes to produce gametes for subsequent fertilization.

SECONDARY MALIGNANCIES

Because many anticancer drugs are known carcinogens, there is concern that the chemotherapy used to induce long-term remission or cure of one cancer may induce second malignancies. Until recently, there had been no reports of increased susceptibility to the development of other malignancies after successful chemotherapy for gestational trophoblastic neoplasia, probably because of the relatively short exposure of these patients to intermittent schedules of methotrexate and dactinomycin and the infrequent use of alkylating agents. However, there have been reports of increased risk of secondary cancers—including acute myelogenous leukemia, colon cancer, melanoma, and breast cancer—developing in patients who received combination chemotherapy regimens containing etoposide for the management of gestational trophoblastic neoplasia.

References

1. Lurain JR. Pharmacotherapy of gestational trophoblastic disease. Expert Opin Pharmacother 2003;11:2005–17.

2. Seckl MJ, Fisher RA, Salerno G, Rees H, Paradinas FJ, Foskett M, et al. Choriocarcinoma and partial hydatidiform moles. Lancet 2000;356:36–9.

3. Smith HO. Gestational trophoblastic disease epidemiology and trends. Clin Obstet Gynecol 2003;46:541–56.

4. Cole LA, Butler S. Detection of hCG in trophoblastic disease: the USA hCG Reference Service experience. J Reprod Med 2002;47:433–44.

5. Bruchim I, Kidron D, Amiel A, Altaras M, Fejgin MD. Complete hydatidiform mole and a coexistent viable fetus: report of two cases and review of the literature. Gynecol Oncol 2000;77:197–202.

6. Wolfberg AJ, Feltmate C, Goldstein DP, Berkowitz RS, Lieberman E. Low risk of relapse after achieving undetectable hCG levels in women with complete molar pregnancy. Obstet Gynecol 2004;104:551–4.

7. van Trommel NE, Massuger LF, Verheijen RH, Sweep FC, Thomas CM. The curative effect of a second curettage in persistent trophoblastic disease: a retrospective cohort survey. Gynecol Oncol 2005;99:6–13.

8. Ngan HY, Bender H, Benedet JL, Jones H, Montruccoli GC, Pecorelli S Gestational trophoblastic neoplasia, FIGO 2000 staging and classification. FIGO Committee on Gynecologic Oncology. Int J Gynecol Obstet 2003;83 (suppl):175–7.

9. Lurain JR. Advances in management of high-risk gestational trophoblastic tumors. J Reprod Med 2002;47:451–9.

10. Newlands ES, Mulholland PJ, Holden L, Seckl MJ, Rustin GJ. Etoposide and cisplatin/etoposide, methotrexate and actinomycin D (EMA) chemotherapy for patients with high-risk gestational trophoblastic tumors refractory to EMA/cyclophosphamide and vincristine chemotherapy and patients presenting with metastatic placental site trophoblastic tumors. J Clin Oncol 2000;18:854–9.

11. Sarwar N, Newlands ES, Seckl MJ. Gestational trophoblastic neoplasia: the management of relapsing patients and other recent advances. Curr Oncol Rep 2004;6:476–82.

12. Osborne R, Covens A, Merchandaui DE, Gerulath A. Successful salvage of relapsed high-risk gestational trophoblastic neoplasia patients using a novel paclitaxel-containing doublet [published erratum appears in J Reprod Med 2005;50:376]. J Reprod Med 2004;49:655–61.

13. Lurain JR, Nejad B. Secondary chemotherapy for high-risk gestational trophoblastic neoplasia. Gynecol Oncol 2005;97:618–23.

14. Lurain JR, Singh DK, Schink JC. Role of surgery in the management of high-risk gestational trophoblastic neoplasia. J Reprod Med 2006;51:773–6.

15. Baergen RN, Rutgers JL, Young RH, Osann K, Scully RE. Placental site trophoblastic tumor: a study of 55 cases and review of the literature emphasizing factors of prognostic significance. Gynecol Oncol 2006;100:511–20.

16. Papadopoulos AJ, Foskett M, Seckl MJ, McNeish I, Paradinas FJ, Rees H, et al. Twenty-five years' clinical experience with placental site trophoblastic tumors. J Reprod Med 2002;47:460–4.

17. Diagnosis and treatment of gestational trophoblastic disease. ACOG Practice Bulletin No. 53. American College of Obstetricians and Gynecologists. Obstet Gynecol 2004;103:1365–77.

18. Matsui H, Iitsuka Y, Suzuka K, Yamazawa K, Tanaka N, Mitsuhashi A, et al. Early pregnancy outcomes after chemotherapy for gestational trophoblastic tumor. J Reprod Med 2004;49:531–4.

Nongynecologic Pelvic Cancers

T. Michael Numnum, MD, and Ronald D. Alvarez, MD

The obstetrician–gynecologist plays an essential role in the counseling, screening, and early detection of cancer in women. Although emphasis is usually placed on detection of gynecologic and breast cancer, the obstetrician–gynecologist should be aware of the manifestations and management of cancers of the pelvis that occur in nonreproductive pelvic organs and of those cancers that occasionally metastasize to the pelvis (see "Cancer Prevention and Screening in Women").

COLORECTAL CANCER

Most patients with colorectal cancer present with gastrointestinal bleeding, abdominal pain, or a change in usual bowel habits. However, 60% of patients with colorectal cancer have no obvious signs of gastrointestinal bleeding. Presenting symptoms usually are associated with the location of the primary site of disease. Left-sided colonic lesions usually produce symptoms of alternating bowel consistency and tenesmus, whereas more proximal lesions usually are accompanied by anemia, weight loss, and fatigue (1). Because many symptoms of colorectal carcinoma are nonspecific, as many as 20% of patients present with advanced-stage disease. Physical examination may be relatively nonspecific, except when there is a large mass in the pelvis signifying advanced disease. The presence of heme-positive stools on rectal examination is a finding that should be considered cancer until proved otherwise.

Evaluation

Colonoscopy is the single best diagnostic tool used to evaluate signs and symptoms of colorectal cancer because it can localize the anatomic location of tumors and provide a tissue diagnosis. Colonoscopy also allows for the removal of any preneoplastic lesions such as polyps and for the evaluation of potential nonmalignant processes. The measurement of carcinoembryonic antigen levels also may be useful in determining the diagnosis. Once a diagnosis of colorectal cancer is established, the extent of disease spread should be determined with radiographic imaging, such as computed tomography (CT). The tumor–node–metastasis (TNM) classification usually is used for staging colorectal cancer.

Treatment

Treatment of patients with colorectal cancer generally depends on the stage of disease and the functional status of the patient. Invasive carcinomas usually are managed surgically with an en bloc colectomy, including mesenteric vessels and lymphatics (2).

Patients with locally advanced colorectal cancer require a multidisciplinary approach using surgical resection with preoperative or postoperative radiation therapy. Newer treatment regimens use a combination of systemic chemotherapy and radiation therapy for locally advanced colorectal cancer. Metastatic colorectal cancer usually is managed with cytotoxic chemotherapy in combination with novel targeted agents such as bevacizumab and cetuximab, although cure rates are generally poor (3–5). Five-year survival rates are dependent on the stage of disease at the time of diagnosis (6).

BLADDER CANCER

Cancer of the bladder is the ninth most common cancer in women, with approximately 17,000 cases per year occurring in the United States and an overall mortality of 25% (7). Approximately 80% of bladder cancers are in people older than 60 years. Bladder cancer is two times more common in whites than African Americans. However, African Americans tend to present with advanced-stage disease more frequently than whites.

Most cases of primary bladder cancer diagnosed in the United States are of the histologically transitional cell type. Adenocarcinomas, squamous cell carcinomas, and bladder sarcomas are far less common in the United States. Because of endemic *Schistosoma haematobium* infections outside the United States, most cases of bladder cancer outside the United States are of squamous cell histology. Primary adenocarcinoma of the bladder is extremely rare and usually associated with a history of bladder exstrophy (8).

RESOURCES

Nongynecologic Pelvic Cancers

American Society of Colon and Rectal Surgeons
http://www.fascrs.org

American Urological Association
http://www.auanet.org

Colon Cancer Alliance
http://www.ccalliance.org/index.html

National Colorectal Cancer Roundtable
http://www.nccrt.org

Risk Factors

Environmental factors are thought to be responsible for most cases of bladder cancer, because the mucosal surfaces of the bladder are constantly exposed to potential toxins excreted in the urine. Most bladder carcinogens are derivatives of aromatic amines. The association between bladder cancer and aromatic amines was first noted in the 19th century in the German aniline dye industry and was later confirmed in British workers in the rubber and textile industries. In total, exposure to chemicals used in the aluminum, dye, rubber, and textile industries may account for up to 20% of all bladder cancers (9).

Tobacco use is now the single most prevalent risk factor for the development of bladder cancer, contributing to more than one half of the cases in the United States. Most studies demonstrate a twofold to threefold increased risk for smokers compared with nonsmokers (10). A history of pelvic irradiation also is associated with an increased risk of bladder cancer (11). Other possible risk factors for the development of bladder cancer may include the prolonged exposure to car exhaust experienced by bus and truck drivers and the prolonged exposure to hair dye experienced by hair stylists (12, 13). The use of the cytotoxic agent cyclophosphamide also carries an increased risk of bladder cancer due to drug-induced hemorrhagic cystitis (14).

History and Physical Examination

A diagnosis of bladder cancer often is delayed because presenting symptoms and signs mimic many benign disorders of the bladder, such as a urinary tract infection or nephrolithiasis. Failure to respond to therapy, such as antibiotics, should prompt evaluation for other causes. Hematuria is the most common presenting symptom, and it is typically described as painless, gross hematuria present throughout micturition. Fifteen percent of patients with asymptomatic hematuria ultimately will be diagnosed with bladder cancer (15). Therefore, any patient with unexplained hematuria requires a full urologic evaluation. Pain is not a common presenting symptom and usually is the result of metastatic disease. Patients with bladder cancer also may report urinary frequency or dysuria. Many patients with these symptoms may have an infectious process. Therefore, prescribing a course of antibiotic therapy is appropriate before considering a full diagnostic workup for bladder cancer, provided that signs and symptoms resolve with therapy.

In general, the physical examination is unremarkable for patients with bladder cancer. However, a full pelvic examination is indicated not only to exclude a gynecologic process but also to evaluate the patient for physical signs of metastatic disease. The rectum also must be examined to rule out gastrointestinal bleeding. The TNM system is used for staging of bladder cancer.

Evaluation

The presence of unexplained hematuria in any patient older than 40 years should be considered urinary tract cancer until proved otherwise. The diagnosis requires a full evaluation, which should consist of urinary cytologic testing, cystourethroscopy, and evaluation of the upper urinary tract with CT, renal ultrasonography, or intravenous pyelography. A urinalysis should include gross and microscopic examination. The sensitivity of urine cytologic testing for the detection of bladder cancer is at least 65% and is largely dependent on the histologic grade of the tumor (16). Accurate interpretation of urine cytologic test findings also requires a skilled cytopathologist.

Cystoscopy is the standard technique for the diagnosis of bladder cancer. It allows detailed visualization of the entire bladder. Cystoscopy also allows for diagnostic biopsies and excision of an obvious bladder tumor. If a diagnosis is confirmed, additional radiographic imaging, such as CT or chest radiography, usually is indicated to rule out metastatic disease.

Treatment

The standard initial treatment for patients with noninvasive bladder cancer is cystoscopic resection of the tumor. Complete cystectomy usually is indicated for patients with multifocal, superficial disease. The use of adjuvant intravesical therapy is dependent upon the number and size of the lesions and the tumor's histologic characteristics. The most commonly used agent for intravesical therapy is Calmette-Guérin bacillus (17).

In general, patients with muscle-invasive tumors require radical cystectomy with bilateral pelvic lymphadenectomy. In women, an anterior pelvic exenteration usually is used to obtain adequate margins. This surgical approach also requires urinary diversion, usually in the form of an ileal conduit. Because of the morbidity of this type of operation, some clinicians are advocating a bladder-conserving approach in the form of partial cystectomy. Patients opting for bladder-conserving surgery usually require adjuvant radiation therapy or chemotherapy postoperatively to produce favorable survival outcomes (18). Consideration also can be given to the use of preoperative neoadjuvant chemotherapy followed by radical resection. Patients with positive lymph nodes or positive margins usually are treated with radiation therapy postoperatively. Patients with advanced and recurrent bladder cancer require systemic therapy, usually platinum-based chemotherapy in combination with other agents (19).

URETHRAL CARCINOMA

Primary urethral cancer makes up less than 1% of all cancer in women (7). Most cases occur between the ages of 50 years and 70 years (20). Histologically, urethral cancer includes squamous cell carcinomas, transitional cell carcinomas, and adenocarcinomas.

Risk Factors

Urethral cancer often is seen in conjunction with transitional cell carcinomas of the proximal urinary tract. In one series, human papillomavirus was identified in 61% of patients with urethral cancer (21). Urethral diverticula also have been implicated as a causative factor because they contribute to chronic infection and urinary stasis.

History and Physical Examination

Most women with urethral cancer present with nonspecific urinary symptoms, such as frequency, dysuria, and hematuria. A patient with an advanced case of urethral cancer may present with a large mass or a urethrovaginal fistula. Physical examination may reveal the presence of an obvious tumor; however, urethral cancer can be mistaken for urethral polyps, diverticula, or prolapse. Cancer of the distal urethra usually is detected at an earlier stage than cancer of the proximal urethra because it is visible and tends to bleed upon inspection. Because the distal urethra primarily drains lymph to the inguinal nodal chain, careful assessment of the inguinal lymph nodes should be performed on physical examination.

Evaluation

Cystoscopy and urethroscopy should be the first step in the evaluation of a urethral mass. Cystoscopy also can aid in identifying either a primary bladder tumor or local extension of a urethral primary tumor into the bladder.

Once a diagnosis has been determined, additional testing should include metastatic assessment. Radiographic imaging will assess the status of the pelvic lymph nodes, which receive lymph drainage from the proximal urethra.

Treatment

The management of urethral cancer depends on the size and anatomic location of the lesion. Small, superficial cancers can be managed with either endoscopic electroresection or laser vaporization. More proximal and larger tumors require a multidisciplinary approach encompassing chemotherapy, radiation therapy, and surgery. Referral to a tertiary medical center usually is necessary to provide the patient access to expertise and clinical trials.

PRESACRAL TUMORS

Presacral tumors are a rare group of tumors originating from tissue that makes up the *presacral space*, also known as the *retrorectal space*, and they often are confused with other pelvic masses. Anatomically, the presacral space is a potential space that lies anterior to the sacrum and posterior to the rectum. Laterally, the space is bounded by the ureters and iliac vessels. The inferior margin of the space is the levator ani muscles, and the superior boundary is the peritoneal reflection. Developmental cysts are the most common types of tumors found in the presacral space. Approximately 50% of presacral tumors ultimately will be malignant (Box 18) (22).

Risk Factors

Because of the rarity and heterogeneity of presacral tumors, risk factors for their development have not been identified. Fifty percent of presacral tumors are congenital.

History and Physical Examination

Because of the hidden anatomy of the presacral space, tumors in this area are difficult to diagnose, and presenting signs and symptoms are relatively nonspecific. As many as 25% of patients with presacral tumors are asymptomatic at the time of diagnosis. The most common symptom associated with a presacral tumor is pain. Other potential symptoms include pelvic pressure, voiding dysfunction, and changes in bowel habits.

On examination, presacral tumors tend to be located in the midline of the pelvis. Most are nontender and mobile.

BOX 18

Histology of Presacral Tumors

Congenital

  Benign

    Developmental tail gut cyst

  Malignant

    Chordoma

Acquired

  Benign

    Leiomyoma

    Schwannoma

    Fibroma

    Angiomyxoma

  Malignant

    Desmoid tumor

    Angiosarcoma

    Chondrosarcoma

    Osteosarcoma

    Fibrosarcoma

    Malignant schwannoma

    Lymphoma

    Squamous cell carcinoma

Malignant tumors tend to be fixed, and invasion into bony structures occasionally can be detected on examination (23).

Evaluation

The evaluation of a presacral mass should include an assessment of the sigmoid colon, ideally with flexible sigmoidoscopy, to detect primary colonic disease and determine if the mass is compressing the colon. Computed tomography or magnetic resonance imaging also can be used to check for metastatic disease and delineate the anatomy of the mass. Because magnetic resonance imaging may show better tissue outlines and evidence of local invasion, it may be a more useful tool for operative planning.

Treatment

Exploratory laparotomy with surgical removal of the mass is the mainstay of treatment for patients with presacral tumors. This treatment will allow for a definitive diagnosis and alleviate symptoms caused by the tumor. Depending on the location of the tumor, a transperineal approach may be feasible. If the tumor proves to be malignant, postoperative radiation therapy may provide some local control (22, 23).

PELVIC LYMPHOMA

Approximately 34,490 women are expected to receive the diagnosis of lymphoma in 2008, and an estimated 10,020 women are expected to die of lymphoma. Non-Hodgkin lymphoma is the fifth most common cause of cancer in U.S. women and the sixth most common cause of cancer death in women (24). Hodgkin lymphoma and non-Hodgkin lymphoma can involve the female genital tract, although this involvement accounts for only 1% of extranodal lymphoma (25). It also is possible, however, for a lymphoma to present as a solitary pelvic mass. Therefore, the obstetrician–gynecologist should be aware of the possibility of encountering this situation and know what to do when it occurs.

History and Physical Examination

Painless lymphadenopathy is the most common presentation of Hodgkin lymphoma and non-Hodgkin lymphoma. Other nonspecific symptoms associated with the disease include fevers, chills, night sweats, anorexia, and weight loss. Physical examination usually is nonspecific but may reveal lymphadenopathy, such as in the supraclavicular and mandibular chain. A patient with ovarian lymphoma may present with pelvic pain and pressure, such as that which occurs with a typical symptomatic pelvic mass. Occasionally, pelvic lymphoma is diagnosed by way of frozen section at the time of laparotomy for a pelvic mass.

If this finding occurs, it is not necessary to perform a staging laparotomy or an extensive debulking procedure. Reproductive organs may be preserved in women who desire future fertility, and in the presence of obvious subcutaneous supraclavicular lymphadenopathy, an open biopsy or fine-needle aspiration may be all that is necessary. A generous excisional biopsy usually is sufficient to confirm the diagnosis and perform appropriate diagnostic tests (25, 26).

Evaluation and Treatment

Once a diagnosis of lymphoma in the female genital tract has been determined, referral to a specialist in hematology and oncology is necessary. Complete staging of non-Hodgkin lymphoma includes a body computed tomographic scan or a positron emission tomography scan followed by a bone marrow biopsy. Positron emission tomography scanning also is useful for surveillance and determining response to treatment (27). Adjuvant chemotherapy usually is prescribed for patients with lymphoma and is based on the stage, grade, and histologic characteristics of the tumor. Long-term survival can be achieved with combination chemotherapy, with or without radiation therapy. Rituximab, a monoclonal antibody directed against the CD20 antigen, has shown promise when used in combination with systemic chemotherapy (28).

NONGYNECOLOGIC CANCER METASTATIC TO THE PELVIS

Nongynecologic cancer metastatic to the pelvis is relatively uncommon. When it does occur, it usually represents metastatic disease to the ovary. Between 5% and 10% of women thought to have a primary ovarian malignancy ultimately will receive the diagnosis of a nongenital tract malignancy (29, 30). Metastatic colon cancer is the most commonly occurring pathologic condition seen in most series, followed by appendiceal, breast, pancreas, and upper gastrointestinal tract cancer (Table 27) (29, 31, 32). Cases of metastatic melanoma, carcinoid tumors, and lymphoma also have been reported. Sometimes, the primary site of malignancy never is identified despite extensive pathologic analysis, including immunohistochemical staining. Tumor markers, such as CA 125, CA 19-9, and carcinoembryonic antigen are rarely useful in this setting. Nongenital ovarian masses tend to have a presentation much like that of primary ovarian cancer, with symptoms such as abdominal pain, early satiety, weight loss, nausea, and vomiting (30, 33, 34).

A detailed history and physical examination should be obtained from any patient presenting with a pelvic mass. Any history of gastrointestinal bleeding should be evaluated before surgical intervention. This evaluation may include upper and lower endoscopy. Chest radiography also may help in the evaluation of metastatic disease.

TABLE 27. Nongenital Primary Cancer Presenting as Ovarian Masses

Study	Colon (%)	Appendix (%)	Breast (%)	Gastric (%)	Lymphoma (%)	Intestinal (%)	Pancreas (%)	Unknown (%)	Other (%)
Moore, et al	32	20	9	7	0	7	5	17	3
Ayhan, et al	21	11	23	21	11	3	1	10	1
Ulbright, et al	34	0	20	9	17	0	6	0	14
Mazur, et al	35	2	41	5	0	2	3	9	3

Data from Ayhan A, Tuncer ZS, Bukulmez O. Malignant tumors metastatic to the ovaries. J Surg Oncol 1995;60:268–76; Mazur MT, Hsueh S, Gersell DJ. Metastases to the female genital tract. Analysis of 325 cases. Cancer 1984;53:1978–84; Moore RG, Chung M, Granai CO, Gajewski W, Steinhoff MM. Incidence of metastasis to the ovaries from nongenital tract primary tumors. Gynecol Oncol 2004;93:87–91; and Ulbright TM, Roth LM, Stehman FB. Secondary ovarian neoplasia: a clinicopathologic study of 35 cases. Cancer 1984;53:1164–74.

A breast examination, including careful assessment of the axillary lymph nodes and recent mammographic findings, is essential to exclude metastatic breast cancer. Because it is unusual for ovarian cancer to metastasize to the liver, any signs or symptoms of liver disease should alert the clinician to the possibility of a nongenital primary malignancy.

The discovery of a nongenital primary malignancy of the ovary at the time of surgery should prompt consultation from a general surgeon. At that time, an assessment can be made about whether to attempt an aggressive debulking procedure. Although it is retrospective, there is some evidence that cytoreductive surgery may have a beneficial effect on survival. Clearly, the type of primary tumor will have a dramatic impact on overall survival. Patients with lymphoma tend to have the best survival, because these tumors are chemosensitive. In contrast, patients with metastatic pancreatic and gastric cancer typically have dismal outcomes (30, 35). Adjuvant therapy, most likely systemic chemotherapy, usually is indicated and is dependent on tumor histologic characteristics and stage of primary disease. Novel targeted agents, such as tyrosine kinase inhibitors and monoclonal antibodies, also may play a role in these metastatic processes (4).

The prognosis for patients with nongenital cancers metastatic to the pelvis is generally poor and depends on the stage of the primary tumor. Other factors associated with survival include size and number of tumors, grade of tumor, and liver and bone involvement (36).

References

1. Speights VO, Johnson MW, Stoltenberg PH, Rappaport ES, Helbert B, Riggs M. Colorectal cancer: current trends in initial clinical manifestations. South Med J 1991;84:575–8.

2. Nelson H, Petrelli N, Carlin A, Couture J, Fleshman J, Guillem J, et al. Guidelines 2000 for colon and rectal cancer surgery. National Cancer Institute Expert Panel. J Natl Cancer Inst 2001;93:583–96.

3. Cunningham D, Humblet Y, Siena S, Khayat D, Bleiberg H, Santoro A, et al. Cetuximab monotherapy and cetuximab plus irinotecan in irinotecan-refractory metastatic colorectal cancer. N Engl J Med 2004;351:337–45.

4. Meyerhardt JA, Mayer RJ. Systemic therapy for colorectal cancer. N Engl J Med 2005;352:476–87.

5. Hurwitz H, Fehrenbacher L, Novotny W, Cartwright T, Hainsworth J, Heim W, et al. Bevacizumab plus irinotecan, fluorouracil, and leucovorin for metastatic colorectal cancer. N Engl J Med 2004;350:2335–42.

6. O'Connell JB, Maggard MA, Ko CY. Colon cancer survival rates with the new American Joint Committee on Cancer sixth edition staging. J Natl Cancer Inst 2004;96:1420–5.

7. Jemal A, Siegel R, Ward E, Murray T, Xu J, Thun MJ. Cancer statistics, 2007. CA Cancer J Clin 2007;57:43–66.

8. Reuter VE. The pathology of bladder cancer. Urology 2006;67(suppl 1):11–7; discussion 17–8.

9. Jung I, Messing E. Molecular mechanisms and pathways in bladder cancer development and progression. Cancer Control 2000;7:325–34.

10. Zeegers MP, Goldbohm RA, van den Brandt PA. A prospective study on active and environmental tobacco smoking and bladder cancer risk (The Netherlands). Cancer Causes Control 2002;13:83–90.

11. Boice JD Jr, Engholm G, Kleinerman RA, Blettner M, Stovall M, Lisco H, et al. Radiation dose and second cancer risk in patients treated for cancer of the cervix. Radiat Res 1988;116:3–55.

12. Czene K, Tiikkaja S, Hemminki K. Cancer risks in hairdressers: assessment of carcinogenicity of hair dyes and gels. Int J Cancer 2003;105:108–12.

13. Boffetta P, Silverman DT. A meta-analysis of bladder cancer and diesel exhaust exposure. Epidemiology 2001;12:125–30.

14. Travis LB, Curtis RE, Boice JD Jr, Fraumeni JF Jr. Bladder cancer after chemotherapy for non-Hodgkin's lymphoma. N Engl J Med 1989;321:544–5.

15. Khadra MH, Pickard RS, Charlton M, Powell PH, Neal DE. A prospective analysis of 1,930 patients with hematuria to evaluate current diagnostic practice. J Urol 2000;163:524–7.

16. Sarnacki CT, McCormack LJ, Kiser WS, Hazard JB, McLaughlin TC, Belovich DM. Urinary cytology and the clinical diagnosis of urinary tract malignancy: a clinicopathologic study of 1,400 patients. J Urol 1971;106:761–4.

17. Martinez-Pineiro JA, Martinez-Pineiro L, Solsona E, Rodriguez RH, Gomez JM, Martin MG, et al. Has a 3-fold decreased dose of bacillus Calmette-Guerin the same efficacy against recurrences and progression of T1G3 and Tis bladder tumors than the standard dose? Results of a prospective randomized trial. Club Urologico Espanol de Tratamiento Oncologico (CUETO). J Urol 2005;174:1242–7.

18. Cookson MS. The surgical management of muscle invasive bladder cancer: a contemporary review. Semin Radiat Oncol 2005;15:10–8.

19. Sternberg CN. Chemotherapy for local treatment of bladder cancer. Semin Radiat Oncol 2005;15:60–5.

20. Amin MB, Young RH. Primary carcinomas of the urethra. Semin Diagn Pathol 1997;14:147–60.

21. Wiener JS, Walther PJ. A high association of oncogenic human papillomaviruses with carcinomas of the female urethra: polymerase chain reaction-based analysis of multiple histological types. J Urol 1994;151:49–53.

22. Lev-Chelouche D, Gutman M, Goldman G, Even-Sapir E, Meller I, Issakov J, et al. Presacral tumors: a practical classification and treatment of a unique and heterogeneous group of diseases. Surgery 2003;133:473–8.

23. Lee RA, Symmonds RE. Presacral tumors in the female: clinical presentation, surgical management, and results. Obstet Gynecol 1988;71:216–21.

24. American Cancer Society. Cancer facts and figures 2008. Atlanta (GA): ACS; 2008. Available at: http://www.cancer.org/downloads/STT/2008CAFFfinalsecured.pdf. Retrieved February 20, 2008.

25. Trenhaile TR, Killackey MA. Primary pelvic non-Hodgkin's lymphoma [letter]. Obstet Gynecol 2001;97:717–20.

26. Allen GW, Forouzannia A, Bailey HH, Howard SP. Non-Hodgkin's lymphoma presenting as a pelvic mass with elevated CA-125. Gynecol Oncol 2004;94:811–3.

27. Lavely WC, Delbeke D, Greer JP, Morgan DS, Byrne DW, Price RR, et al. FDG PET in the follow-up management of patients with newly diagnosed Hodgkin and non-Hodgkin lymphoma after first-line chemotherapy. Int J Radiat Oncol Biol Phys 2003;57:307–15.

28. Coiffier B. New treatment strategies in lymphomas: aggressive lymphomas. Ann Hematol 2004;83(suppl):S73–4.

29. Ulbright TM, Roth LM, Stehman FB. Secondary ovarian neoplasia: a clinicopathologic study of 35 cases. Cancer 1984;53:1164–74.

30. Moore RG, Chung M, Granai CO, Gajewski W, Steinhoff MM. Incidence of metastasis to the ovaries from nongenital tract primary tumors. Gynecol Oncol 2004;93:87–91.

31. Ayhan A, Tuncer ZS, Bukulmez O. Malignant tumors metastatic to the ovaries. J Surg Oncol 1995;60:268–76.

32. Mazur MT, Hsueh S, Gersell DJ. Metastases to the female genital tract: analysis of 325 cases. Cancer 1984;53:1978–84.

33. Petru E, Pickel H, Heydarfadai M, Lahousen M, Haas J, Schaider H, et al. Nongenital cancers metastatic to the ovary. Gynecol Oncol 1992;44:83–6.

34. Dietrich CS 3rd, Desimone CP, Modesitt SC, Depriest PD, Ueland FR, Pavlik EJ, et al. Primary appendiceal cancer: gynecologic manifestations and treatment options. Gynecol Oncol 2007;104:602–6.

35. Ayhan A, Guvenal T, Salman MC, Ozyuncu O, Sakinci M, Basaran M. The role of cytoreductive surgery in nongenital cancers metastatic to the ovaries. Gynecol Oncol 2005;98:235–41.

36. Culine S, Kramar A, Saghatchian M, Bugat R, Lesimple T, Lortholary A, et al. Development and validation of a prognostic model to predict the length of survival in patients with carcinomas of an unknown primary site. French Study Group on Carcinomas of Unknown Primary. J Clin Oncol 200;20:4679–83.

Cancer in Pregnancy

Kim A. Boggess, MD, and John F. Boggess, MD

Cancer is among the leading causes of nonaccidental death in the United States in women aged 20–39 years, accounting for approximately 17% of all deaths in 2004 (1). Of these deaths, 1,225 were caused by breast cancer; 462, cervical cancer; 386, leukemia; 346, colorectal cancer; and 312, cancer of the brain and other areas of the nervous system (1). Given these statistics, it is not surprising that cancer can complicate pregnancy.

Cancer complicates approximately 1 in 1,000 pregnancies, and it is estimated that approximately 3,500 new cases of cancer are diagnosed annually in pregnant women or women who recently have experienced childbirth in the United States (2). Cancers of the breast, thyroid, and cervix, malignant melanoma, and Hodgkin lymphoma account for two thirds of all cases reported (2).

The diagnostic and therapeutic management of the pregnant patient with cancer is especially complex because it necessitates consideration of the mother and the fetus. Some diagnostic modalities and therapies pose risk to the developing fetus; however, in most cases, the cancer and the pregnancy can be managed concurrently with a good outcome for the baby and without compromising maternal prognosis.

It has been speculated that the immunologic and physiologic alterations of pregnancy may modify the biologic behavior of cancer. To date, there is no objective evidence that the risk of developing cancer increases with pregnancy, that cancer in remission will recur more frequently during pregnancy, or that the prognosis for patients with cancer diagnosed during pregnancy will be worse than that for cancer patients who are not pregnant.

Many signs and symptoms associated with malignancy may be confused with signs and symptoms of normal pregnancy, so a cancer diagnosis may be delayed or perhaps completely overlooked. A treatment plan formulated by an interdisciplinary team of health care providers is critical to the successful management of a pregnant woman with cancer. As the trend for delaying pregnancy into the later reproductive years continues, physicians can expect to see more cases of cancer complicating pregnancy.

RESOURCE

Cancer in Pregnancy

Society of Maternal–Fetal Medicine
http://www.smfm.org/index.cfm?zone=publicintro

DISEASE SITES

Cervix

Cervical cancer is the most common reproductive tract cancer associated with pregnancy. The incidence of cervical cancer complicating pregnancy is reported to be 1 per 1,000–2,500 deliveries (3). Additionally, carcinoma in situ is estimated to affect approximately 1 in 750 pregnancies.

Cervical cytologic screening is equivalent in reliability for pregnant and nonpregnant women and should be performed routinely for all women seeking prenatal care. An endocervical brush and spatula can be used safely in pregnancy; referral for colposcopy should be made according to standard guidelines (4). When cervical cytologic abnormalities are detected in the pregnant woman, the primary responsibility of the obstetrician–gynecologist is to exclude the possibility of an invasive cervical cancer (Fig. 23). Therefore, all diagnostic and treatment decisions are balanced with this goal in mind.

Minimally abnormal Pap test results require colposcopy to exclude the presence of malignant-appearing lesions of the cervix. If no lesion is detected, biopsy can be avoided. Other abnormal Pap test results that indicate visible lesions and or possible lesions require colposcopy and biopsy, and any suspicion of invasive disease requires conization. The colposcopic appearance of the cervix is different in pregnancy because of cervical hypertrophy, eversion of the transformation zone, and redundancy of adjacent tissues. If the obstetrician–gynecologist is unable to complete an adequate examination, the patient should be referred to an obstetrician–gynecologist with advanced surgical training, experience, and demonstrated competence, such as a gynecologic oncologist; delay in establishing a diagnosis of cervical cancer during pregnancy may have a profound effect on a woman's treatment choices.

Cervical biopsies in pregnant patients are associated with heavier bleeding than in nonpregnant patients. The bleeding generally can be controlled with silver nitrate or Monsel solution. Endocervical curettage is not recommended in pregnant patients and can be replaced by obtaining a cytologic specimen using an endocervical brush. If preinvasive disease is confirmed and invasive disease excluded, further therapy may be delayed until after delivery (3). Progression after delivery to a higher grade of dysplasia has been shown to occur in approximately 7% of women, and no progression to a microinvasive or invasive lesion has been reported. If results of the examination suggest microinvasion, cervical conization is necessary to rule out invasive cancer. In pregnant patients with nonin-

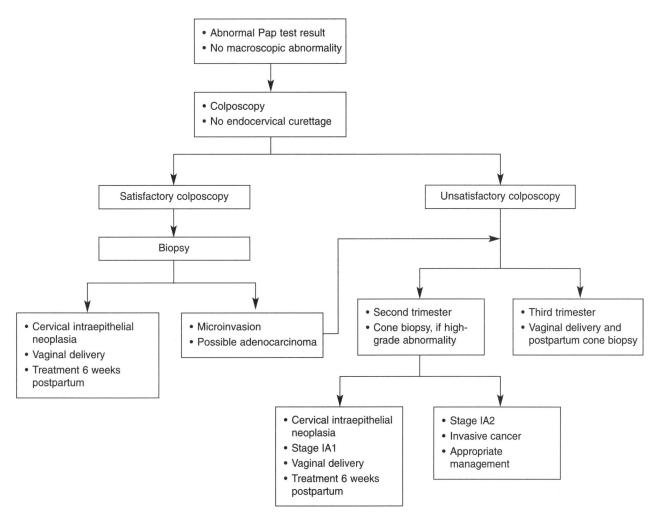

■ **FIG. 23.** Algorithm for the management of an abnormal Pap test result in pregnancy. Hacker NF. Cervical cancer. In: Berek JS, Hacker NF. Practical gynecologic oncology. 4th ed. Philadelphia (PA): Lippincott Williams and Wilkins; 2005. p. 380.

vasive cervical intraepithelial neoplasia (CIN) or carcinoma in situ of the cervix, it is widely accepted that with careful surveillance with repeated cytology and colposcopy testing, pregnancy can be allowed to proceed to term. A modest therapeutic delay in patients with early microinvasive carcinoma of the cervix does not appear to adversely affect maternal prognosis (5).

A cervical cone biopsy in pregnancy is associated with significant bleeding (approximately 500 mL) in nearly 10% of patients and is associated with spontaneous abortion rates as high as 18% in the first trimester. For this reason, conization should typically be delayed until after the first trimester of pregnancy. Pregnancy loss rates after conization in the second trimester have been reported to be approximately 4% (6). Overall, pregnant patients with cervical intraepithelial neoplasia who undergo cervical conization during pregnancy do not appear to be at increased risk of adverse pregnancy outcome (6). Cerclage placement can be performed at the time of cone biopsy in an attempt to decrease morbidity. In addition, the cerclage can reduce bleeding if placed before the cervix is incised.

Some clinicians prefer a wedge resection through the affected portion of the cervix, which is believed to provide the necessary information without the morbidity associated with classic conization (3).

When the diagnosis of invasive cervical carcinoma is established during pregnancy, gestational age, stage of disease, and maternal desire to continue pregnancy are critical considerations in treatment planning (Fig. 24). Traditionally, the recommendation has been that at less than 20 weeks of gestation, the disease should be treated definitively; at 20 weeks or later, treatment should be delayed until fetal maturity is achieved. Many women, however, decline therapy in favor of continuing the pregnancy. If the patient's decision is to delay treatment, discussion between the patient, perinatologist, obstetrician, and gynecologic oncologist should be thorough and well documented to arrive at the safest outcome for the mother and fetus. Modern neonatal intensive care settings report nearly 100% survival for infants born at 28 weeks of gestation, with less than 10% long-term morbidity and 60% survival for infants born at 24 weeks of gestation. These

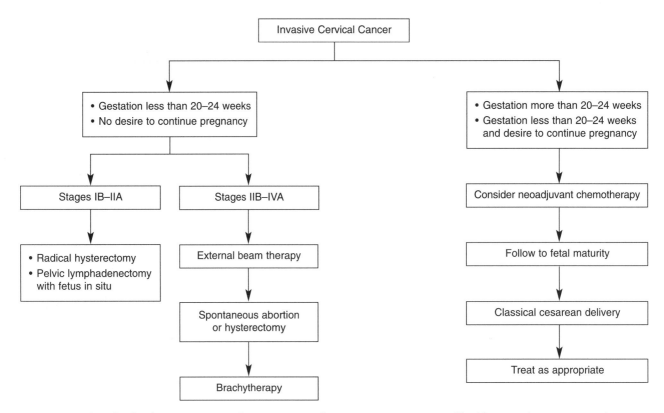

■ **FIG. 24.** Algorithm for the management of invasive cervical cancer in pregnancy. Modified from Hacker NF. Cervical cancer. In: Berek JS, Hacker NF. Practical gynecologic oncology. 4th ed. Philadelphia (PA): Lippincott Williams and Wilkins; 2005. p. 381.

results challenge the traditional standard for early definitive therapy. Before planned delivery, determination of fetal pulmonary maturity may be useful.

Newborn infants of patients with exophytic cervical tumors generally undergo cesarean delivery to decrease the possibility of maternal hemorrhage from a friable tumor. With small cervical tumors, no adverse maternal effects of vaginal delivery (hemorrhage, sepsis, or decreased survival) have been reported (7). There are reports, however, of episiotomy site recurrence after vaginal delivery; thus, follow-up visits should monitor the perineum (8).

When a patient decides in favor of definitive therapy, the options of radical surgery compared with chemoradiotherapy should be presented. The patient and her family should be counseled regarding the option of termination of the pregnancy before initiation of therapy, as well as the possibility of fetal loss. Women can experience significant grief at a pregnancy loss even in the first trimester, so caregivers should be sensitive to signs of depression and bereavement.

Patients with small stage IB lesions (IB1 lesions) or IIA lesions have the option of radical hysterectomy with lymphadenectomy or chemoradiotherapy, whereas patients with bulky and advanced lesions (stages IB2, IIB, III, and IV) are treated with chemoradiotherapy. Radical surgery facilitates ovarian preservation. If the decision has been made to proceed with irradiation in early pregnancy,

spontaneous abortion usually will occur when approximately 40 Gy have been delivered (after approximately 3–5 weeks of therapy).

Because pregnancy does not appear to influence disease progression, a planned delay in therapy for cervical cancer may be justified to improve the neonatal outcome. In one case series, 28 women with stage I cervical cancer who received the diagnosis during (or immediately after) pregnancy underwent successful planned treatment delay for up to 25 weeks of gestation to improve fetal maturity with no apparent adverse effect on mother or fetus (5).

Ovary

The presence of an adnexal mass in a pregnant woman is not uncommon, with an estimated incidence between 0.2% and 2% (9–12). The rate of malignant transformation among persistent masses ranges from 2% to 3% but has been reported to be as high as 13% (9). Most ovarian cysts discovered during pregnancy will resolve spontaneously.

The detection of adnexal masses during pregnancy has become more common with the frequent use of ultrasonography. In one series of 7,996 pregnant women who underwent ultrasound examination for various indications, 4.1% of women had at least one detectable adnexal mass (13). No masses were malignant, and most (82%) of these masses were smaller than 3 cm in diameter. Estimates of malignancy derived from surgical exploration of adnexal masses cluster around 1 in 1,000 pregnancies (9, 14). Ovarian cancer diagnosed during pregnancy is rare, occurring in only 1–2% of ovarian masses.

The management of a persistent adnexal mass during pregnancy is a challenge for the obstetrician–gynecologist because the specter of malignancy provokes significant anxiety in the patient. In addition, the risk of rupture or torsion may be as high as 7% (9).

Most adnexal masses during pregnancy are identified as incidental findings of ultrasonography. Ultrasound criteria can be used to assess risk of malignancy. Unilocular, simple cysts smaller than 5 cm have a low risk of cancer; complex or solid masses, masses with nodules or thick septations, and masses larger than 5 cm have a higher risk of malignant transformation (15). Color-flow Doppler ultrasonography has been suggested as a tool to differentiate between benign and malignant ovarian masses. However, significant overlap exists in blood flow patterns, so Doppler ultrasonography does not offer a significant advantage over ultrasonography alone (16).

Magnetic resonance imaging (MRI) can be used safely to evaluate adnexal masses in a pregnant woman. The primary advantages of MRI are the capacity to develop three-dimensional planar images, delineate tissue planes, and characterize pelvic structures. The use of MRI probably adds to the diagnostic evaluation of an adnexal mass when the diagnosis after ultrasonography is uncertain and a radiologist experienced in interpreting of adnexal masses in pregnancy is available (16). Three-dimensional and four-dimensional ultrasonography allow for enhanced imaging of pelvic structures and masses and evaluation of tumor vascularity, and these modalities may allow for improved distinction between benign and malignant processes as the technology is developed (17).

Decision making regarding the management of a persistent adnexal mass in a pregnant woman involves weighing the risks of expectant management with the risks of immediate surgical intervention (18). The risks of expectant management include delay in diagnosis of malignancy, ovarian torsion, cyst rupture, or obstruction of labor. As noted previously, ultrasound criteria can stratify women based on risk of cancer. In selected cases, close observation is a reasonable alternative to surgical treatment in pregnant women with an adnexal mass. Women with ultrasound findings suggestive of malignancy should not be considered candidates for expectant management (16).

Indications for the surgical management of an ovarian mass in a pregnant woman include 1) strong suspicion for malignancy, large size, or both; 2) symptoms; or 3) increased risk of torsion, rupture, or obstruction of labor (16). Torsion has been reported in 9–12% of masses; rupture, in 9% of masses; and labor obstruction, in 17% of cases (16). Later studies report lower rates of complications, likely reflecting a higher proportion of asymptomat-

ic, incidental ovarian masses detected by routine prenatal ultrasonography. Surgery typically is delayed until the early second trimester, to reduce the risk of miscarriage and fetal exposure to anesthetics during organogenesis.

The surgical management of ovarian tumors in pregnant women is similar to that in nonpregnant women. The surgical approach may involve open laparotomy or laparoscopy. The benefits of laparoscopic surgery include shorter hospital stay, earlier return to normal activity, and reduced postoperative pain (19). However, laparoscopic surgery requires insufflation of the peritoneal cavity with carbon dioxide to distend the abdomen and displace the bowel upward to allow for visualization of pelvic structures. Serious complications, such as hypercarbia and perforation of internal organs—including the uterus—have been reported. The authors of a recent review concluded that the evidence for the magnitude of the benefits and risks of laparoscopic surgery for ovarian tumors during pregnancy is drawn from case series studies that are associated with potential bias, so results and conclusions should be interpreted with caution (19). Several case series demonstrate promising use of laparoscopy for the management of ovarian masses during pregnancy (20, 21).

There are scant data regarding pregnant women treated for ovarian cancer, so controversy exists surrounding management. Surgery with adequate staging remains the standard for ovarian cancer therapy during pregnancy. The prognosis for patients with epithelial ovarian cancer diagnosed during pregnancy is similar to that for non-pregnant women (22). Because the patient group is of reproductive age, germ cell tumors (primarily dysgerminomas) and epithelial tumors of low malignant potential are the most commonly encountered ovarian malignancies in pregnancy (22). Surgical staging and unilateral salpingo-oophorectomy are recommended. Stage IA dysgerminomas, stage IA, grade 1 immature teratomas, and epithelial tumors of low malignant potential do not require adjuvant chemotherapy. No evidence suggests that adjuvant chemotherapy in patients with early-stage disease or patients with optimal cytoreduction of advanced disease improves survival with tumors of low malignant potential. All other germ cell tumors require combination chemotherapy with bleomycin, etoposide, and cisplatin; its use in the second and third trimesters has been associated with successful outcomes for mother and infant.

Epithelial ovarian malignancies grossly confined to the ovary require full surgical staging. For patients with advanced disease, the extent of cytoreduction requires prudent individualization based on gestational age and maternal desires. The postoperative management of ovarian cancer includes chemotherapy. A combination of cyclophosphamide and cisplatin or carboplatin has been administered in the second and third trimesters reportedly without adverse effects on the fetus (18).

Leukemia and Lymphoma

Recent advances in the management of leukemia, Hodgkin disease, and non-Hodgkin lymphoma have substantially improved the prognosis for patients with these malignancies. Most patients are able to achieve complete remission. Hodgkin disease presents at a median age of 30 years. However, leukemia rarely complicates pregnancy, occurring in approximately 1 in 75,000 pregnancies (23). Chronic leukemia and non-Hodgkin lymphoma generally occur in postmenopausal women and are extremely rare in pregnancy, whereas acute leukemias are more likely during the reproductive years. Given the likelihood of remission or cure with aggressive management of these diseases, treatment delays are not advised.

Evaluation of patients with lymphoma begins with history gathering to identify constitutional symptoms (for example, weight loss, night sweats, and fever) and clinical node evaluation by lymph node biopsy and excision to determine the histopathologic subclassification of disease. Fine-needle aspiration is not adequate. Bone marrow biopsy and other laboratory tests usually are necessary. A staging laparotomy to evaluate subdiaphragmatic disease no longer is performed. Nonpregnant patients are evaluated by chest radiography; computed tomographic scanning of the chest, abdomen, and pelvis; and bipedal lymphangiography in some instances. In the pregnant patient, MRI with ultrasonographic evaluation when necessary can provide sufficient information for treatment planning.

As in the nonpregnant patient, in the pregnant patient early-stage (stage I or II) nonbulky disease can be treated by mantle irradiation, followed by treatment to the paraaortic and splenic areas. Alternatively, these patients can be treated with chemotherapeutic regimens, such as doxorubicin, bleomycin, vinblastine, and dacarbazine or nitrogen mustard, vincristine, procarbazine, and prednisone in the second and third trimesters, followed by irradiation to involved fields. Requisite fetal irradiation precautions are essential. Patients wishing to continue their pregnancies may consider deferring subdiaphragmatic irradiation until after delivery. Several case series described successful outcomes for mother and fetus when chemotherapy, or irradiation, or both were appropriately individualized (23, 24).

Non-Hodgkin lymphoma often is disseminated at the time of diagnosis and is generally managed with aggressive chemotherapy, such as cyclophosphamide, doxorubicin, vincristine, and prednisone. Supradiaphragmatic irradiation with abdominal shielding is useful for patients with symptomatic disease. Although experience in managing non-Hodgkin lymphoma in pregnant women is less extensive, favorable outcomes have been reported after aggressive treatment (25).

Combination chemotherapy is the treatment of choice for patients with leukemia (26). When it is clinically necessary to treat a woman in the first trimester of pregnancy, extensive counseling by a multidisciplinary health care team regarding possible adverse outcomes for both mother and fetus is essential. Acute lymphocytic leukemia is managed with prednisone, vincristine, and daunorubicin. Induction therapy for acute myelogenous leukemia includes daunorubicin and cytarabine. Although successful pregnancy outcomes have been reported with the use of multiagent chemotherapy in the first trimester, it frequently is associated with a risk of teratogenesis, prematurity, stillbirth, and miscarriage; thus, the option of therapeutic abortion should be considered. Combination chemotherapy in the second and third trimesters is less frequently associated with adverse fetal outcome; when possible, treatment should be delayed until that time (25, 27).

Patients undergoing treatment for leukemia or lymphoma in pregnancy should be counseled to consider having umbilical cord stem cells collected in the event that maternal stem cell transplantation becomes necessary. Many medical–ethical issues related to this practice are unresolved, however (28).

Skin

The incidence of cutaneous malignant melanoma has been increasing over the past decade. The effect of pregnancy on the course of women with malignant melanoma is still a matter of debate, although two recent studies report that there is no appreciable difference in outcome and survival rate between pregnant and nonpregnant women with melanoma (29, 30). In a large, population-based study of pregnant women over a 10-year period, no difference in the distribution of tumor stage or thickness or lymph node metastases was found (30). A limitation of the study was the inability to capture data on women who did not continue their pregnancy beyond 20 weeks of gestation; this limitation may have biased the results if women who terminated their pregnancies or miscarried had more advanced tumors, a poorer prognosis, or both.

Breast

Breast cancer is the most common malignancy associated with pregnancy, with an incidence of 1 in 10,000 to 1 in 3,000. It is speculated that with the increase in delayed childbearing, breast carcinoma diagnosed during pregnancy may become more frequent (31). As many as 3% of women with breast cancer are pregnant or lactating at the time of receiving the diagnosis. The physiologic changes associated with a pregnant woman's breast, such as engorgement and hypertrophy, may obscure a breast mass so that the diagnosis of breast cancer may be delayed up to several months in pregnant women (32). This delay likely contributes to the more advanced disease at presentation in this group of women. Significantly more pregnant women than their nonpregnant counterparts have lymph node metastases (61% versus 38%, $P<.05$), and pregnant women have a lower percentage of stage I disease than do their nonpregnant counterparts (45% versus 58%, *P*=.015) (33, 34). Despite these differences, stage for stage, no differences in survival are found between these groups.

A thorough breast examination is recommended at the initial prenatal care visit, when pregnancy-associated breast changes are minimal. Diagnostic mammography can be performed with minimal risk to the fetus with the use of abdominal shielding, but information may be limited by pregnancy-associated breast changes.

Ultrasonography is another important tool to provide a rapid and accurate method of differentiating cystic lesions from solid lesions in the breast. Fine-needle aspiration, core biopsy, and even excisional biopsy should be performed when clinically indicated to establish a diagnosis. In the diagnosis of breast cancer in pregnant women, fine-needle aspiration was shown to be highly accurate in a study of more than 300 pregnant and lactating women (35). Although procedures performed on the breast during pregnancy are associated with a higher risk of infection and of milk fistula formation in the lactating breast, a persistent breast mass warrants further investigation without delay.

Once diagnosis has been established, breast cancer treatment should not be delayed because of pregnancy. The multidisciplinary team should outline treatment options, with consideration of guidelines for nonpregnant patients and modification to protect the fetus. Because pregnancy has not been demonstrated to decrease survival, abortion should not be recommended on that basis alone. Some women may choose to terminate their pregnancies after weighing treatment options, potential risk to the fetus, and their long-term prognosis.

Treatment strategies for pregnant women do not differ from treatment strategies for nonpregnant patients. The role of sentinel lymph node biopsy in treatment planning is discussed separately in a later discussion. Modified radical mastectomy with axillary lymphadenectomy if deemed appropriate can be performed safely in pregnancy with minimal risk to the mother or fetus. Breast reconstruction surgery, if desired, should be delayed until after delivery. Breast-conserving surgery (lumpectomy with axillary lymphadenectomy) is equally effective and technically feasible; however, it requires postoperative radiotherapy, which exposes the fetus to the unnecessary risk of ionizing radiation. Delaying postoperative radiation therapy could increase the risk of local cancer recurrence. If the diagnosis of breast cancer is made late in pregnancy, definitive surgical treatment can be carried out immediately and radiation therapy deferred until after delivery (32).

Adjuvant chemotherapy is offered in node-positive disease or tumors with adverse biologic characteristics. When possible, chemotherapy should be delayed until the second or third trimester, when organogenesis is complete. Typically, doxorubicin, cyclophosphamide, and 5-fluorouracil are the agents of choice. Many case reports document the relative safety of chemotherapeutic agents in pregnancy; however, there are no large studies or long-term follow-up series (32). Methotrexate and paclitaxel are other agents often considered for adjuvant therapy; however, the former generally is avoided because of its teratogenic effects and the latter deferred because of a paucity of data on its use in pregnancy. The use of tamoxifen in pregnancy is controversial but has been reported without adverse fetal outcome (36).

SENTINEL LYMPH NODE BIOPSY DURING PREGNANCY

Regional lymph node status continues to be the most important prognostic factor for patients with melanoma and breast cancer. Sentinel lymph node biopsy has become an acceptable alternative to routine staging with regional lymphadenectomy (37). The sentinel lymph node biopsy technique relies on injection of a radioactive colloid, or a vital dye, or both in the proximity of the primary lesion.

The role of sentinel lymph node biopsy in the treatment of pregnant women with breast cancer or malignant melanoma is not clear. The radiation from the procedure might harm the fetus, and the breast lymphatic pathways may be altered in pregnancy. The agents used for the identification of the sentinel lymph node are blue dye and radiocolloid technetium. The blue dye might be methylene blue, isosulfan blue, or patent blue. Blue dyes such as isosulfan blue (a class C drug) have not been tested in pregnant animals or humans and, thus, should not be used in pregnant or breast-feeding patients. Methylene blue has been known to cause fetal methemoglobinemia when injected intravenously or into amniotic fluid and thus theoretically could pose a risk during pregnancy. Radiocolloids include technetium sulfur colloid and technetium-labeled albumin, which are considered safer agents. Biologic pharmacokinetic data show that a very small amount of injected radiocolloid circulates in the blood pool. The amount of radioactivity involved in sentinel lymph node biopsy is very low compared with standard radionuclide procedures, and most injected radiocolloid stays at the injection site or moves to the sentinel lymph nodes, both of which are excised during the procedure. This situation, plus the fact that the rapid physical decay of the radiotracer results in negligible amounts detected at sites distant from injection, suggests minimal risk of fetal exposure (38).

In a study of nine pregnant women, six with melanoma and three with breast cancer, investigators found that sentinel lymph node mapping was feasible in pregnancy, with no adverse reaction noted and no impact on fetal outcome (39). Despite these promising data, caution should be exercised in the use of sentinel lymph node biopsy for pregnant women. Sentinel lymph node biopsy should be used after the period of organogenesis, and because small quantities of the radioactive colloid can be excreted into breast milk, breast-feeding should be avoided for 2–3 days after a sentinel lymph node biopsy.

THERAPEUTIC RADIATION EXPOSURE

The benefits of radiation therapy as part of a treatment regimen for cancer must be weighed against the potential risk of harm to the patient and, in the pregnant patient, the risk to the developing fetus. Radiation therapy plays a major role in the definitive treatment of patients with cervical and breast carcinomas, Hodgkin disease, and non-Hodgkin lymphoma. Physicians caring for a pregnant woman who requires radiation therapy may be inclined to advocate termination of pregnancy for fear of fetal injury. Radiation doses used in cancer treatment usually range between 4,000 cGy and 7,000 cGy, which is approximately 10^4–10^5 times the exposure that occurs with diagnostic radiologic procedures. Also, iodine 131 administered to a woman with hyperthyroidism after 10–12 weeks of gestation, when the fetal thyroid becomes capable of trapping iodine, may accumulate in the fetal thyroid and cause partial or complete thyroid ablation.

Fetal risk is dependent on gestational age at the time of exposure, dose, field size, distance between the edges of the radiation field and the fetus, amount of radiation leakage and scatter, and energy source. For example, a distance of more than 30 cm from the field edges yields a fetal exposure of only 4–20 cGy. Thus, many areas distant from the pelvis, such as the head, neck, and breast, can be treated with radiation therapy without significant fetal exposure. Lead shielding over the uterus also can reduce fetal exposure. Although the absolute safe level of ionizing radiation to the fetus is unknown, most authors agree that a fetal dose of less than 0.1 Gy should not result in gross malformations or growth restriction (40, 41). Higher doses and exposure during the first trimester have been associated with a significant risk of spontaneous abortion in the first trimester, fetal malformation, and growth restriction (40, 42).

Animal studies document a wide variety of organ system malformations from radiation exposure during organogenesis. Studies of human exposure report that central nervous system (CNS) effects (microcephaly and retardation), growth abnormalities, and ocular abnormalities predominate. In humans, the CNS and growth effects persist well into the fetal stage (20–25 weeks of gestation), beyond which CNS effects become less severe and abnormalities such as anemia, pigment changes, and erythema become more frequent (40).

Patients whose disease will be managed by irradiation require careful treatment planning and extensive counseling regarding possible pregnancy outcomes, including consultation with a qualified medical physicist to deter-

mine dose levels to the fetus. Appropriate techniques for fetal dose reduction are well documented and should be included in treatment planning (42).

Most types of cancer remote from the pelvis can be managed safely with radiation therapy. Pregnancy is not an absolute contraindication to radiation therapy in patients with breast cancer, supradiaphragmatic Hodgkin disease, brain tumors, and head and neck cancers. The decision to give radiation therapy to a pregnant woman with cancer should be made by the patient and her physician after careful consideration of the risks (42).

DIAGNOSTIC RADIATION EXPOSURE

Most diagnostic radiologic studies expose the mother and fetus to very low doses of radiation. Fetal exposure varies based on the procedure, the site to be imaged, and the possibility for abdominal shielding. Nonionizing forms of imaging, such as ultrasonography or MRI, often are preferred for use in pregnancy over ionizing forms of imaging, such as chest radiography, computed tomography, positron emission tomography, gallium scanning, and bone scanning. Although ultrasonography and MRI provide images using nonionic radiation, the theoretical possibility of fetal damage through thermal effects (ultrasonography or MRI) or cavitation (ultrasonography) has been raised. To date there have been no confirmed adverse fetal outcomes associated with standard diagnostic ultrasonography or MRI (40). The use of gadolinium-based contrast medium for MRI, however, is not recommended (U.S. Food and Drug Administration pregnancy category C drug) because it can cross the placenta, be filtered by the fetal kidney, and be reingested through the amniotic fluid. Generally, cancer in a pregnant woman can be evaluated adequately and safely by nonionizing studies and carefully selected ionizing imaging studies when necessary for appropriate therapeutic decision making and staging.

EFFECTS OF CHEMOTHERAPY ON THE FETUS AND BREASTFEEDING

Fetal effects of chemotherapeutic agents depend on the mechanism of action and tissue distribution of the drug, as well as the gestational age at which the fetus is exposed. Most cytotoxic agents exert their effect by interfering with some stage of DNA or RNA synthesis, by interrupting essential metabolic pathways, or by destroying macromolecules. Many agents are thought to be teratogenic if administered during the period of organogenesis. Exposure during the second and third trimesters is not associated with fetal malformations but may be linked to fetal growth restriction, microcephaly, and neonatal pancytopenia. Long-term effects discovered during childhood also are being recognized.

Drugs in pregnancy are assigned a risk factor (A, B, C, D, or X) according to definitions provided by the U.S. Food and Drug Administration. Chemotherapeutic agents generally fall into category C or D. Category C drugs are drugs for which human risk cannot be ruled out; animal studies are either lacking or reveal adverse (embryocidal, teratogenic, or other) effects on the fetus, but controlled studies in women are not available. However, potential benefit may justify the potential risk. Category D drugs demonstrate positive evidence of risk; investigational or postmarketing data show fetal risk. However, potential benefits to the mother may outweigh fetal risk. Category X drugs are contraindicated in pregnancy; studies in animals or humans or investigational or postmarketing reports have shown fetal risk that clearly outweighs any possible benefit to the mother. No chemotherapeutic agents have been proved safe for breast-feeding. Some are excreted in breast milk, a fact that leads to legitimate concerns regarding potential neonatal adverse effects.

Breast, hematologic, and cervical cancers are the most frequent malignancies that require chemotherapy during pregnancy. A retrospective cohort study of 29 pregnant women with cancer found a higher rate of prematurity and fetal death among pregnancies of women treated with chemotherapy compared with those of women not similarly exposed (43). In general, management of cancer in pregnancy should be individualized and may differ depending on the trimester of diagnosis. Chemotherapy should be used, but with caution, when indicated in pregnancy.

METASTASES OF MATERNAL TUMORS TO THE PLACENTA AND FETUS

Vertical transmission of maternal cancer is exceptionally rare. The rarity of this complication is likely caused by the placental barrier and the fetal immune system. From 1866 to 1989, only 53 cases of metastasis to the products of conception were reported. Of these 53 cases, 45 were metastatic to the placenta (27% melanoma) and 12 to the fetus (7 melanoma, 4 leukemia or lymphoma, and 1 hepatocellular carcinoma) (26). The likely mechanism of dissemination is hematogenous. The placenta of a woman recently treated or undergoing treatment for cancer should be sent for thorough histopathologic evaluation. Additionally, careful examination and close follow-up of the infant are necessary, particularly if the maternal tumor was melanoma because 70% of reported metastatic tumors reaching the fetus were melanomas.

MATERNAL–FETAL CONFLICT

The presence of the fetus in a patient with cancer may complicate therapeutic decisions when the interests of the fetus are in conflict with the interests of the mother. Pregnant women with cancer may have particularly diffi-

cult choices. Potentially lifesaving therapy for themselves may be potentially detrimental to the health and well-being of the fetus. Delaying therapy may favor fetal well-being, but to the disadvantage of the mother.

Two ethical principles should guide the health care team as they navigate treatment options with the pregnant woman with cancer: autonomy and beneficence. The pregnant woman will have her own perspective on her own best interests and well-being and therefore should be given the freedom to choose therapies based on personal beliefs and values. The fetus does not yet possess the capacity to express personal beliefs; therefore, the physician has no autonomy-based obligation to the fetus. The principle of beneficence (which includes nonmaleficence) requires the physician to assess objectively the various therapeutic options and implement those with the greatest balance of benefit and risk. However, the physician also must consider the well-being of the fetus and try to offer the fetus the greatest balance of benefit and risk.

Another important principle that should be considered is the principle of justice, which requires that individuals (in this case, both pregnant and nonpregnant patients) be treated fairly. A woman's right to refuse invasive medical treatment that would benefit another should not be diminished because she is pregnant. Justice requires that pregnant and nonpregnant individuals be afforded similar rights (44).

PRECONCEPTION AND REPRODUCTIVE IMPLICATIONS OF CANCER TREATMENT

The most common types of cancer in women younger than 40 years are breast cancer, melanoma, cervical cancer, non-Hodgkin lymphoma, and leukemia. Aggressive chemotherapy and radiotherapy or radical surgery in young women with cancer has improved life expectancy, but these treatments often cause infertility or premature ovarian failure because of massive destruction of the ovarian reserve. All chemotherapeutic agents act by disrupting vital cell processes and arresting normal cell growth. The risk of chemotherapy-induced amenorrhea depends on a woman's age, the specific agent used, and the total dose given. Older women have a higher incidence of complete ovarian failure and permanent infertility compared with younger women. Alkylating agents severely affect fertility by causing ovarian fibrosis and follicular and oocyte depletion. Cisplatin causes ovarian failure, and vinca alkaloids are known aneuploidy inducers (45).

Many women undergoing cancer treatment desire to retain fertility. Fertility preservation options for female cancer patients include ovarian transposition, ovarian suppression, oocyte preservation, and embryo cryopreservation. To date, the most effective approach is embryo cryopreservation. This approach requires in vitro fertilization, which may not be appropriate for all women.

For women undergoing gonadotoxic radiotherapy, transposition of the ovaries out of the field of irradiation can maintain ovarian function. The most common indications are Hodgkin disease, cervical cancer, and pelvic sarcomas. Reported rates of ovarian function and ability to conceive after radiation therapy and ovarian transposition range from 16% to 90% (45).

Ovarian suppression with either a gonadotropin-releasing hormone agonist or the oral contraceptive pill to keep the ovaries quiescent during chemotherapy in an effort to preserve fertility has been studied. Contradictory results on the effects of gonadotropin-releasing hormone agonists have been reported. Oral contraceptive pills have been shown to have a possible protective effect in younger women. Further studies are needed to define the optimal ovarian suppression regimen.

Oocyte preservation is being studied as a means of maintaining fertility, although oocytes are very sensitive to cooling (45). Exposure to cytoprotective agents causes hardening of the zona pellucida. Women with cancer may have only one opportunity for oocyte harvesting before undergoing potentially sterilizing treatment, because a cycle of controlled ovarian stimulation requires several weeks, and there is a delay of a few months before treatment cycles. The success of the method also depends on the total number of eggs harvested (fewer than 10 oocytes harvested reduces the chance of pregnancy). The overall live birthrate per cryopreserved oocyte is approximately 2%, which is much lower than that achieved with in vitro fertilization and fresh oocytes (45).

Cancer as a complication of pregnancy is relatively uncommon. When cancer is suspected or diagnosed in a pregnant woman, however, the health care team and the patient and her family face many complex medical, ethical, and emotional decisions. The goal of care for a patient with a cancer in pregnancy is to balance optimal maternal outcome and fetal well-being. Contemporary management considers the age of the fetus; the type, extent, and growth potential of the tumor; and a treatment plan formulated by an interdisciplinary team of health care providers.

References

1. Jemal A, Seigel R, Ward E, Murray T, Xu J, Thun MJ. Cancer statistics, 2007. CA Cancer J Clin 2007;57:43–66.

2. Smith LH, Danielsen B, Allen ME, Cress R. Cancer associated with obstetric delivery: results of linkage with the California Cancer Registry. Am J Obstet Gynecol 2003; 189:1128–35.

3. Creasman WT. Cancer and pregnancy. Ann NY Acad Sci 2001;943:281–6.

4. Wright TC Jr, Massad LS, Dunton CJ, Spitzer M, Wilkinson EJ, Solomon D. 2006 consensus guidelines for the management of women with abnormal cervical screening tests. J Low Genit Tract Dis 2007;11:201–22.

5. Takushi M, Moromizato H, Sakumoto K, Kanazawa K. Management of invasive carcinoma of the uterine cervix associated with pregnancy: outcome of intentional delay in treatment. Gynecol Oncol 2002;87:185–9.

6. Demeter A, Sziller I, Csapo Z, Szantho A, Papp Z. Outcome of pregnancies after cold-knife conization of the uterine cervix during pregnancy. Eur J Gynaecol Oncol 2002; 23:207–10.

7. van der Vange N, Weverling GJ, Ketting BW, Ankum WM, Samlal R, Lammes FB. The prognosis of cervical cancer associated with pregnancy: a matched cohort study. Obstet Gynecol 1995;85:1022–6.

8. Cliby WA, Dodson MK, Podratz KC. Cervical cancer complicated by pregnancy: episiotomy site recurrences following vaginal delivery. Obstet Gynecol 1994;84:179–82.

9. Sherard GB 3rd, Hodson CA, Williams HJ, Semer DA, Hadi HA, Tait DL. Adnexal masses and pregnancy: a 12-year experience. Am J Obstet Gynecol 2003;189:358–62; discussion 362–3.

10. Zanetta G, Mariani E, Lissoni A, Ceruti P, Trio D, Strobelt N, et al. A prospective study of the role of ultrasound in the management of adnexal masses in pregnancy. BJOG 2003;110:578–83.

11. Schmeler KM, Mayo-Smith WW, Peipert JF, Weitzen S, Manuel MD, Gordinier ME. Adnexal masses in pregnancy: surgery compared with observation. Obstet Gynecol 2005;105:1098–103.

12. Leiserowitz GS, Xing G, Cress R, Brahmbhatt B, Dalrymple JL, Smith LH. Adnexal masses in pregnancy: how often are they malignant? Gynecol Oncol 2006;101:315–21.

13. Hill LM, Connors-Beatty DJ, Nowak A, Tush B. The role of ultrasonography in the detection and management of adnexal masses during the second and third trimesters of pregnancy. Am J Obstet Gynecol 1998;179:703–7.

14. Whitecar P, Turner S, Higby K. Adnexal masses in pregnancy: a review of 130 cases undergoing surgical management. Am J Obstet Gynecol 1999;181:19–24.

15. Lerner JP, Timor-Tritsch IE, Federman A, Abramovich G. Transvaginal ultrasonographic characterization of ovarian masses with an improved, weighted scoring system. Am J Obstet Gynecol 1994;170:81–5.

16. Leiserowitz GS. Managing ovarian masses during pregnancy. Obstet Gynecol Surv 2006;61:463–70.

17. Fleischer AC. Gynecologic sonography: past, present, and future. J Ultrasound Med 2003;22:759–63.

18. Giuntoli RL 2nd, Vang RS, Bristow RE. Evaluation and management of adnexal masses during pregnancy. Clin Obstet Gynecol 2006;49:492–505.

19. Bunyavejchevin S, Phupong V. Laparoscopic surgery for presumed benign ovarian tumor during pregnancy. Cochrane Database Syst Rev 2006:CD005459.

20. Mathevet P, Nessah K, Dargent D, Mellier G. Laparoscopic management of adnexal masses in pregnancy: a case series. Eur J Obstet Gynecol Reprod Biol 2003;108:217–22.

21. Tinelli FG, Tinelli R, La Grotta F, Tinelli A, Cicinelli E, Schonauer MM. Pregnancy outcome and recurrence after conservative laparoscopic surgery for borderline ovarian tumors. Acta Obstet Gynecol Scand 2007;86:81–7.

22. Machado F, Vegas C, Leon J, Perez A, Sanchez R, Parilla JJ, et al. Ovarian cancer during pregnancy: analysis of 15 cases. Gynecol Oncol 2007;105:446–50.

23. Chelghoum Y, Vey N, Raffoux E, Pigneux A, Witz B, et al. Acute leukemia during pregnancy: a report on 37 patients and a review of the literature. Cancer 2005;104:110–7.

24. Dilek I, Topcu N, Demir C, Bay A, Uzun K, Gul A, et al. Hematological malignancy and pregnancy: a single-institution experience of 21 cases. Clin Lab Haematol 2006; 28:170–6.

25. Hurley TJ, McKinnell JV, Irani MS. Hematologic malignancies in pregnancy. Obstet Gynecol Clin North Am 2005; 32:595–614.

26. Pavlidis NA. Coexistence of pregnancy and malignancy [published erratum appears in Oncologist 2002;7:585]. Oncologist 2002;7:279–87.

27. Safdar A, Johnson N, Gonzalez F, Busowski JD. Adult T-cell leukemia-lymphoma during pregnancy. N Engl J Med 2002;346:2014–5.

28. Wagner JE. Umbilical cord blood stem cell transplantation. Am J Pediatr Hematol Oncol 1993;15:169–74.

29. Silipo V, De Simone P, Mariani G, Buccini P, Ferrari A, Catricala C. Malignant melanoma and pregnancy. Melanoma Res 2006;16:497–500.

30. O'Meara AT, Cress R, Xing G, Danielsen B, Smith LH. Malignant melanoma in pregnancy: a population-based evaluation. Cancer 2005;103:1217–26.

31. Gwyn K, Theriault R. Breast cancer during pregnancy. Oncology (Williston Park) 2001;15:39–46; discussion 46, 49–51.

32. Keleher AJ, Theriault RL, Gwyn KM, Hunt KK, Stellin CB, Singletary SE, et al. Multidisciplinary management of breast cancer concurrent with pregnancy. J Am Coll Surg 2002;194:54–64.

33. Zemlickis D, Lishner M, Degendorfer P, Panzarella T, Burke B, Sutcliffe SB, et al. Maternal and fetal outcome after breast cancer in pregnancy. Am J Obstet Gynecol 1992;166:781–7.

34. Petrek J, Seltzer V. Breast cancer in pregnant and postpartum women. J Obstet Gynaecol Can 2003;25:944–50.

35. Gupta RK, McHutchison AG, Dowle CS, Simpson JS. Fine-needle aspiration cytodiagnosis of breast masses in pregnant and lactating women and its impact on management. Diagn Cytopathol 1993;9:156–9.

36. Gonzalez-Angulo AM, Walters RS, Carpenter RJ Jr, Ross MI, Perkins GH, et al. Paclitaxel chemotherapy in a pregnant patient with bilateral breast cancer. Clin Breast Cancer 2004;5:317–9.

37. Scoggins CR, Chagpar AB, Martin RC, McMasters KM. Should sentinel lymph-node biopsy be used routinely for staging melanoma and breast cancers? Nat Clin Pract Oncol 2005;2:448–55.

38. Gentilini O, Cremonesi M, Trifiro G, Ferrari M, Baio SM, Caracciolo M, et al. Safety of sentinel node biopsy in pregnant patients with breast cancer. Ann Oncol 2004;15: 1348–51.

39. Mondi MM, Cuenca RE, Ollila DW, Stewart JH 4th, Levine EA. Sentinel lymph node biopsy during pregnancy: initial clinical experience. Ann Surg Oncol 2007;14:218–21.

40. Kal HB, Struikmans H. Radiotherapy during pregnancy: fact and fiction. Lancet Oncol 2005;6:328–33.

41. Hall EJ. Radiation, the two-edged sword: cancer risks at high and low doses. Cancer J 2000;6:343–50.

42. Greskovich JF Jr, Macklis RM. Radiation therapy in pregnancy: risk calculation and risk minimization. Semin Oncol 2000;27:633–45.

43. Peres RM, Sanseverino MT, Guimaraes JL, Coser V, Giuliani L, Moreira RK, et al. Assessment of fetal risk associated with exposure to cancer chemotherapy during pregnancy: a multicenter study. Braz J Med Biol Res 2001;34: 1551–9.

44. American College of Obstetricians and Gynecologists. Ethics in obstetrics and gynecology. 2nd ed. Washington, DC: ACOG; 2004. p. 35.

45. Maltaris T, Seufert R, Fischl F, Schaffrath M, Pollow K, Koelbl H, et al. The effect of cancer treatment on female fertility and strategies for preserving fertility. Eur J Obstet Gynecol Reprod Biol 2007;130:148–55.

Long-Term Quality of Life and Symptom Management for Women With Cancer

Richard T. Penson, MD, and Don S. Dizon, MD

Quality of life is a subjective, multidimensional concept that includes the performance of everyday activities taken in the context of one's culture, value systems, goals, standards, and concerns. Although understanding quality of life can illuminate the meaning of the experience of illness, it is clear that it also can inform an appreciation of the complexity of medical issues. In clinical research, quality-of-life data can accurately describe a population, predict outcomes, guide clinical decisions, screen for disease or dysfunction, and inform the allocation of resources.

Quality-of-life considerations are especially important in gynecologic cancer patients. For example, 20–40% of patients are reported to have significant distress, yet only 10% of them are identified and referred for psychosocial evaluation (1). Toxic effects and symptoms that can diminish quality of life are varied and include pain, emotional distress, neuropathy, alopecia, nausea and vomiting, anemia, and fatigue (2). All these issues can be present across the treatment spectrum, from sequelae of adjuvant therapy to symptoms at the end of life.

Psychosocial support, therefore, remains a prominent feature of contemporary cancer care. The input of appro-priate members of an interdisciplinary team is critical in addressing the many issues that patients and their families face. In addition to medical specialties involved in gynecologic cancer care, other critical components may include social workers, patient advocates, nursing coordinators, and spiritual counselors. Only by forging relationships across disciplines and specialties can cancer care providers support services aimed at addressing the emotional, nutritional, and genetic concerns of women; assist in financial counseling; and provide general information on cancer diagnosis and treatment options.

SURVIVORSHIP

For patients diagnosed with malignancies, survivorship starts at the time of diagnosis and continues to the end of life. In the past 30 years the number of people living in the United States who have had cancer has tripled, to more than 10 million, yet the physical and psychosocial burden of ongoing issues remains underappreciated (3). As well as understanding the challenges to their physical, psychologic, and sexual functioning, survivors need to appreciate the experience of their illness, their need for empathetic affirmation, and the importance of mourning losses (4).

Most gynecologic cancer survivors (90%) report supportive care needs, and approximately one third experience posttraumatic stress disorder (5). The initial keys to improving this situation include better awareness and coordination between primary and specialty care. At present, the need for survivor-specific care is not recognized by payers, but clearly this care goes beyond surveillance for recurrence and must encompass a more comprehensive approach to all aspects of rehabilitation (6). Typical oncologic follow-up often fails to attend to primary care issues of health and screening, including such vital issues as smoking cessation and lifestyle modifications such as diet and exercise (7).

Approximately 20% of cancer survivors report limitations in their ability to work, and 1 in 10 is unable to maintain employment (8). Whereas there is legal protection against discrimination, survivors often need their physicians to act as their advocates.

Finally, the National Cancer Institute estimates that as many as 24% of adults with cancer are parents of children younger than 18 years. Patients and survivors are very concerned about the effect their illness has on their children and are grateful for guidance at challenging times (9).

SPECIFIC PROBLEMS

Psychologic Distress

Psychologic distress ranges from common normal feelings of vulnerability, sadness, and fears to problems that can become disabling, such as depression, anxiety, panic, social isolation, and spiritual crisis. In one series of more than 200 women undergoing treatment or postsurveillance for ovarian cancer, 33% reported an overall heightened level of psychologic distress, with 21% meeting the clinical criteria for a diagnosis of depression and 29% scoring above the 75th percentile for anxiety (10). For women with advanced disease who required continued therapy, lower scores on emotional well-being have been demonstrated; a comparison of these scores with the scores of women with early-stage disease demonstrated that women with advanced disease also had more problems related to depression and anxiety (11).

Management begins even before the initial referral to a gynecologic oncologist. In a study of 151 women referred to a gynecologic oncologist for evaluation, severe depressive symptoms were seen in 42% of this group and moderate to severe anxiety in 29%, with no differences noted among women who ultimately received a diagnosis of cancer and those with benign conditions (12). Because of the degree of distress noted among women referred to a gynecologic oncologist, it is important that the general obstetrician–gynecologist participate in the screening for distress at the time a referral is considered. The prompt identification of patients experiencing psychologic or emotional problems enables these women to access psychologic and therapeutic interventions early on and, therefore, helps reduce suffering.

For women with a diagnosis of cancer, factors that may place them at risk for distress include young age, having children at home, being single or nonpartnered, previous psychiatric history, and previous history of alcohol or drug use (13). The use of brief questionnaires also can assist the practitioner in screening. For example, the Hospitalized Anxiety and Depression Scale questionnaire is a brief, 14-item scale that contains 7-item subscales that assess for depression and anxiety. Other assessment tools include the Center for Epidemiologic Studies Depression Scale and the Beck Anxiety Inventory (14, 15).

Managing depression in cancer patients often requires the use of antidepressants, and many agents are available (Table 28). Of these, the selective serotonin reuptake inhibitors generally are tolerated well and can improve the symptoms of depression within 2–4 weeks. The tricyclic antidepressants have a slightly longer onset of action but can be useful for patients with appreciable sleep disturbances. Newer agents target multiple neurotransmitters in the brain. For example, bupropion is thought to block the reuptake of norepinephrine while inhibiting the absorption of dopamine.

TABLE 28. Commonly Used Antidepressants

Drug Class	Agents (Daily Dose)	Common Adverse Effects
SSRI	Citalopram, 20–60 mg	Nausea
	Escitaprolam, 10–20 mg	Heartburn
	Paroxetine, 20–50 mg	Drowsiness
	Fluvoxamine, 50–300 mg	Sexual dysfunction
	Sertraline, 25–200 mg	Sleep disturbances
TCA	Amitriptyline, 150–300 mg	Xerostomia
	Nortriptyline, 50–150 mg	Constipation
	Amoxapine, 150–400 mg	Tachycardia
	Clomipramine, 100–150 mg	Orthostasis
	Desipramine, 100–300 mg	Sexual dysfunction
	Doxepin, 75–300 mg	Hypotension
	Imipramine, 150–300 mg	
	Maprotiline, 75–150 mg	
	Protriptyline, 15–60 mg	
	Trimipramine, 50–150 mg	
MAOI	Phenelzine, 45–90 mg	Orthostasis
	Tranylcypromine, 30–60 mg	Dizziness
	Isocarboxazid, 20–60 mg	Sleep disturbances
	Selegiline patch, 6–12 mg/24 h	Weight gain
		Headaches
		Sexual dysfunction
Atypical	Duloxetine, 40–60 mg	Nausea
	Mirtazapine, 15–45 mg	Nervousness
	Bupropion, 300–450 mg	Xerostomia
	Trazodone, 75–400 mg	Fatigue
	Venlafaxine, 75–375 mg	Sleep disturbances
	Nefazodone, 300–600 mg	Weight gain
		Diplopia

Abbreviations: MAOI indicates monoamine oxidase inhibitor; SSRI, selective serotonin reuptake inhibitor; TCA, tricyclic antidepressant.

Patients with cancer can manifest anxiety in many ways. In severe cases, reactions can disrupt relationships, normal routines, and even subsequent treatment. Severe anxiety disorders fall into one of six categories (Table 29). Gynecologists and oncologists should promptly recognize when symptoms have surpassed the normal level of anxiety and moved on to severe states such that activities of

TABLE 29. Manifestations of Anxiety in Patients With Cancer

Anxiety Disorder	Characterization	Treatment
Panic	Intense anxiety that lasts for several minutes to hours; autonomic symptoms—including palpitations, sweating, and nausea—are common	Anxiolytics
Adjustment	Anxiety associated with an identified stressor (for example, diagnosis, results of laboratory tests, relapse)	Counseling, education, anxiolytics
Phobia	Fears or avoidance related to a specific situation (for example, magnetic resonance imaging examinations) or circumstance (for example, needles related to placement of intravenous lines)	Counseling, anxiolytics
Obsessive–compulsive	Persistent thoughts accompanied by repetitive behaviors	Counseling, antidepressants
Posttraumatic stress	Extreme anxiety that recurs, stemming from the diagnosis and treatment of cancer	Counseling
Generalized anxiety	Excessive worrying, inability to relax, startling easily	Antidepressants, anxiolytics, psychotherapy

daily living and normal interactions are affected. Medical treatment may require supportive counseling and medication, such as antidepressants and anxiolytics (Table 30). For patients experiencing extreme symptoms not relieved by the care afforded in the scope of routine practice, referral to mental health specialists should be prompt.

Pain

Pain is one of the more prevalent and feared symptoms among gynecologic cancer survivors (16). It can be manifested in a variety of ways stemming from differing pathophysiologic mechanisms and inciting etiologies (Table 31). The World Health Organization has sponsored a three-step analgesic ladder that builds from the use of nonsteroidal agents and acetaminophen for mild pain to weak and then strong opioids if control is not achieved (17). However, this classification oversimplifies the management of cancer-related pain. The National Comprehensive Cancer Network has established guidelines built on several principles that are useful in guiding the management of cancer pain (Box 19).

Pain therapy involves appropriate pharmacologic treatment (Table 32). Patients experiencing severe, uncontrolled pain may require treatment in a controlled setting with short-acting intravenous pain medications. This strategy allows a rapid onset to peak control and titration to desired effects. A common means to accomplish these goals is the use of patient-controlled analgesia. It provides

TABLE 30. Commonly Used Anxiolytics

Agent	Indications
Clonazepam	Social phobia, generalized anxiety disorder
Lorazepam	Panic disorder
Alprazolam	Panic disorder, generalized anxiety disorder
Buspirone	Generalized anxiety disorder
Propanolol	Social phobia

continuous pain relief and allows the patient to determine when additional, breakthrough medication is required. Once control has been established, the total analgesic dose required over 24 hours can be converted to an outpatient regimen and schedule using oral or subcutaneous medications (Table 33). If a patient requires an outpatient regimen, titration with oral short-acting opioids can be performed, but careful short-term follow-up is necessary.

For patients experiencing little or no relief of cancer-related pain, other measures may become necessary; these measures include patient-controlled analgesia delivered via the spine, nerve blocks, and nonmedical treatments. The need to discuss these modalities may necessitate referral to a specialized pain clinic.

Adverse effects of pain management also must be anticipated and managed aggressively (Table 34). Opioids

TABLE 31. Pain Classifications in Patients With Malignancy

Pathophysiology	Characteristics	Etiology
Somatic	Well-localized and described as aching, constant, rarely sharp or stabbing	Fracture, burn, incision, and trauma
Visceral	Poorly localized, can be sharp and stabbing but mostly aching or dull, referred to skin in intraabdominal processes	Bowel obstruction or perforation, metastatic tumor, and constipation
Neuropathic	Numbness or tingling and burning, can be sharp paroxysmal	Chemotherapy, cord compression, and metabolic causes

BOX 19

The National Comprehensive Cancer Network Components of Pain Management

1. Quantify the pain using a numeric value that corresponds to severity.
2. Use routine and regular formal pain assessments.
3. Evaluate response to treatment by routine reassessment of pain intensity.
4. Provide educational materials on pain management.
5. Offer psychosocial support and resources for patients.

frequently disrupt bowel function, causing constipation and nausea. Immediate use of laxatives and stool softeners is recommended as prophylaxis, along with instructions to increase fluids and to exercise whenever possible. Severe constipation warrants further evaluation to ensure that the patient has not developed a bowel obstruction or ileus. Respiratory depression is another adverse effect of therapy, so careful attention to the level of sedation and respiratory rate is crucial. For severe respiratory depression resulting in altered consciousness and reduced respiratory rate, the use of naloxone may be indicated. However, the decision to use naloxone must be made with extreme caution because it can precipitate extreme pain, cardiac irritability, hypertension, pulmonary edema, and cardiac arrest.

Intimacy and Sexual Function

Sexual dysfunction encompasses a broad spectrum of issues, including the psychologic, physical, interrelational, and physiologic realms. All these realms can be affected by the diagnosis of, and treatment for, cancer. Therefore, it is not surprising that sexual dysfunction affects nearly all women treated for a gynecologic cancer (18). Despite these reports, sexual dysfunction remains an often-neglected part of the survivor experience. A recent survey of the New England Association of Gynecologic Oncologists reported that less than one half of health care providers gathered a sexual history, with 80% of them citing time constraints as the most common barrier against further discussion (19). Some cancer centers have addressed these issues in the context of a broader survivorship initiative through the establishment of sexual medicine programs. These specialized centers often employ a multidisciplinary approach to sexuality and sexual health, encompassing gynecology, internal medicine, sex therapy, social work, pharmacology, and psychology.

The cornerstone of treatment, whether it be in a private office or in a specialized program, involves open-ended communication, patient education, and support. For the practicing obstetrician–gynecologist, it may be useful to bring up these issues using the PLISSIT framework for sexual assessment and rehabilitation, which involves permission, limited information, specific suggestions, and intensive therapy (20).

Therapeutic options are vast and allow a tailored approach to each woman. The options may include hormonal agents, dilator therapy, lubricants, education on alternative expressions of intimacy, sexual positioning, and counseling (Table 35) (18). The comfort level and expertise of the individual practitioner will determine which problems can be treated in the office and which problems require referral.

Fertility Considerations

Approximately 4% of all cancer cases occur in patients younger than 35 years, and breast cancer and cervical cancer are among the most commonly diagnosed types of cancer in this population (21). For women who receive the diagnosis of cancer in their reproductive years, cancer therapy represents a threat to future fertility. In 2006, the American Society of Clinical Oncology put forward recommendations on fertility preservation in patients with cancer (21). Among the recommendations were the counseling of patients about the risks to future fertility associated with all aspects of cancer treatment, from surgery to

TABLE 32. Pain Medications in Common Clinical Use

Patient Status	Regimen	Agent	Dose	Order
Inpatient	Nonnarcotic	Ketorolac	15–30 mg IV	Every 6 hours as needed
	Patient-controlled analgesia	Morphine (IV)	50 mg in 50 mL 5% glucose (1 mg/mL)	Bolus: 0.5–1.0 mg Infusion: 0–0.2 mg/h Lockout: 5–15 minutes
		Hydromorphone (IV)		Bolus: 0.2 mg Infusion: 0.1–1.0 mg/h Lockout: 5–20 minutes
		Morphine SC patient-controlled analgesia	50 mg in 20 mL 0.9% sodium chloride (25 mg/mL)	Bolus: 5–10 mg Infusion: 0–2.5 mg/h Lockout: 5–15 minutes
Outpatient	Nonnarcotic	Acetaminophen	Tablets: 325–650 mg	
		Ibuprofen	Tablets: 400–800 mg	
	Short-acting narcotics	Morphine	Tablets: 15 mg, 30 mg Capsules: 15 mg, 30 mg Immediate release oral solution: 10–20 mg/5 mL Immediate release oral concentrate: 20 mg/mL Suppositories: 5 mg, 10 mg, 20 mg, 30 mg	
		Oxycodone	Tablets: 5 mg, 15 mg, 30 mg Caplets: 5 mg Oral solution: 5 mg/5 mL Oral concentrate: 20 mg/mL	
		Hydromorphone	Tablets: 1 mg, 2 mg, 3 mg, 4 mg, 8 mg Oral solution: 5 mg/5 mL Oral concentrate: 20 mg/mL	
		Codeine	Tablets: 15 mg, 30 mg, 60 mg Solution: 5 mg/5 mL	
		Fentanyl	Lozenges: 200 micrograms, 400 micrograms, 600 micrograms, 800 micrograms, 1,200 micrograms, 1,600 micrograms	
	Long-acting narcotics	Morphine	Tablets: 15 mg, 30 mg, 60 mg, 100 mg, 200 mg (every 12 hours)	
		Oxycodone	Tablets: 10 mg, 20 mg, 40 mg, 60 mg (every 12 hours)	
		Fentanyl	Patches: 12.5 micrograms per hour, 25 micrograms per hour, 50 micrograms per hour, 75 micrograms per hour, 100 micrograms per hour (every 3 days)	

Abbreviations: IV indicates intravenous; SC, spinal cord.

chemotherapy to radiotherapy. Patients interested in fertility preservation should be counseled regarding embryo cryopreservation and be advised about emerging technologies, including oocyte or ovarian tissue cryopreservation. In an effort not to delay the treatment, these issues should be addressed promptly, and if necessary, referral to a reproductive specialist should be expedited.

For women with early gynecologic cancers, techniques that offer fertility preservation may be reasonable. Such options include trachelectomy for early-stage cervical cancer, medical therapy for well-differentiated endometrial cancer, and fertility-sparing surgery for ovarian cancers—in particular, for tumors of low malignant potential.

For women who desire pregnancy after treatment of cancer and are unable to reproduce, education should be offered on alternative choices of parenthood, including egg donation, gestational surrogacy, and adoption.

Fatigue

Fatigue is probably the most prevalent symptom in patients with cancer and is best characterized as a persistent lack of energy. It may be present at the time of diagnosis, during therapy, or after treatment. It is nearly ubiquitous among cancer survivors and can disrupt routine activities, causing a negative impact on quality of life. It is a common cause of long-term disability in this population and, thus, has social and economic implications. As such, health care providers often are thrust into the role of patient advocate as patients work to attain benefits from employers, insurers, and local and state agencies.

The differential diagnosis of cancer-related fatigue is difficult, because it can be secondary to other medical problems, treatment related, or due to the cancer itself. The workup must start with screening for fatigue and a medical evaluation to rule out other causes. Standard history taking in the cancer patient should include screening questions for fatigue, because some patients may not bring up the issue for fear it could cause changes in the treatment plans or that they could be labeled as "difficult."

Cancer-related anemia is a well-known cause of fatigue; other causes include hypothyroidism, poor nutrition, being sedentary, or other medical problems such as congestive heart failure, diabetes, or chronic obstructive pulmonary disease. Cancer treatments, including surgery, contemporary chemotherapy, chemoradiation protocols, and radiation therapy, are associated with the onset or worsening of fatigue, which can last beyond the end of treatment. Once fatigue has been identified, coexisting conditions should be addressed because resolving them can improve fatigue considerably. Studies have shown that exercise intervention both increases energy and improves mood (22). In addition, multiple studies show that improvement of anemia in cancer patients can improve fatigue and quality of life (23). Although transfusions can provide immediate relief, prophylaxis against severe anemia (hemoglobin levels less than 10 g/dL) is possible with the use of erythropoietin-stimulating agents. However, caution is recommended because of recent findings that correction of cancer-related anemia not attributable to chemotherapy was associated with an increased mortality rate in one randomized trial of darbepoetin compared with placebo (24).

Much of this evaluation can be initiated by the primary gynecologist or gynecologic oncologist. However, in a busy clinical practice, the evaluation may require consul-

TABLE 33. Equianalgesic Dosage Conversion

Drug	Equianalgesic Dose (mg)	
	Oral*	Intravenous
Morphine	30	10
Hydromorphone	7.5	1.5
Fentanyl transdermal patch (25 micrograms per 3 days)	50 per day (morphine)	0.7 per hour
Codeine (30 mg)	200	130
Oxycodone	20	–

*Common dose ratio between oral and subcutaneous dose is 2:1.

TABLE 34. Management of Adverse Effects of Pain Medication

Symptom	Management
Constipation	Docusate sodium, 100 mg two–three times per day
	Bisacodyl, 10 mg every day as needed
	Polyethylene glycol, 17g/d
	Magnesium citrate, 150–300 mL/d
Respiratory depression	Decrease or stop opiate, depending on level of sedation and respiratory rate; support ventilation; administer naloxone, 0.04 mg/mL, by way of intravenous pyelography, if severe
Nausea	Promethazine, 12.5 mg intravenously every 4 hours as needed
Pruritus	Diphenhydramine, 25 mg orally or intravenously every 6 hours as needed

TABLE 35. Sexual Problems in Cancer Survivors

Symptom (frequency)	Etiology	Therapy
Lack of desire	Changes in the hormonal milieu, non-malignant chronic diseases (for example, diabetes or hypertension), psychologic distress, lifestyle factors	Endocrine therapy (estrogen or testosterone), couples counseling, sex therapy, and relaxation techniques
Arousal disorder	Anxiety and vaginal dryness	Anxiolytics, water-based lubricants, estrogen therapy, and counseling
Anorgasmia	Psychologic distress, medications, non-malignant chronic diseases, and prior trauma	Counseling, sex therapy, prostaglandin E inhibitors, and clitoral stimulation devices
Dyspareunia	Vaginal stenosis, vaginal dryness, and surgical scars	Vaginal dilators and water-based lubricants

tation with experts in cancer survivorship and mental health as well as nutritionists and patient advocates.

Nausea and Vomiting

Nausea and vomiting are significant problems for cancer patients. They can result in decreased compliance with treatment and multiple complications, including metabolic derangements, anorexia, poor surgical healing, and death. Patients with gynecologic cancer may present with nausea and vomiting related to their disease or report these problems as a postoperative complication. In the former patients, surgery often provides relief; in the latter patients, the nausea and vomiting often are limited to the immediate postoperative period and are rarely a long-term issue. In patients receiving chemotherapy, nausea and vomiting can occur during or immediately after chemotherapy is administered, or they can be delayed—with symptoms occurring more than 24 hours after the patient is treated. Previous experiences with diagnosis or treatment also can result in a conditioned response, known as anticipatory nausea and vomiting.

For gynecologic cancer patients receiving chemotherapy, the emetic potential of agents has been classified as low, moderate, or high (Table 36), and drugs are available to assist in their treatment (Table 37) (25). The addition of the NK-1 receptor antagonists, which act centrally to block the binding of substance P to the NK-1 receptor, as well as the serotonin (5HT-3) receptor antagonists, helps control symptoms in patients receiving chemotherapy. Table 38 shows the pharmacologic management according to the emetogenicity of the regimen. Commonly employed adjuvant therapies to control nausea and vomiting include sea bands, acupuncture, relaxation, and cognitive–behavioral therapy, although the medical literature contains a paucity of data on their effectiveness.

For patients with nausea and vomiting not related to chemotherapy, the use of dopamine receptor antagonists, prochlorperazine, or metoclopramide often can provide relief. However, for patients with protracted symptoms unrelated to chemotherapy, an evaluation of other causes is essential. Physicians must rule out anatomic reasons for protracted symptoms, such as bowel obstruction, hepatic or renal dysfunction, and brain metastases. For patients nearing the end of life, sedation with midazolam can be effective in the relief of nausea and vomiting, as well as anxiety.

Neurotoxicity

Cancer-related neurotoxic effects can be caused by the malignancies themselves and the treatment modalities we use to manage them. Pelvic tumors may abut the sacral plexus or cause nerve root compression and thus pain and loss of function. Surgical resection may result in injuries to the lumbosacral nerve plexus. For gynecologic cancer patients, chemotherapy-related neurotoxic effects remain a challenging and common problem.

TABLE 36. Emetogenic Potential of Common Gynecologic Cancer Regimens

Emetogenic Potential	Regimen
High (risk greater 90%)	Cisplatin and doxorubicin, then cyclophosphamide
	High-dose cisplatin (50 mg/m^2 or greater)
	Adriamycin and cisplatin
Moderate (risk 30–90%)	Carboplatin
	Carboplatin and paclitaxel
	Low-dose cisplatin (less than 50 mg/m^2)
	Oral cyclophosphamide
	Doxorubicin
	Oral etoposide
	Ifosfamide
	Methotrexate (250 mg/m^2 or greater)
Low (risk 10–30%)	Capecitabine
	Docetaxel
	Liposomal doxorubicin
	5-Fluorouracil
	Gemcitabine
	Paclitaxel
	Nanoparticle albumin-bound paclitaxel
	Topotecan
	Methotrexate (greater than 50–250 mg/m^2)
Minimal (risk less than 10%)	Bevacizumab
	Bleomycin
	Methotrexate (50 mg/m^2 or less)
	Sorafenib
	Vinorelbine

Chemotherapy-induced neurotoxicity generally manifests as sensory symptoms such as numbness and tingling in a "stocking-and-glove" distribution. It also can involve a motor component, though it is not as common. Of the agents used in management of gynecologic cancer, cisplatin and the taxanes are implicated, as are the vinca alkaloids (vinorelbine) and podophyllotoxins (etoposide). Typically, symptoms will develop in a dose-dependent manner and worsen as treatment continues. Taxane-induced neuropathy generally is not long term, and most patients can expect eventual resolution. However, neural injury from cisplatin may not be reversible.

Administration of glutamine or tricyclic antidepressants may be helpful in patients with paclitaxel-induced

TABLE 37. Drugs Used in Relief of Nausea and Vomiting

Drug Class	Agent	Dosage
NK-1 receptor antagonist	Aprepitant	125 mg PO day 1, then 80 mg daily on days 2–3
Corticosteroid	Dexamethasone	12 mg PO day 1, then 8 mg daily on days 2–4
5HT-3 receptor antagonist	Ondansetron	8–12 mg IV day 1, then 8 mg PO two times per day on days 2–4
	Granisetron	2 mg PO or 0.01 mg/kg (maximum: 1 mg) IV on day 1
	Dolasetron	100 mg PO or IV on day 1
	Palonosetron	0.25 mg on IV day 1
Benzodiazepine	Lorazepam	0.5–2 mg PO every 4–6 hours on days 1–4
Dopamine-receptor antagonist	Metoclopramide	5–10 mg PO/IM/IV every 6–8 hours as needed
	Prochlorperazine	5–10 mg PO every 6–8 hours as needed

Abbreviations: 5HT-3, indicates 5-hydroxytryptamine-3; IM, intramuscularly; IV, intravenously; NK-1, neurokinin-1; PO, orally.

TABLE 38. Example of a Schedule for Nausea Control

Emetic Potential	Suggested Management
Low	Prochlorperazine orally every 6 hours
Moderate	Aprepitant, days 1–3 or dexamethasone, days 1–4
	Ondansetron, days 1–4
	Lorazepam, days 1–4
High	Aprepitant, days 1–3
	Ondansetron, day 1
	Dexamethasone, days 1–4
	Lorazepam, days 1–4

neuropathy, and amifostine may provide protection from cisplatin-induced neuropathy (26, 27). Gabapentin also has been used to help alleviate neuropathic pain related to neurotoxicity (28). However, there appears to be no drug available to prevent or cure chemotherapy-induced neuropathy reliably (29).

Prevention often is the best treatment strategy. For patients at risk for neuropathy (ie, patients with long-standing diabetes or neuropathy of other causes) or patients undergoing treatment with therapies known to carry a risk of neuropathy, patient education about symptoms is important, as is frequent monitoring by the treating physician for evolving symptoms during therapy. Emerging signs of neurotoxicity may warrant dose delays or reduction of planned therapy, which can help prevent the signs from worsening. For patients who develop worsening or late-onset neurotoxic effects, especially after chemotherapy has ended, referral to a neurologist is recommended.

Lymphedema

Lymphedema is a chronic, progressive condition in which protein-rich fluid accumulates in the superficial tissues of the body (30). Surgical removal of pelvic lymph nodes and radiation therapy are risk factors for the development of lower extremity lymphedema (31). A study of 487 women with a history of gynecologic cancer found an incidence of symptomatic lymphedema of 36%, with the highest rates occurring in women receiving treatment for vulvar cancer (32). Other etiologies include advanced cancer, poor nutrition status, obesity, and delayed wound healing.

Patients at high risk for developing lymphedema should be educated as to its signs and symptoms and should recognize that it can occur well beyond the post-treatment period (Box 20). Patients who develop lymphedema should be referred for complex decongestive therapy to specialty programs encompassing physical therapy and massage. Usually offered through lymphedema clinics, complex decongestive therapy is a four-part program consisting of nail care, manual lymphatic drainage, compression bandaging, and therapeutic exercise. At least one prospective trial in breast cancer patients demonstrated that it was effective in the decreasing girth and volume, reducing pain scores, and achieving modest gains in quality of life (33).

Diarrhea

For cancer survivors, diarrhea can be a challenging and difficult symptom. All facets of treatment may predispose patients to diarrhea. Surgical excision of pelvic cancers may require bowel resection, which can cause changes in bowel absorption; if a large amount of bowel is resected, malabsorption results and causes large-volume diarrhea (also known as the short gut syndrome). Many chemotherapeutic agents used in the management of gynecologic malignancies also cause diarrhea; among the most notori-

BOX 20

Patient Instructions for the Prevention of Lymphedema

- Keep legs elevated when possible.
- Keep skin clean and well moisturized.
- Guard against injury to the extremities—wear shoes when outdoors, and maintain nail hygiene.
- Avoid constrictive pressure on the extremities—wear loose-fitting clothing and avoid elastic stockings.
- Be vigilant about the signs of infection—redness, warmth, pain, or fever.
- Exercise regularly.

ous are 5-fluorouracil and cisplatin. In addition, irradiation can result in acute and delayed injury to the bowel that causes painful and hemorrhagic diarrhea (radiation enteritis).

Therapy is multifactorial and includes nutrition counseling, patient education, and medication. Although there is no standard diet, recommendations usually include low fiber intake and use of high-calorie, electrolyte-replacing drinks. Avoidance of agents that may increase gastrointestinal motility, such as alcohol and caffeine, also is recommended. Many agents can reduce diarrhea, mostly by affecting gut opioid receptors to reduce peristalsis (Table 39). However, they should not be used if a bowel obstruction is suspected.

Constipation

Constipation is a common problem in the cancer survivor and may be accompanied by anorexia, pain, and malnutrition. In women with gynecologic cancer, constipation may be a sequela of the original surgery, be the presenting symptom of an ileus or bowel obstruction, or be caused by chemotherapy or pain medication. Constipation should be evaluated to rule out an anatomic cause that might necessitate surgical intervention. Otherwise, a bowel regimen should be initiated early—even before symptoms arise—in women receiving treatment for cancer or for cancer-related pain. For patients who require treatment, lifestyle and dietary modifications can help maintain normal bowel function, and medications are available to help stimulate bowel movements (Table 34).

Bowel Obstruction

Bowel obstruction may be present at the time of diagnosis of advanced gynecologic malignancies. In these patients, resection with curative intent often will require bowel resection of the obstructed area, which may result

in a colostomy. Bowel obstruction in patients with recurrent disease often accompanies a diagnosis of disease progression. Although surgery can be performed, the intent is not curative, and the risks of reoperation should be weighed against the potential benefits to the patient.

If an operation does not appear to be helpful, nonsurgical choices may be a reasonable alternative for palliation. Percutaneous endoscopic gastric tube placement is highly effective; one informative series reported that more than 90% of patients with advanced ovarian cancer achieved symptomatic relief (no nausea and vomiting) within a week (34). Total parenteral nutrition may prolong life, but it comes at the cost of edema, thrombosis, and infection. Chemotherapy typically is ineffective in restoring bowel function in heavily pretreated patients with recurrent disease (35). Octreotide, a synthetic somatostatin analogue, reduces secretions and may improve obstruction; a preparation with long-acting release is available (36). Finally, colonic stenting may provide effective palliation in patients with gastric outlet or colon obstruction, but it can be painful. Stents also have other risks, including the potential for migration, perforation, or ultimate failure resulting in reobstruction (37).

Fistula Formation

Fistulae are abnormal channels connecting two organs or locations that generally do not communicate. In gynecologic cancer patients, fistulae can form between the bowels and skin (enterocutaneous fistulae), bladder and vagina (vesicovaginal fistulae), and bowel and bladder (enterovesicular fistulae), although other connections also occur. Fistulae involving the vagina are generally painless but problematic. Intermittent positional leakage is typically a sign of a ureterovesical fistula, and continuous urine loss is more characteristic of a vesicovaginal fistula.

It is important to define the exact nature of the connection using radiographic tests (for example, barium enema or computed tomography). Treatment usually includes sur-

TABLE 39. Antidiarrheal Agents

Agent	Dosage	Mode of Action
Loperamide	Initial dosage of 4 mg orally, then 2 mg orally after each loose stool	Decreases peristalsis and increases anal sphincter tone
Diphenoxylate–atropine	2 tablets orally four times per day 5–10 mL orally two to four times a day Use as needed for symptoms	Decreases peristalsis
Tincture of opium (10%)	0.3–1.0 mL every 2–6 hours as needed	Decreases peristalsis

gical intervention aimed at correction of the tract by the creation of ostomies. Repair alone may be successful, and ostomies may be avoided. For patients who are not surgical candidates, treatment is aimed at palliation and may require pain medication and prophylactic antibiotics.

Radiation Cystitis

A complication of radiation therapy known as *radiation cystitis* can occur immediately after radiotherapy or years later. It involves changes in bladder function manifested by dysuria, urinary retention, urinary frequency, and in more severe cases, hematuria. The exclusion of other possible etiologies, including urinary tract infections, fistula formation, and primary tumors of the genitourinary system, is required before establishing the diagnosis of radiation cystitis. Mild symptoms can be treated medically with antibiotics (if an infection is suspected or diagnosed), analgesics, and patient education. More serious manifestations, including hemorrhage, may require further interventions. Available options have not been tested rigorously for efficacy in randomized trials. These options include hyperbaric oxygen therapy, which may stimulate angiogenesis in the injured area; ladder irrigation using agents to sclerose or contract superficial vessels, such as alum (aluminum); and aminocaproic acid, which inhibits plasminogen activation to help alleviate bleeding. Given the complex nature of the diagnosis and treatment, referral to a urologist may be required.

Urethral Obstruction

Urinary tract obstruction occurs as the result of tumor obstruction or scarring related to previous pelvic surgery or radiation therapy. If untreated, it will lead to renal failure and death. However, it is readily relieved by percutaneous nephrostomy or cystoscopic stenting. For patients diagnosed with obstruction at diagnosis, stents are usually temporary and can be removed at the end of adjuvant treatment. For women with advanced or recurrent disease, stents are permanent and must be replaced at regular intervals (usually every 3 months).

Neutropenia

The use of chemotherapy and pelvic radiation therapy is common in the treatment of patients with gynecologic cancer. Both modalities can have a negative impact on the bone marrow. Successive or concomitant treatments are often used in the management of endometrial and cervical cancers, and lowering of blood counts is not uncommon. Of the three cell lineages (red blood cells, white blood cells, and platelets), the one of most concern is neutropenia—a total absolute neutrophil count below 1,500 cells/mm^3. Chemotherapy-induced neutropenia continues to be a major risk factor for fever and infection, which remains a chief reason for hospitalization and treatment-related mortality. Fortunately, the advent of myeloid colony–stimulating factors has reduced the incidence of febrile neutropenia and infection-related mortality.

The American Society of Clinical Oncology guidelines strongly recommend the use of prophylactic colony-stimulating factors in susceptible patients (38). Characteristics of patients considered to be at high risk for febrile neutropenia are given in Box 21. Agents include filgrastim and pegfilgrastim. Each agent should be administered for 1–3 days by way of a subcutaneous injection after chemotherapy. Pegfilgrastim is available as a 6-mg subcutaneous injection and requires one dose per treatment cycle; filgrastim is dosed by weight, at 5 mg/kg, and requires daily administration until bone marrow recovery is documented, which usually requires a 5-day course.

Anemia

As noted earlier, anemia can lead to disruptions in quality of life and can contribute to cancer-related fatigue. The etiology of anemia is multifactorial, and a medical evaluation should be performed to identify other causes beyond cancer, such as nutritional deficiencies, active bleeding,

---

BOX 21

Considerations for the Use of Prophylactic Myeloid Colony-Stimulating Factors

Patient Specific
  Age older than 65 years
  Medical history
    Poor performance status
    Anorexia or cachexia
    Active infection
    Open wounds
    Other serious medical problems
    Cancer history
    Advanced stage of disease
    Extensive treatment history
    Chemoradiation therapy
    Bone marrow transplant
    Previous episode of fever with neutropenia
Treatment Specific
  High-risk regimens
    Topotecan
    Paclitaxel
    Docetaxel
    Combination regimens

alcoholism, and thyroid disorders. The easiest way to manage anemia is through blood transfusions. For patients with cancer, two erythropoietin-stimulating agents are available in the United States: epoetin and darbepoetin alpha.

Clinical trials have supported the use of erythropoietin-stimulating agents in the management of anemia in cancer patients. In a notably successful investigation of quality of life, 2,370 cancer patients undergoing chemotherapy for a solid tumor malignancy received epoetin alfa therapy. Treatment was associated with an improvement in quality of life that was statistically correlated to correction in hemoglobin levels (39).

The use of erythropoietin-stimulating agents to correct hemoglobin levels in patients not receiving chemotherapy should be avoided. One recently completed trial evaluating darbepoetin alpha compared with placebo showed that despite a reduced need for transfusions in patients receiving darbepoetin, there was an increase in the risk of death associated with its use (24). This finding has prompted the U.S. Food and Drug Administration to issue a black-box warning for epoetin and darbepoetin.

Cachexia

Beyond fatigue, the cachexia–anorexia syndrome is associated with increased cancer-related mortality rates. Pharmacologic interventions include progestogens (megestrol), cannabinoids (dronabinol), corticosteroids (dexamethasone), and anabolic agents (oxandrolone). Megestrol acetate is perhaps most often used to improve appetite and increase weight in cancer-associated anorexia, and it appears to offer superior palliation compared with dronabinol (40).

PALLIATIVE CARE: MORE THAN HOSPICE

Palliative (Greek, "to cloak") care involves the relief of suffering by treating symptoms. Often the best way to palliate is to manage the underlying condition effectively, and palliative care increasingly has been integrated earlier into cancer care in an aggressive and comprehensive approach. Whereas there is no objective way to delineate palliative care from end-of-life care, it is essential to recognize that when symptoms are present, they must be addressed early and repeatedly, especially when the goal is no longer cure (Box 22).

Patients should be engaged in advanced care planning early in treatment. A survey to determine whom patients named in the advanced care planning as their emergency contact and health care proxy, as well as their primary support (41), showed that more than 40% of patients did not name the same person to all three roles, and even among women in relationships, 46% did not name their partners to these roles. Physicians need to understand

whom patients want involved in their care. Many centers have addressed this challenge by forming palliative care services that incorporate an interdisciplinary approach to end of life.

BOX 22

End-of-Life Issues

- Define dreams and responsibilities.
- Jointly decide on the do-not-resuscitate status early in the discussion of goals of care.
- Discuss place of death preference.
- Treat pain to at least a score of 5 out of 10.
- Challenge fear and isolation.

References

1. Kadan-Lottick NS, Vanderwerker LC, Block SD, Zhang B, Prigerson HG. Psychiatric disorders and mental health service use in patients with advanced cancer: a report from the Coping With Cancer Study. Cancer 2005;104:2872–81.

2. Wenzel L, Huang HQ, Monk BJ, Rose PG, Cella D. Quality-of-life comparisons in a randomized trial of interval secondary cytoreduction in advanced ovarian carcinoma: a Gynecologic Oncology Group study. J Clin Oncol 2005;23:5605–12.

3. Wenzel L, Cella D. Quality of life issues in gynecologic cancer. In: Hoskins WJ, Perez CA, Young RC, Barakat RR, Markman M, Randall ME, editors. Principles and practices of gynecologic oncology. 4th ed. Philadephia (PA): Lippincott Williams & Wilkins; 2005. p. 1333–42.

4. Swenson MM, MacLeod JS, Williams SD, Miller AM, Champion VL. Quality of life after among ovarian germ cell cancer survivors: a narrative analysis. Oncol Nurs Forum 2003;30:380.

5. Hodgkinson K, Butow P, Fuchs A, Hunt GE, Stenlake A, Hobbs KM, et al. Long-term survival from gynecologic cancer: psychosocial outcomes, supportive care needs and positive outcomes. Gynecol Oncol 2007;104:381–9.

6. Rowland JH, Hewitt M, Ganz PA. Cancer survivorship: a new challenge in delivering quality cancer care. J Clin Oncol 2006;24:5101–4.

7. Demark-Wahnefried W, Pinto BM, Gritz ER. Promoting health and physical function among cancer survivors: potential for prevention and questions that remain. J Clin Oncol 2006;24:5125–31.

8. Short PF, Vargo MM. Responding to employment concerns of cancer survivors. J Clin Oncol 2006;24:5138–41.

9. Rauch PK, Muriel AC. Raising an emotionally healthy child when a parent is sick. New York (NY): McGraw-Hill; 2005.

10. Bodurka-Bevers D, Basen-Engquist K, Carmack CL, Fitzgerald MA, Wolf JK, de Moor C, et al. Depression, anx-

iety, and quality of life in patients with epithelial ovarian cancer. Gynecol Oncol 2000;78:302–8.

11. Lutgendorf SK, Anderson B, Rothrock N, Buller RE, Sood AK, Sorosky JI. Quality of life and mood in women receiving extensive chemotherapy for gynecologic cancer. Cancer 2000;89:1402–11.

12. Fowler JM, Carpenter KM, Gupta P, Golden-Kreutz DM, Andersen BL. The gynecologic oncology consult: symptom presentation and concurrent symptoms of depression and anxiety. Obstet Gynecol 2004;103:1211–7.

13. Holland JC, Bultz BD. The NCCN guideline for distress management: a case for making distress the sixth vital sign. J Natl Compr Canc Netw 2007;5:3–7.

14. Zigmond AS, Snaith RP. The hospital anxiety and depression scale. Acta Psychiatr Scand 1983;67:361–70.

15. Beck AT, Epstein N, Brown G, Steer RA. An inventory for measuring clinical anxiety: psychometric properties. J Consult Clin Psychol 1988;56:893–7.

16. Ross JR, Riley J, Quigley C, Welsh KI. Clinical pharmacology and pharmacotherapy of opioid switching in cancer patients. Oncologist 2006;11:765–73.

17. World Health Organization. Cancer pain relief: with a guide to opioid availability. 2nd ed. Geneva: WHO; 1996.

18. Krychman ML. Sexual rehabilitation medicine in a female oncology setting. Gynecol Oncol 2006;101:380–4.

19. Wiggins DL, Wood R, Granai CO, Dizon DS. Sex, intimacy, and the gynecologic oncologist: survey results of the New England Association of Gynecologic Oncologists. J Psychosoc Oncol 2007;25:61–70.

20. Stausmire JM. Sexuality at the end of life. Am J Hosp Palliat Care 2004;21:33–9.

21. Lee SJ, Schover LR, Partridge AH, Patrizio P, Wallace WH, Hagerty K, et al. American Society of Clinical Oncology recommendations on fertility preservation in cancer patients [published erratum appears in J Clin Oncol 2006;24:5790]. J Clin Oncol 2006;24:2917–31.

22. Pinto BM, Frierson GM, Rabin C, Trunzo JJ, Marcus BH. Home-based physical activity intervention for breast cancer patients. J Clin Oncol 2005;23:3577–87.

23. Wenzel L, Vergote I, Cella D. Quality of life in patients receiving treatment for gynecologic malignancies: special considerations for patient care. Int J Gynaecol Obstet 2003; 83(suppl 1):211–29.

24. Glaspy J, Smith R, Aapro M, Ludwig H, Pinter T, Smakal M, et al. Results from a phase III, randomized, double-blind, placebo-controlled study of darbepoetin alfa for the treatment of anemia in patients not receiving chemotherapy or radiotherapy [abstract]. In: American Association for Cancer Research Annual Meeting: Proceedings; 2007 Apr 14–18; Los Angeles, CA. Philadelphia (PA): AACR; 2007. Available at: http://www.abstractsonline.com/viewer/view Abstract.asp?CKey={0F449D11-0E8D-43DF-85E7-77E5F4589E7D}&MKey={E3F4019C-0A43-4514-8F66-B86DC90CD935}&AKey={728BCE9C-121B-46B9-A8EE-

DC51FDFC6C15}&SKey={FA30AEE6-5964-4270-8253-C16F6E2F75DA}. Retrieved October 18, 2007.

25. Kris MG, Hesketh PJ, Somerfield MR, Feyer P, Clark-Snow R, Koeller JM, et al. American Society of Clinical Oncology guideline for antiemetics in oncology: update 2006 [published erratum appears in J Clin Oncol 2006; 24:5431–2]. J Clin Oncol 2006;24:2932–47.

26. Lorusso D, Ferrandina G, Greggi S, Gadducci A, Pignata S, Tateo S, et al. Phase III multicenter randomized trial of amifostine as cytoprotectant in first-line chemotherapy in ovarian cancer patients. Multicenter Italian Trialsin Ovarian Cancer investigators. Ann Oncol 2003;14:1086–93.

27. Hilpert F, Stahle A, Tome O, Burges A, Rossner D, Spathe K, et al. Neuroprotection with amifostine in the first-line treatment of advanced ovarian cancer with carboplatin/paclitaxel-based chemotherapy—a double-blind, placebo-controlled, randomized phase II study from the Arbeitsgemeinschaft Gynakologische Onkologoie (AGO) Ovarian Cancer Study Group. Arbeitsgemeinschaft Gynakologische Onkologoie (AGO) Ovarian Cancer Study Group. Support Care Cancer 2005;13:797–805.

28. Backonja M, Glanzman RL. Gabapentin dosing for neuropathic pain: evidence from randomized, placebo-controlled clinical trials. Clin Ther 2003;25:81–104.

29. Annas GJ. Informed consent, cancer, and truth in prognosis [published erratum appears in N Engl J Med 1994;330: 651]. N Engl J Med 1994;330:223–5.

30. Badger C, Preston N, Seers K, Mortimer P. Physical therapies for reducing and controlling lymphoedema of the limbs. The Cochrane Database of Systematic Reviews 2004, Issue 4. Art. No. D003141. DOI:10.1002/14651858. CD003141.pub2.

31. Gaarenstroom KN, Kenter GG, Trimbos JB, Agous I, Amant F, Peters AA, et al. Postoperative complications after vulvectomy and inguinofemoral lymphadenectomy using separate groin incisions. Int J Gynecol Cancer 2003;13: 522–7.

32. Ryan M, Stainton MC, Jaconelli C, Watts S, MacKenzie P, Mansberg T. The experience of lower limb lymphedema for women after treatment for gynecologic cancer. Oncol Nurs Forum 2003;30:417–23.

33. Mondry TE, Riffenburgh RH, Johnstone PA. Prospective trial of complete decongestive therapy for upper extremity lymphedema after breast cancer therapy. Cancer J 2004;10: 42–8; discussion 17–9.

34. Pothuri B, Montemarano M, Gerardi M, Shike M, Ben-Porat L, Sabbatini P, et al. Percutaneous endoscopic gastrostomy tube placement in patients with malignant bowel obstruction due to ovarian carcinoma. Gynecol Oncol 2005; 96:330–4.

35. Abu-Rustum NR, Barakat RR, Venkatraman E, Spriggs D. Chemotherapy and total parenteral nutrition for advanced ovarian cancer with bowel obstruction. Gynecol Oncol 1997;64:493–5.

36. Matulonis UA, Seiden MV, Roche M, Krasner C, Fuller AF, Atkinson T, et al. Long-acting octreotide for the treatment

and symptomatic relief of bowel obstruction in advanced ovarian cancer. J Pain Symptom Manage 2005;30:563–9.

37. Baron TH. Expandable metal stents for the treatment of cancerous obstruction of the gastrointestinal tract. N Engl J Med 2001;344:1681–7.

38. Smith TJ, Khatcheressian J, Lyman GH, Ozer H, Armitage JO, Balducci L, et al. 2006 update of recommendations for the use of white blood cell growth factors: an evidence-based clinical practice guideline. J Clin Oncol 2006;24: 3187–205.

39. Demetri GD, Kris M, Wade J, Degos L, Cella D. Quality-of-life benefit in chemotherapy patients treated with epoet-

in alfa is independent of disease response or tumor type: results from a prospective community oncology study. Procrit Study Group. J Clin Oncol 1998;16:3412–25.

40. Jatoi A, Windschitl HE, Loprinzi CL, Sloan JA, Dakhil SR, Mailliard JA, et al. Dronabinol versus megestrol acetate versus combination therapy for cancer-associated anorexia: a North Central Cancer Treatment Group study. J Clin Oncol 2002;20:567–73.

41. Dizon DS, Gass JS, Bandera C, Weitzen S, Clark M. Does one person provide it all? Primary support and advanced care planning for women with cancer. J Clin Oncol 2007; 25:1412–6.

Integrative Medicine

Shelley W. Wroth, MD, and Tracy Gaudet, MD

In 2006, the National Center for Complementary and Alternative Medicine published a systematic review of more than 500 articles on the motivation for use of complementary and alternative medicine in cancer. Powerful motivators to choose these modalities included a perceived beneficial response, a desire for control, and a strong belief in complementary and alternative therapies, but they did not include a disappointment with conventional medicine (1). In studies of patients with gynecologic cancer in the United States since 2000, the use of complementary and alternative practices ranged from 48% to 66% (2–7). Therefore, at least one half of patients use or have used these modalities. Consequently, it is important that physicians understand what these modalities entail, how they work, how likely they may be to cure a condition or relieve symptoms, and how they may interact with the treatments the physicians prescribe.

This discussion will define the terms *complementary medicine* and *alternative medicine*, as well as the more current and comprehensive term *integrative medicine*; discuss use patterns in the United States, focusing on women with gynecologic cancers; and discuss the potential risks and benefits of the most popular therapies and lifestyle interventions in light of current medical knowledge.

A variety of terms have been used to describe these practices, including *complementary medicine*, *alternative medicine*, and *unconventional medicine*. These terms do not capture the goal of best-practice medicine, which involves taking the safest and most effective practices from traditional Western medicine and other medical systems and traditions to best care for patients. The term that is now used to describe this inclusive approach is *integrative medicine*. Integrative medicine is grounded in the importance of caring for the well-being of the whole person, encompassing not only her physical health but also her spiritual and emotional health. In addition, it emphasizes patient partnership in maintaining the body's health through lifestyle practices of diet, exercise, and stress management.

Complementary and alternative practices have been defined as "medical interventions not taught widely at U.S. medical schools or generally available at U.S. hospitals" (8). The spectrum of therapies, practitioners, and products within this category is extremely broad and spans everything from botanical approaches to magnet therapy. The National Institutes of Health has categorized complementary and alternative therapies into five domains:

1. Biologically based therapies: botanicals, supplements, and vitamins
2. Manipulative-based therapies: chiropractic, osteopathic manipulation, and massage
3. Mind-body–based therapies: relaxation techniques, hypnosis, and imagery
4. Energy-based therapies: healing and therapeutic touch, Reiki, and magnet therapy
5. Therapies based on complete systems: Oriental medicine and acupuncture, homeopathy, and Ayurveda.

According to a survey assessing the use of integrative medicine in the United States, most users are women, and most individuals do not inform their physicians of their use. The use of these approaches also is associated with higher education levels, higher socioeconomic status, younger age, and greater health consciousness (8). In recent surveys of U.S. women with gynecologic cancers, the same patient characteristics held true, with only 12–39% of patients getting guidance for the use of these interventions from a physician, nurse, or complementary and alternative therapy practitioner. Most women chose complementary and alternative approaches for an improved sense of well-being, control of adverse effects from treatment, and anticancer effects (6). This discussion first will examine lifestyle interventions including diet, exercise, and spirituality, and then each of the five categories of complementary and alternative practices as defined by the National Institutes of Health.

LIFESTYLE INTERVENTIONS

Diet and Nutrition

Multiple studies have investigated the role of diet in cancer risk and survivorship. As is well known, anorexia and cachexia can be adverse effects of cancer and chemotherapy, and dietary counseling, nutritional support, and pharmacologic management (such as megestrol) are critical for adequate nutrition and improved outcome (9, 10). However, it also is well established that obesity is a risk factor for breast and endometrial cancer (11); therefore, many patients who seek treatment are obese, and 71% of cancer survivors are overweight or obese (12). Studies also have documented that obesity at the time of diagnosis was associated with increased cancer mortality in patients with breast and cervical cancer, as well as cancers across the board (13). A large study of 5,204 breast cancer survivors showed an increased risk ratio of recurrence and a higher all-cause mortality in patients with increased weight gain compared with survivors with stable weight (14).

Therefore, nutrition counseling and weight management are critical to decrease recurrence and mortality (15). Five studies have attempted to determine the most effective methods of weight management in breast cancer survivors (16–20). Individual dietary counseling, alone or combined with a structured dietary program, was the most effective intervention. Until more is known, the same guidelines for weight management for the general population should be used for cancer survivors, including dietary, exercise, and behavioral treatment.

A study of 2,619 breast cancer survivors in the Nurses' Health Study showed significantly lower mortality from nonbreast cancer causes in patients reporting high proportional intakes of fruit, vegetables, whole grains, and low-fat dairy products than in patients reporting high intake of meat, refined grains, dairy products with high fat content, and desserts (21). There has been a great deal of controversy about the role of fat intake and its relationship to cancer, especially breast cancer. Preliminary results from the Women's Intervention Nutrition Study (22) and the ongoing Women's Healthy Eating and Living Study (23) suggest that women in the low-fat-diet group (less than 15% of total energy intake from fat) showed a 24% relative risk reduction in recurrence; patients with estrogen receptor–negative disease had a 42% relative risk reduction for recurrence. The general recommendations for levels of fat in the diet are 20–35% of total energy intake, with less than 10% from saturated fat and less than 3% from trans fatty acids (24). These levels may be lowered for breast cancer patients following the outcomes of the aforementioned studies.

Few studies have been done on the role of protein or carbohydrate intake. Studies have shown an increase in recurrence of disease in breast cancer survivors with increased intake of red meat, bacon, and liver (25). Current recommendations for protein intake are 0.8 g per kilogram of body weight, or 10–35% of total energy intake from protein (26). Protein sources with lower saturated fat and more monounsaturated fat include chicken, fish, and legumes. Because there also are few data on optimal carbohydrate intake for cancer patients, it is recommended that they follow the guidelines for prevention of chronic disease. Carbohydrate intake should be 45–65% of total energy intake, including 3–4 g of fiber per 1,000 kJ (24). Carbohydrates should come chiefly from nutrient-dense foods such as vegetables, whole fruits, and whole grains. The American Cancer Society guidelines for carbohydrates recommend at least five servings of fruit and vegetables daily (24).

Another area of dietary controversy is the role of soy in cancer risk and prevention. Soybeans contain phytoestrogens. Phytoestrogens exert estrogenic and antiestrogenic effects, depending on their concentration in the diet, levels of endogenous estrogens, and individual characteristics of the consumer, such as gender and menopausal status (27). Phytoestrogens in soybeans inhibit breast cancer cell proliferation in vitro and breast cancer development in animal models (28). However, 13 human studies have failed to support the hypothesis that a soy-rich diet in adult women is protective against the development of breast cancer (29). The safety of phytoestrogens in women with breast cancer also is controversial. One review found that adult consumption of soy does not appear to affect the survival of breast cancer patients (30). However, two studies—one in vitro (31) and one animal study (32)—demonstrated that genistein, a component of the isoflavones in soybeans, inhibited the antiproliferative effect of tamoxifen and increased the expression of estrogen-responsive genes, raising questions about isoflavone use in women taking tamoxifen. In summary, there is no clear evidence that soy intake in an adult is protective against breast cancer or that it affects breast cancer survivorship. However, women using tamoxifen may want to avoid soy foods, and women with a history of breast cancer probably should defer taking supplements containing isolated high-concentration isoflavones (27).

Exercise

Multiple systematic reviews were published in 2005 and 2006, including 16 investigations into exercise and cancer survivorship (33–35). Most of these studies involved patients with breast cancer and included endurance training or mixed training (endurance and strength training) of moderate to vigorous intensity (50–75% of baseline capacity) at least 3 days per week for 10–60 minutes per session. The patients were monitored for 2–15 weeks. All studies concluded that there was a consistent, positive effect on vigor and vitality, cardiopulmonary fitness, quality of life, depression, anxiety, and fatigue. No adverse effects were reported. Three studies in breast and colon cancer survivors suggest that individuals with a routine exercise regimen had a decreased risk of recurrence and death. The American Cancer Society, Centers for Disease Control and Prevention, American College of Sports Medicine, and World Health Organization recommend at least 30 minutes of moderate-intensity activity at least 5 days per week (24, 36, 37).

SPIRITUAL HEALING

Spiritual healing is a broad classification of approaches involving "the intentional influence of one or more persons upon another living system without using known physical means of intervention" (38). It may be an important source of coping and strength for many patients with cancer. However, this area is not addressed often in end-of-life care, nor is it easy to study. Definitions of spirituality and religion and their impact on individuals' lives vary widely. One meta-summary of qualitative literature on the spiritual perspectives of adults, most of whom had cancer, at the end of life focused on themes of spiritual despair (alienation, loss of self, and dissonance), spiritual work (forgiveness, self-exploration, and search for balance), and spiritual well-being (connection, self-actualization, and consonance) (39). Another recent systematic review included 17 studies focused on the question of whether spiritual coping strategies affect illness adjustment in patients with cancer. This review found seven studies showing positive effects of religious coping, three studies showing religious coping to be harmful, and seven studies having nonsignificant results. However, many studies failed to control for important variables such as stage of disease and social support (40). Religiosity has been associated with delays in seeking care in some populations, such as African-American women with breast cancer (41).

Spiritual healing is a part of a larger system of strategies that purport to heal through some exchange or channeling of supraphysical energy. Such approaches include therapeutic touch, Reiki healing, external Qigong, and prayer. Proponents of these energy-field therapies claim that some of these techniques can act across long distances—hence the collective name *distant healing* (42). The power of *distant healing* was examined in a meta-analysis of 23 clinical studies, with 10 positive studies evaluating therapeutic touch compared with sham control, two positive studies evaluating distant intercessory prayer, and four positive studies evaluating other forms of distant healing. Only one study included patients with cancer. However, in an update to this review that included 17 additional studies, no effect greater than placebo was noted (43). In summary, spirituality and cancer care is an area in which more research is needed. To assess this aspect of care, a simple series of questions may provide valuable information for supportive care to patients. The questions should determine whether spirituality is an important source of strength, whether patients believe that spirituality affects their medical care, and whether they need any support in this area.

INTEGRATIVE THERAPIES

Biologically Based Therapies

BOTANICALS

Biologically based therapies are the greatest concern for many physicians in integrative cancer care because of unknown interactions between herbal therapies and prescription medications, chemotherapy, and radiation therapy. Botanical therapies, supplements, and vitamins are regulated as foods, not as drugs, by the U.S. Food and Drug Administration. Botanical manufacturing companies may not claim to treat a disease, but they can make structure and function claims on their labels. There is now only voluntary compliance by these companies with good manufacturing practices for the proper identification of the ingredients and dosage of their products and for solubility standards.

However, the large numbers of patients using alternative therapies are most likely to use these interventions during active treatment, frequently in an attempt to minimize side effects of therapy. The benefit of any intervention always should be weighed against its potential for harm, with a higher level of evidence required given the greater potential for harm. Table 40 includes important potential interactions between herbal preparations and prescription medications. Table 41 lists herbal products with potential serious toxic effects. Table 42 lists integrative therapies commonly used to control adverse effects of disease and treatment, such as stomatitis, peripheral neuropathy, nausea and vomiting, depression and anxiety, insomnia, constipation, and fatigue.

Extracts of medicinal mushrooms have been used as adjuvant cancer therapy in China. The best studied mushrooms are shiitake (*Lentinus edodes*), reishi (*Ganoderma lucidum*), maitake (*Grifola frondosa*), and *Coriolus versicolor*. Multiple studies have looked at in vitro and animal models of the effects of medicinal mushrooms on immune functioning, but few clinical trials exist. Most research has focused on isolated pharmaceutically active mushroom compounds, such as the glucans lentinan from *L edodes*, schizophyllan (sonifilan) from *Schizophyllum commune*, grifolan from *G frondosa*, and sodium stibogluconate from *Sclerotinia sclerotiorum*.

The available evidence indicates that the anticarcinogenic properties of these polysaccharides are caused by enhancement of the numbers or functions of macrophages, natural killer cells, and subsets of T cells—that is, by the modulation of innate and adaptive immunity (44). Clinical trials that have been conducted in Japan since the 1970s studied two components of *C versicolor*, polysaccharide K and polysaccharide peptide. Polysaccharide K extended 5-year survival rates in patients with cancer of the stomach, colon, rectum, nasopharynx, and lung (non–small cell type), as well as HLA-B40–positive breast cancer. In phase 2 and 3 trials in China of polysaccharide peptide, increased

TABLE 40. Important Potential Interactions Between Herbal Preparations and Prescription Medications

Category	Drug	Herb	Potential Problem
Anticoagulants and antiplatelets	Warfarin, enoxaparin, dipyridamole, clopidogrel, aspirin, and heparin	Aloe, black cohosh, bromelain, capsicum, chamomile, dandelion, dong quai, fenugreek, feverfew, garlic, ginger, ginkgo biloba, ginseng, goldenseal, licorice, and red clover	Increased bleeding
Nonsteroidal antiinflammatory drugs	Rofecoxib and naproxen	None	None
Benzodiazepines	Alprazolam	Chamomile, ginkgo biloba, kava kava, St. John's wort, and valerian	Increased sedative effects
Barbiturates	Phenobarbital	Kava kava and valerian	Additive or synergistic effects
Antidepressants	Venlafaxine, paroxetine, and amitriptyline	Kava kava and valerian	Additive or synergistic effects
Immunosuppressants	Cyclosporin, tacrolimus, and corticosteroids	Astragalus and echinacea	Antagonistic effects
Chemotherapeutic agents	Irinotecan	St. John's wort	Decreased effects of irinotecan
Monoamine oxidase inhibitors	Phenelzine, and tranylcypromine	Ephedra, ginseng, guarana, licorice, and mate	Hypertension additive effects
Antidiabetic agents	Glipizide, glyburide, insulin, metformin, and rosiglitazone	Aloe, fenugreek, ginseng, and karela	Alteration in blood glucose levels
Antihypertensive agents	Captopril, propranolol, and diltiazem	Ephedra, guarana, and mate	Antagonistic effects
Cardiac glycosides	Digoxin	Aloe, ginseng, hawthorn, kyushin, and licorice	Increased risk of cardiac toxicity
Potassium-sparing diuretics	Spironolactone	Licorice	Antagonistic diuretic effects
Lithium	Lithium carbonate	Green tea and guarana	Increased lithium levels
Thyroid hormones	Levothyroxine	Kelp	Interference with thyroid replacement
Estrogens	Conjugated estrogen	Black cohosh, dong quai, ginseng, licorice, red clover, and soy isoflavones	Additive effects
Antiestrogens	Tamoxifen	Soy isoflavones, kudzu, and dong quai	Antagonistic effects
Central nervous system stimulants	Methylphenidate, modafinil, and caffeine	Ephedra, green tea, guarana, and mate	Additive stimulation effects
Iron supplements	Ferrous sulfate	Saw palmetto and St. John's wort	Limiting of iron absorption
Anticonvulsants	Carbamazepine	Borage and evening primrose	Lowered seizure threshold
Angiotensin-converting enzyme inhibitors	Enalapril	Capsicum	Increased incidence and severity of cough
Nonnucleoside reverse-transcriptase inhibitors	Saquinavir	Cat's claw, chamomile, echinacea, garlic, goldenseal, and St. John's wort	Alteration of drug metabolism

Data from Memorial Sloan-Kettering Cancer Center. About herbs, botanicals and other products. MSKCC Integrative Medicine. New York (NY): MSKCC; 2007. Available at: http://www.mskcc.org/mskcc/html/11570.cfm. Retrieved January 18, 2008.

TABLE 41. Herbal Products With Serious Toxic Effects

Herbal Product	Effects
Chaparral tea	Promoted as an antioxidant and pain reliever, has caused liver failure requiring liver transplantation (1)
Chaste tree berry	Used to treat premenstrual syndrome, can interfere with dopamine-receptor antagonists (2)
Coltsfoot expectorant and other alkaloids	Have been linked to liver failure (3)
Comfrey	Ingested or used on bruises, can obstruct blood flow to the liver and possibly lead to death (4)
Feverfew (used for migraines and premenstrual syndrome), garlic (has many preventive and therapeutic uses), ginger (used to relieve nausea), and ginkgo (dilates arteries)	Can interact with anticoagulants and increase bleeding; anticoagulant effects are possible in unusually high doses or when these substances are used in combination (5)
Jin bu huan	A sedative and analgesic containing morphinelike substances, can cause hepatitis and dangerously slow heart rate (6)
Kava kava	A sedative and hypnotic, can cause hepatotoxicity and liver failure (7)
Laxatives such as senna, cascara, and aloe	Can cause potassium loss when used repeatedly over time, particularly dangerous when used with digitalis or prescription diuretics (8)
Licorice (used to treat peptic ulcers and as an expectorant)	Contraindicated with cardiac glycosides (9)
Lobelia	An emetic that may cause coma and death at high doses; lesser effects include rapid heartbeat and breathing problems (10)
Ma-huang, or ephedra	Herbal form of the central nervous system stimulant commonly known as speed; sold with names such as Herbal Ecstasy, Cloud 9, and Ultimate Xphoria; also in many herbal weight loss products; can cause hypertension, heart attack, and stroke (11)
Siberian ginseng capsules	Some contain instead a weed with male hormonelike chemicals (12)
St. John's wort	Antidepressant of proven effectiveness in management of mild depression; increases metabolism of many prescription medications and, thus, reduces their efficacy (13)
Yohimbe (bodybuilder, "enhances male performance")	Has caused seizures, kidney failure, and death (14)

1. Sheikh NM, Philen RM, Love LA. Chaparral-associated hepatotoxicity. Arch Intern Med 1997;157:913-9.
2. Sliutz G, Speiser P, Schultz AM, Spona J, Zeillinger R. Agnus castus extracts inhibit prolactin secretion of rat pituitary cells. Horm Metab Res 1993;25:253-5.
3. Chitturi S, Farrell GC. Herbal hepatotoxicity: an expanding but poorly defined problem. J Gastroenterol Hepatol 2000;15:1093-9.
4. Ridker PM, McDermott WV. Comfrey herb tea and hepatic veno-occlusive disease. Lancet 1989;1:657-8.
5. Groenewegen WA, Heptinstall S. A comparison of the effects of an extract of feverfew and parthenolide, a component of feverfew, on human platelet activity in-vitro. J Pharm Pharmacol 1990;42:553-7.
6. Horowitz RS, Feldhaus K, Dart RC, Stermitz FR, Beck JJ. The clinical spectrum of jin bu huan toxicity. Arch Intern Med 1996;156:899-903.
7. Wooltorton E. Herbal kava: reports of liver toxicity. CMAJ 2002;166:777.
8. Chin RL. Laxative-induced hypokalemia [letter]. Ann Emerg Med 1998;32:517-8.
9. Eriksson JW, Carlberg B, Hillorn V. Life-threatening ventricular tachycardia due to liquorice-induced hypokalaemia. J Intern Med 1999;245:307-10.
10. Brinker F. Herb contraindication and drug interactions: with extensive appendices addressing specific conditions, herb effects, critical medications and nutritional supplements. 3rd ed. Sandy (OR): Eclectic Medical Publications; 2001.
11. Haller CA, Benowitz NL. Adverse cardiovascular and central nervous system events associated with dietary supplements containing ephedra alkaloids. N Engl J Med 2000;343:1833-8.
12. Awang DV. Siberian ginseng toxicity may be case of mistaken identity [letter]. CMAJ 1996;155:1237.
13. Izzo AA. Ernst E. Interactions between herbal medicines and prescribed drugs: a systematic review. Drugs 2001;61:2163-75.
14. Favreau JT, Ryu ML, Braunstein G, Orshansky G, Park SS, Coody GL, et al. Severe hepatotoxicity associated with the dietary supplement LipoKinetix. Ann Intern Med 2002;136:590-5.

Adapted from Cassileth BR. Questionable cancer therapies. In: Holland JF, Frei E, Bast R, Kufe D, Pollock RE, Weichselbaum RR, editors. Holland and Frei's cancer medicine. 5th ed. Hamilton (Ont): BC Decker; 2000. p. 1045-54.

TABLE 42. Integrative Therapies to Relieve Common Symptoms During Cancer Treatment and Recovery

Symptom	Intervention	Comment
Anxiety	Music therapy	Relief of anxiety and stress, for relaxation.
	Kava kava	U.S. Food and Drug Administration issued a warning to physicians and consumers because of 30 cases of liver damage in Europe; available in the United States but not recommended until studied further.
	Relaxation techniques	Supportive data, but they include multiple modalities such as group therapy and audiotapes.
	Yoga	Decreased stress and anxiety when practiced several times weekly in healthy patients; not recommended if patient is at increased risk of fracture.
	Aromatherapy	Lavender aromatherapy is associated with decreased stress.
Pain	Acupuncture	One randomized controlled trial and one case study showed statistically significant pain improvement with acupuncture.
	Guided imagery	Improvement of quality of life in cancer patients.
	Hypnosis	In 1995 the National Institutes of Health issued a statement "Evidence supporting the efficacy of hypnosis in alleviating chronic pain associated with cancer seems strong."*
	Music therapy	Helpful in a variety of pain conditions because of the ability to improve mood, encourage relaxation, and increase pain threshold; positive evidence for treatment of cancer pain.
	Physical therapy	Used to treat a wide variety of pain conditions; improves shoulder range of motion in patients with breast cancer after mastectomy.
	Therapeutic touch	Studies suggest improved well-being.
Constipation	Aloe vera	Combination product of aloe vera, 150 mg, celandine, 300 mg, and psyllium, 50 mg, found effective in research.
	Phosphorus	Approved by U.S. Food and Drug Administration for occasional constipation; oral or rectal delivery available for adults and children.
	Flax seed	One to two tablespoons ground seed (not oil) in liquid up to three times per day; do not use for patients with prostate cancer.
	Psyllium	Divided doses of 2–45 g administered in studies; do not use after bowel surgery, strictures, or impaired motility.
Depression	Music therapy	Mood enhancement; positive systematic review; small-magnitude effect.
	St. John's wort	Many small studies over 20 years showed same effectiveness as tricyclic antidepressants with 1–3 months of treatment for mild to moderate depression; controversial data exist compared with data on use of selective serotonin reuptake inhibitors; two studies showed no benefit of St. John's wort; other data showed equal efficacy with fewer adverse effects with doses of 300–600 mg three times per day; St. John's wort has multiple drug interactions.
	Relaxation techniques	Positive small studies.
	Yoga	Positive small studies; avoid in patients at risk for fracture.
	5-Hydroxytryptophan	Precursor of serotonin; studied doses of 200–300 mg daily; related cases of eosinophilia myalgia syndrome, possibly due to contaminant.
	Dehydroepiandrosterone	Endogenous steroid hormone; studied doses of 30–90 mg; do not use in hormonally sensitive types of cancer, such as breast, prostate, ovarian, or hepatic cancer.
Fatigue	Acupressure and Shiatsu	Finger pressure at acupoints used in China since 2000 BC; may increase alertness.
	Physical therapy	Inconclusive results; additional studies needed.
	Yoga	Preliminary studies show yoga may decrease fatigue in adults.

(continued)

TABLE 42. Integrative Therapies to Relieve Common Symptoms During Cancer Treatment and Recovery (*continued*)

Symptom	Intervention	Comment
Insomnia	Melatonin	Studied doses of 0.5–50 mg; quick-release form more effective taken 30–60 minutes before bedtime; reduced sleep latency in older patients.
	Music therapy	Better sleep quality, longer duration, greater sleep efficiency, shorter sleep latency, less sleep disturbance, and less daytime dysfunction in older adults.
	Valerian	Approved by German Commission E; studied doses of 400–600 mg taken 30–60 minutes before bedtime; frequently combined with lemon balm and hops.
	Acupuncture	Commonly used in traditional Chinese medicine; positive small studies.
	Aromatherapy	Preliminary small studies show hypnotic effect of lavender and chamomile aromatherapy.
	Guided imagery	Early research supports combined guided imagery and pharmacologic treatment of insomnia; avoid in preexisting psychosis and personality disorders.
	Kundalini Yoga	Case study supportive of improved sleep; no adverse effects.
	Relaxation techniques	Several human trials showed decreased sleep latency; meditation appears to be more effective than progressive muscle relaxation.
Nausea and vomiting	Acupuncture	Two systematic reviews of acupuncture for chemotherapy-induced nausea and vomiting supportive, one showing electroacupuncture more effective; 11–12 high-quality studies in review showed significant benefit; two systematic reviews and one meta-analysis showed decreased nausea and vomiting postoperatively with acupuncture.
	Music therapy	Decreased nausea and vomiting in patients taking cyclophosphamide preparing for bone marrow transplant.
	Ginger	One randomized controlled trial and one open label study showed decreased severity and duration of chemotherapy-induced nausea and vomiting; may increase effectiveness of prochlorperazine
	Hypnosis	Mixed results; no studies comparing it with antiemetics or other relaxation therapies.
Neuropathy	γ-Linolenic acid	Evidence for use in diabetic neuropathy; studied up to 480 mg daily; may increase effects of multiple chemotherapeutic agents, including doxorubicin, cisplatin, carboplatin, docetaxil, epirubicin, idarubicin, mitoxantrone, paclitaxel, tamoxifen, vincristine, vinblastine, and vinorelbine.
Stomatitis	Povidone–iodine	Mouth rinses with 10–20 mL as often as four times per day decreased severity of mucositis secondary to chemotherapy and radiation therapy in clinical trials.

*Integration of Behavioral and Relaxation Approaches into the Treatment of Chronic Pain and Insomnia. NIH Technol Assess Statement 1995 Oct 16-18:1–34.

Natural Standard. Natural Standard databases. Cambridge (MA): Natural Standard. Available at: http://www.naturalstandard.com. Retrieved September 19, 2007.

5-year survival rates were found in patients with esophageal cancer, and increased immune states were found in 70–97% of patients with cancers of the stomach, esophagus, lung, ovary, and cervix. Two trials of *C versicolor* extract in breast cancer patients were found. One showed no effect in patients with estrogen receptor–negative disease. The other study of 540 patients with estrogen receptor–positive disease randomized patients after mastectomy and lymphadenectomy to chemotherapy or chemotherapy plus polysaccharide K. This study showed statistically significantly increased 5-year survival rates, as well as decreased recurrence rates (45).

Further research is needed on the biologic activity of mushrooms after oral administration to humans and ani-

mals, although a case–control study did find lower rates of stomach cancer in patients with dietary mushroom intake (46). The high tolerability and absence of interactions noted with chemotherapeutic agents make this area a rich one for continued study. These promising results are tempered by possible contamination of products with metals, including arsenic, lead, cadmium, and mercury, so patients using these products need to be aware of the variation in manufacturing practices (44).

Essiac is an herbal formula that contains at least four herbs, including burdock root, Indian rhubarb, sheep sorrel, and the inner bark of slippery elm. It was developed by Rene Caisse, who used it to treat hundreds of cancer patients for more than 40 years. There are no published complete reports of laboratory or clinical studies that prove the effectiveness of Essiac as a treatment for patients with cancer (47). In fact, a recent study showed that Essiac stimulated the in vitro growth of human breast cancer cells (48). No significant adverse side effects have been documented, but there is no current evidence to recommend its use.

SUPPLEMENTS

Like botanical therapies, supplements also have been used in cancer therapy. Melatonin has shown promise for further study as adjuvant therapy and in the improvement of common side adverse effects of disease and treatment. In a review of 10 clinical trials of melatonin in cancer treatment or supportive care, despite differences in tumor type and dosing of melatonin, use of melatonin showed decreased mortality rate at 1 year with no serious adverse effects (49). Melatonin in lower doses also may be useful in the management of insomnia, which frequently is seen in patients with cancer. Melatonin is metabolized by way of the cytochrome p450 system, so increased adverse effects may be noted with common drugs such as anastrozole, cimetidine, ciprofloxacin, and interferon; decreased therapeutic effects may occur with drugs such as insulin, nafcillin, omeprazole, and ritonavir. Melatonin should be avoided in patients who have clotting abnormalities or use anticoagulants, but it is promising for future studies (50).

Shark cartilage has been a popular supplement to cancer therapy because of the observation that sharks' bodies are primary composed of cartilage and they rarely have been known to get cancer. However, there have been two trials on the safety and efficacy of the use of shark cartilage in patients with advanced cancer—one a randomized, placebo-controlled trial of patients with breast or colorectal cancer. Neither trial showed any difference in survival or quality of life (51, 52). No data support the use of shark cartilage in the treatment of patients with cancer.

Laetrile, sometimes called vitamin B$_{17}$, is another supplement that has been used popularly to manage cancer. A recent systematic review of clinical evidence—including 36 reports, none of which were controlled clinical trials—showed no published proven effectiveness for laetrile as a treatment for cancer (53). No sound clinical data support its use for cancer therapy.

VITAMINS

Megadoses of vitamins have been used by some patients for supportive therapy for cancer. The U.S. Preventive Services Task Force published its recommendations for vitamin supplements to prevent cancer and cardiovascular disease in 2003. It found the evidence for or against supplements of vitamins A, C, and E, multivitamins with folic acid, or antioxidant combinations for cancer prevention to be insufficient. The task force specifically recommended against supplementation with beta carotene because of the

evidence of increased lung cancer in some studies (54). In a large prospective cohort study of 97,275 California teachers, 280 of whom developed ovarian cancer, women who consumed more than 3 mg of isoflavones daily in the diet had a relative risk of ovarian cancer of 0.56 (95% confidence interval, 0.33; 0.96) compared with women whose intake was less than 1 mg daily. No other dietary associations were found (55).

The role of dietary supplements during cancer therapy is an area that needs further study in order to develop evidence-based guidelines. Challenges of designing trials include the fact that no causal risk factors are known for many cancers; the time between causal events of disease occurrence is probably long; there is no known optimal age, dosing, or duration for therapy; and baseline nutrition status and easy availability of vitamin supplements are confounding factors. Current recommendations for cancer patients undergoing therapy are that a daily multivitamin supplement at the level of current Dietary Reference Intakes can be taken safely as part of a program of healthy nutrition (56).

Manipulative-Based Therapies

CHIROPRACTIC

Chiropractic focuses on the relationship between structure (primarily the spine) and function, and how that relationship affects the preservation and restoration of health. It uses manipulative therapy as an integral treatment tool. Chiropractors legally may do more than manipulate and align the spine. They also may gather medical histories, perform physical examinations, and order laboratory and radiographic tests to arrive at diagnoses. Chiropractors complete 4-year chiropractic college programs of study accredited by the Council on Chiropractic Education and are nationally licensed.

The most significant risk factor associated with chiropractic is stroke. Vertebrobasilar accidents occur chiefly after a cervical manipulation with a rotatory component. Estimates of vertebrobasilar accidents range from 1 per 20,000 cervical manipulations to 1 per 1 million cervical manipulations. The second most common complication of spinal manipulation is cauda equina syndrome related to progression of disk herniation. The incidence of cauda equina syndrome is estimated to be less than 1 per 1 million treatments.

MASSAGE

Massage therapy involves manipulation of the soft tissues of the body to normalize them. A wide variety of approaches are available, including deep tissue massage, Swedish massage, reflexology, and Rolfing. Massage is a therapeutic technique used by various practitioners, including physicians, physical therapists, osteopathic physicians, chiropractors, acupuncturists, nurses, and massage therapists. The American Massage Therapy Association accredits 25% of massage training schools. The National Certification Board for Therapeutic Massage and Bodywork administers a certification examination used by 24 states. Certification requires passing this examination and completing a minimum of 500 in-class hours of formal education and training. Licensure is offered at the state level in 30 states. Because of the heterogeneity of this field, when working with a massage therapist, it is important to ask for qualifications, including education, licensing, certification, and experience.

In a 2005 review of the safety and efficacy of massage therapy for patients with cancer (57), massage was found in studies to cause blood vessel dilation, increased skin temperature, decreased heart rate, and relaxation of mind and body. Studies have shown acute increases in natural killer cell number and activity after massage; however, the clinical importance of claims of increased immunity remains unproven (58–59). Massage is widely used by cancer patients; 26% of 453 adult patients surveyed at MD Andersen Cancer Center reported its use (60). The most promising use for massage found in the systematic review of the Cochrane Collaborative Group (61) was for anxiety reduction, with a 19–32% reduction rate in anxiety noted in cancer patients. Weaker evidence was noted for improvement of fatigue, pain, nausea and vomiting, sleep problems, and depression (57).

Statements about the effects of massage on constipation, wound healing, or decreased scar tissue formation cannot be made because of the insufficient number of studies. Deep tissue massage should be avoided in patients with increased risk of complications, including patients with bleeding disorders; patients taking anticoagulation therapy; patients with edema caused by heart or kidney failure, deep vein thrombosis, or phlebitis; patients with fever or infection that can be spread by blood or lymph circulation; and patients with leukemia or lymphoma. Massage should not be performed on or near malignant tumors or bone metastases; over bruises, unhealed scars, or open wounds; on or near recent fracture sites; or over joints or other tissues that are acutely inflamed.

Mind-Body–Based Therapies

Patients' emotional health, as well as physical health, can suffer greatly after a diagnosis of cancer. In patients with cancer, mind-body–based therapies have been shown to have great benefit in controlling anxiety, depression, and pain related to procedures.

RELAXATION TECHNIQUES

Meditation is a self-directed practice for relaxing the body and calming the mind. Mindfulness-based stress reduction is based on Vipassana meditation from India, which has been practiced for more than 2,500 years. Mindfulness-based stress reduction is a structured, 8-week didactic program developed by Jon Kabat-Zinn at the University of Massachusetts. It incorporates sitting, walking, and loving–kindness meditation, as well as body scanning and mindful movement. It has been studied extensively, and benefits have been noted in multiple health conditions. Studies in cancer patients show decreased anxiety, total mood disturbance, depression, anger, confusion, and total stress, as measured before and after completing the 8-week course (62–64).

Transcendental meditation involves sitting comfortably with the eyes closed for 15–20 minutes twice daily. With this technique, the individual's awareness relaxes, and he or she experiences an unusual state of restful alertness. Transcendental meditation has been shown to decrease emotional and physical response to stress. Data on its use in cancer patients and cancer symptom management is sparse, but there is weak evidence that it may help reduce anxiety and stress (65). In rare cases meditation may lead to a "spiritual emergency," which is defined as a crisis during which the process of growth and change becomes chaotic and overwhelming as individuals enter new realms of spiritual experience.

Yoga is part of the Ayurvedic medical system developed in India, which incorporates breath awareness and control, meditation, movement, and chanting. Studies including yoga as part of a multidisciplinary intervention for cancer patients support its benefits for stress management, anxiety, and insomnia (66). There are no studies in cancer patients with yoga as a lone intervention. It is likely safe, because a primary teaching of yoga is to do no harm and follow the current limits of your body; an exception is the patient with bony metastases, who would be at increased risk for fracture (67).

HYPNOSIS AND GUIDED IMAGERY

Hypnosis involves the induction of trance states and the use of therapeutic suggestions. The American Society of Clinical Hypnosis Certification in Clinical Hypnosis ensures that the certified individual is a health care professional who is licensed in that state or province to provide medical, dental, or psychotherapeutic services. Hypnosis has documented value for decreasing pain and anxiety in patients with cancer. Hypnosis was found to be valuable for improving quality of life and decreasing physical distress, anxiety, and pain associated with procedures in pediatric and adult patients (68–71). A study of women receiving hypnotherapy before breast biopsy showed less postsurgical pain and distress (72). Hypnosis can have long-lasting effects as well. In a randomized, controlled trial of women with breast cancer who underwent weekly group therapy with or without hypnosis, the use of group therapy resulted in statistically significant reductions in pain and suffering over a 10-month follow-up, and the addition of hypnosis further decreased pain sensation (73).

Hypnotized individuals occasionally report unanticipated negative effects during and after hypnosis. These effects usually are transient and minor, such as headaches, dizziness, or nausea. Rarely people have symptoms of anxiety or panic, unexpected reactions to a suggestion, and difficulties awakening from hypnosis. Hypnosis is not recommended for patients with dissociative personality disorders.

EXPRESSIVE ART AND MUSIC THERAPY

Art therapy involves the use of the creative arts to give expression to emotions and experiences that may be difficult to access and deal with in order to improve self-understanding and quality of life. Art therapy has been studied in cancer patients as a strategy to improve coping with disease and pain, as well as to enhance quality of life. A randomized, controlled trial of women with breast cancer who were undergoing radiation therapy showed improved coping at 2 months and 6 months after radiation treatment (74). Other studies in cancer patients showed appreciable changes (decreased distress and increased health-related quality of life) (75, 76).

Music therapy also has been investigated for its ability to mitigate distress and pain in patients with cancer. A recent systematic review for the Cochrane Database of 51 studies showed that listening to music reduces pain intensity levels and opioid requirements. However, the magnitude of benefit was small, and the clinical significance is unclear.

Energy-Based Therapies

Energy-based therapies involve the use of energy fields. There are two types: biofield therapy and bioelectromagnetic-based therapy. Biofield therapies are intended to affect energy fields that purportedly surround and penetrate the human body. The existence of such fields has not been proved scientifically. Some forms of energy therapy manipulate biofields by applying pressure or manipulating the body by placing the hands in or through these fields. Examples include Qigong, Reiki, and therapeutic touch. Bioelectromagnetic-based therapies involve the unconventional use of electromagnetic fields, such as pulsed fields, magnetic fields, or alternating current or direct current fields.

HEALING TOUCH AND THERAPEUTIC TOUCH

Healing Touch is an energy-based therapy that began in the 1980s as a nursing continuing education program. Therapeutic Touch is an energy-based therapy from the Krieger–Kunz method. A review of 30 studies of Healing Touch included three randomized trials with cancer patients. The largest study of 164 patients undergoing chemotherapy showed statistically significant improvement in decreased blood pressure and pain and improved

mood and fatigue. Two smaller studies showed no significant differences in interpersonal well-being, function, mood, or fatigue between intervention and control groups (77). A more recent randomized, controlled trial of Healing Touch showed improved quality of life in 62 breast cancer and gynecologic cancer patients receiving radiation therapy, with increased scores in overall function, vitality, pain, physical function, emotional role function, mental health, and health transition (78). Healing Touch may be an important adjuvant therapy for patients undergoing cancer treatment and end-of-life care.

REIKI

Reiki is an energy-based therapy described by the Reiki Regulatory Working Group as "a method of natural healing that originates with Mikao Usui in Japan in the early 20th century. The ability to heal oneself and others is passed on through initiation or attunement." A Reiki treatment involves a fully clothed patient, with the practitioner's hands over or lightly touching the patient's body, which is in a seated or lying position (79). A phase 2 clinical trial of Reiki in cancer patients found decreased pain and increased quality of life, but no change in opioid use compared with rest and standard care (80). No specific contraindications are known.

MAGNET THERAPY

Clinical data on the use of bioelectromagnetic-based therapy are scarce. Furthermore, they do not show that this therapy is effective in the management of cancer.

Therapies Based on Complete Systems

ACUPUNCTURE

Acupuncture is a therapeutic intervention that is used in many Asian systems of medicine. It is based on the theory that energy channels, called meridians, run throughout the body and that disease results from blockages of this energy. Acupuncture, which involves stimulating specific anatomic points in the body along these meridians by puncturing the skin with a very fine (32-gauge or smaller) needle, is one approach to release these blockages. There are many distinct styles of acupuncture, including Oriental medicine, Japanese Manaka style, Korean hand acupuncture, and the Worsley 5-element method. Training in acupuncture consists of a 3- to 4-year program at a school of Oriental medicine. Forty states license or register acupuncturists. The National Certification Commission for Acupuncture and Oriental Medicine offers a written, point location, and clean needle technique examination. To retain certification and licensure, an acupuncturist must pass this examination and meet continuing education requirements every 4 years. Medical doctors may be certified by the American Board of Medical Acupuncture by taking a minimum 300 hours of training in acupuncture.

The 1997 National Institutes of Health Consensus Development Conference on Acupuncture established that evidence based on clinical trials suggested beneficial roles for acupuncture in managing chemotherapy-induced nausea and vomiting and dental pain. Acupuncture also may have a therapeutic role in managing persistent fatigue in cancer patients, with a randomized, controlled trial showing a 31% improvement over 2 years (81). In addition, acupuncture may help control cancer pain. A study of auricular acupuncture in 90 cancer patients showed a statistically significant 36% decrease in pain at 2 months in the acupuncture group compared with 2% in the control group (82). Finally, acupuncture showed promise in the management of vasomotor symptoms in cancer patients. In a trial of 194 patients with breast and prostate cancer who received 6 weekly acupuncture treatments, 79% obtained greater than a 50% reduction in hot flushes, and 21% gained less than a 50% reduction in hot flushes (83).

Minor bleeding and bruising are the most common complications of acupuncture. These complications rarely necessitate treatment other than local pressure to the needle site for minor bleeding and occur in approximately 2% of all needles placed. The most significant risk of acupuncture is infection with hepatitis if needles are reused. Many states require that only disposable needles be used. Pneumothorax is the second most appreciable risk of acupuncture. Acupuncture is not recommended in patients with thrombocytopenia, bleeding disorders, or aplasia or in patients taking anticoagulative agents.

HOMEOPATHY

Homeopathic medicine is another complete medical system. It is based on the "law of similars"—that small, highly diluted quantities of medicinal substances are given to cure symptoms, when the same substances given at higher or more concentrated doses actually would cause those symptoms in a healthy person. In a recent systematic review of homeopathic therapy in cancer treatment, six studies met the inclusion criteria and showed insufficient evidence for homeopathy in cancer care (84). Homeopathic preparations continue to be tested in vitro for their effects on growth and gene expression in cellular and animal models in prostate and breast cancer patients. A prospective study of 100 cancer patients referred for homeopathic care found that 75% of patients reported the approach to be helpful or very helpful (85). Further research is needed in this area, but currently no compelling evidence exists for the use of homeopathy in cancer care (84, 86).

AYURVEDA

Ayurveda is a complete medical system developed in India based on ancient Sanskrit texts. Ayurveda incorporates spirituality, emotions, individual characteristics, family history, seasons, and age to determine balance and, therefore, health in an individual. Treatments include diet, yoga, breathing exercises, meditation, herbal therapies, and cleansing regimens. Multiple Ayurvedic herbal therapies are being examined for cytotoxic effects in vitro and possible applications in cancer care.

References

1. Verhoef MJ, Balneaves LG, Boon HS, Vroegindewey A. Reasons for and characteristics associated with complementary and alternative medicine use among adult cancer patients: a systematic review. Integr Cancer Ther 2005;4: 274–86.

2. Vapiwala N, Mick R, Hampshire MK, Metz JM, DeNittis AS. Patient initiation of complementary and alternative medical therapies (CAM) following cancer diagnosis. Cancer J 2006;12:467–74.

3. von Gruenigen VE, Frasure HE, Jenison EL, Hopkins MP, Gil KM. Longitudinal assessment of quality of life and lifestyle in newly diagnosed ovarian cancer patients: the roles of surgery and chemotherapy. Gynecol Oncol 2006; 103:120–6.

4. Navo MA, Phan J, Vaughan C, Palmer JL, Michaud L, Jones KL, et al. An assessment of the utilization of complementary and alternative medication in women with gynecologic or breast malignancies. J Clin Oncol 2004;22:671–7.

5. Powell CB, Dibble SL, Dall'Era JE, Cohen I. Use of herbs in women diagnosed with ovarian cancer. Int J Gynecol Cancer 2002;12:214–7.

6. Swisher EM, Cohn DE, Goff BA, Parham J, Herzog TJ, Rader JS, et al. Use of complementary and alternative medicine among women with gynecologic cancers. Gynecol Oncol 2002;84:363–7.

7. von Gruenigen VE, White LJ, Kirven MS, Showalter AL, Hopkins MP, Jenison EL. A comparison of complementary and alternative medicine use by gynecology and gynecologic oncology patients. Int J Gynecol Cancer 2001;11:205–9.

8. Eisenberg DM, Kessler RC, Foster C, Norlock FE, Calkins DR, Delbanco TL. Unconventional medicine in the United States: prevalence, costs, and patterns of use. N Engl J Med 1993;328:246–52.

9. Brown JK. A systematic review of the evidence on symptom management of cancer-related anorexia and cachexia. Oncol Nurs Forum 2002;29:517–32.

10. Ravasco P, Monteiro-Grillo I, Vidal PM, Camilo ME. Dietary counseling improves patient outcomes: a prospective, randomized, controlled trial in colorectal cancer patients undergoing radiotherapy. J Clin Oncol 2005;23: 1431–8.

11. International Agency for Research in Cancer. Weight control and physical activity. IARC handbook of cancer prevention No. 6. Lyon: IARC; 2002.

12. Demark-Wahnefried W, Aziz NM, Rowland JH, Pinto BM. Riding the crest of the teachable moment: promoting long-term health after the diagnosis of cancer. J Clin Oncol 2005;23:5814–30.

13. Calle EE, Rodriguez C, Walker-Thurmond K, Thun MJ. Overweight, obesity, and mortality from cancer in a prospectively studied cohort of US adults. N Engl J Med 2003;348:1625–38.

14. Kroenke CH, Chen WY, Rosner B, Holmes MD. Weight, weight gain, and survival after breast cancer diagnosis. J Clin Oncol 2005;23:1370–8.

15. Jones LW, Demark-Wahnefried W. Diet, exercise, and complementary therapies after primary treatment for cancer. Lancet Oncol 2006;7:1017–26.

16. Demark-Wahnefried W, Kenyon A, Eberle P, Skye A, Kraus WE. Preventing sarcopenic obesity among breast cancer patients who receive adjuvant chemotherapy: results of a feasibility study. Clin Exerc Physiol 2002;4:44–9.

17. de Waard F, Ramlau R, Mulder Y, de Vries T, van Waveren S. A feasibility study on weight reduction in obese postmenopausal breast cancer patients. Eur J Cancer Prev 1993;2:233–8.

18. Djuric Z, DiLaura NM, Jenkin I, Darga L, Jen CK, Mood D, et al. Combining weight-loss counseling with the Weight Watchers plan for obese breast cancer survivors. Obes Res 2002;10:657–65.

19. Goodwin P, Esplen MJ, Butler K, Winocur J, Pritchard K, Brazel S, et al. Multidisciplinary weight management in locoregional breast cancer: results of a phase II study. Breast Cancer Res Treat 1998;48:53–64.

20. Loprinzi CL, Athmann LM, Kardinal CG, O'Fallon JR, See JA, Bruce BK, et al. Randomized trial of dietician counseling to try to prevent weight gain associated with breast cancer adjuvant chemotherapy. Oncology 1996;53:228–32.

21. Kroenke CH, Fung TT, Hu FB, Holmes MD. Dietary patterns and survival after breast cancer diagnosis. J Clin Oncol 2005;23:9295–303.

22. Chlebowski RT, Blackburn GL, Elashoff RE, Thomson C, Goodman MT, Shapiro A, et al. Dietary fat reduction in postmenopausal women with primary breast cancer; phase III Women's Intervention Nutrition Study (WINS). The WINS Investigators [abstract]. J Clin Oncol 2005;23(suppl 16):10.

23. Pierce JP, Faerber S, Wright FA, Rock CL, Newman V, Flatt SW, et al. A randomized trial of the effect of a plant-based dietary pattern on additional breast cancer events and survival: the Women's Healthy Eating and Living (WHEL) Study. Women's Healthy Eating and Living (WHEL) study group. Control Clin Trials 2002;23:728–56.

24. World Health Organization. Global strategy on diet, physical activity and health. Geneva: WHO; 2007. Available at: http://www.who.int/dietphysicalactivity/en. Retrieved September 19, 2007.

25. Hebert JR, Hurley TG, Ma Y. The effect of dietary exposures on recurrence and mortality in early stage breast cancer. Breast Cancer Res Treat 1998;51:17–28.

26. Institute of Medicine. Dietary reference intakes for energy, carbohydrates, fiber, fat, fatty acids, cholesterol, protein, and amino acids. Washington, DC: The Institute; 2005.

27. Low Dog TL, Micozzi MS. Women's health in complementary and integrative medicine: a clinical guide. St. Louis (MO): Elsevier Churchill Livingstone; 2005.

28. Barnes S, Grubbs C, Setchell KD, Carlson J. Soybeans inhibit mammary tumors in models of breast cancer. In: Pariza MW, Felton JS, Aeschebacher HU, Sato S, editors. Mutagens and carcinogens in the diet: proceedings of a satellite symposium of the Fifth International Conference on Environmental Mutagens, held in Madison, Wisconsin, July 5–7, 1989. New York (NY): Wiley–Liss; 1990. p. 239–53.

29. Adlercreutz H. Phytoestrogens and breast cancer. J Steroid Biochem Mol Biol 2002;83:113–8.

30. Messina MJ, Loprinzi CL. Soy for breast cancer survivors: a critical review of the literature. J Nutr 2001;131(suppl): 3095S–108S.

31. Jones JL, Daley BJ, Enderson BL, Zhou JR, Karlstad MD. Genistein inhibits tamoxifen effects on cell proliferation and cell cycle arrest in T47D breast cancer cells. Am Surg 2002;68:575–7; discussion 577–8.

32. Ju YH, Doerge DR, Allred KF, Allred CD, Helferich WG. Dietary genistein negates the inhibitory effect of tamoxifen on growth of estrogen-dependent human breast cancer (MCF-7) cells implanted in athymic mice. Cancer Res 2002;62:2474–7.

33. McNeely ML, Campbell KL, Rowe BH, Klassen TP, Mackey JR, Courneya KS. Effects of exercise on breast cancer patients and survivors: a systematic review and meta-analysis. CMAJ 2006;175:34–41.

34. Schmitz KH, Holtzman J, Courneya KS, Masse LC, Duval S, Kane R. Controlled physical activity trials in cancer survivors: a systematic review and meta-analysis. Cancer Epidemiol Biomarkers Prev 2005;14:1588–95.

35. Knols R, Aaronson NK, Uebelhart D, Fransen J, Aufdemkampe G. Physical exercise in cancer patients during and after medical treatment: a systematic review of randomized and controlled clinical trials. J Clin Oncol 2005;23:3830–42.

36. Brown JK, Byers T, Doyle C, Courneya KS, Demark-Wahnefried W, Kushi LH, et al. Nutrition and physical activity during and after cancer treatment: an American Cancer Society guide for informed choices. CA Cancer J Clin 2003;53:268–91.

37. Warburton DE, Nicol CW, Bredin SS. Prescribing exercise as preventive therapy. CMAJ 2006;174:961–74.

38. Benor D. Survey of spiritual healing research. Complementary Medical Research 1990;4:9–33.

39. Williams AL. Perspectives on spirituality at the end of life: a meta-summary. Palliat Support Care 2006;4:407–17.

40. Thune-Boyle IC, Stygell JA, Keshtgar MR, Newman SP. Do religious/spiritual coping strategies affect illness adjustment in patients with cancer? A systematic review of the literature. Soc Sci Med 2006;63:151–64.

41. Gullatte MM, Phillips JM, Gibson LM. Factors associated with delays in screening of self-detected breast changes in

African-American women. J Natl Black Nurses Assoc 2006;17:45–50.

42. National Center for Complementary and Alternative Medicine. Energy medicine: an overview. No. D235. Available at: http://nccam.nih.gov/health/backgrounds/energymed.htm. Retrieved October 15, 2007.

43. Astin JA, Harkness E, Ernst E. The efficacy of "distant healing": a systematic review of randomized trials. Ann Intern Med 2000;132:903–10.

44. Borchers AT, Keen CL, Gershwin ME. Mushrooms, tumors, and immunity: an update. Exp Biol Med (Maywood) 2004;229:393–406.

45. Kidd PM. The use of mushroom glucans and proteoglycans in cancer treatment. Altern Med Rev 2000;5:4–27.

46. Hara M, Hanaoka T, Kobayashi M, Otani T, Adachi HY, Montani A, et al. Cruciferous vegetables, mushrooms, and gastrointestinal cancer risks in a multicenter, hospital-based case-control study in Japan. Nutr Cancer 2003;46:138–47.

47. Kaegi E. Unconventional therapies for cancer, I: Essiac. The task Force on Alternative Therapies of the Canadian Breast Cancer Research Initiative. CMAJ 1998;158:897–902.

48. Kulp KS, Montgomery JL, Nelson DO, Cutter B, Latham ER, Shattuck DL, et al. Essiac and Flor-Essence herbal tonics stimulate the in vitro growth of human breast cancer cells. Breast Cancer Res Treat 2006;98:249–59.

49. Mills E, Wu P, Seely D, Guyatt G. Melatonin in the treatment of cancer: a systematic review of randomized controlled trials and meta-analysis. J Pineal Research 2005;39:360–6.

50. Lee CO. Complementary and alternative medicines patients are talking about: melatonin. Clin J Oncol Nurs 2006;10:105–7.

51. Loprinzi CL, Levitt R, Baron DL, Sloan JA, Atherton PJ, Smith DJ, et al. Evaluation of shark cartilage in patients with advanced cancer: a North Central Cancer Treatment Group trial. North Central Cancer Treatment Group. Cancer 2005;104:176–82.

52. Miller DR, Anderson GT, Stark JJ, Granick JL, Richardson D. Phase I/II trial of the safety and efficacy of shark cartilage in the treatment of advanced cancer. J Clin Oncol 1998;16:3649–55.

53. Milazzo S. Lejeune S, Ernst E. Laetrile for cancer: a systematic review of the clinical evidence. Support Care Cancer 2007;15:583–95.

54. U.S. Preventive Services Task Force. Routine vitamin supplementation to prevent cancer and coronary vascular disease. Nutr Clin Care 2003;6:102–7.

55. Chang ET, Lee VS, Canchola AJ, Clarke CA, Purdie DM, Reynolds P, et al. Diet and risk of ovarian cancer in the California Teachers Study Cohort. Am J Epidemiol 2007;165:802–13.

56. Norman HA, Butrum RR, Feldman E, Heber D, Nixon D, Picciano MF, et al. The role of dietary supplements during cancer therapy. J Nutr 2003;133(suppl 1):3794S–9S.

57. Corbin L. Safety and efficacy of massage therapy for patients with cancer. Cancer Control 2005;12:158–64.

58. Ironson G, Field T, Scafidi F, Hashimoto M, Kumar M, Kumar A, et al. Massage therapy is associated with enhancement of the immune system's cytotoxic capacity. Int J Neurosci 1996;84:205–17.

59. Zeitlin D, Keller SE, Shiflett SC, Schleifer SJ, Bartlett JA. Immunological effects of massage therapy during academic stress. Psychosom Med 2000;62:83–4.

60. Richardson MA, Sanders T, Palmer JL, Greisinger A, Singletary SE. Complementary/alternative medicine use in a comprehensive cancer center and the implications for oncology. J Clin Oncol 2000;18:2505–14.

61. Fellowes D, Barnes K, Wilkinson S. Aromatherapy and massage for symptom relief in patients with cancer (Cochrane Review). In: The Cochrane Library, Issue 3, 2004. Oxford: Update Software.

62. Speca M, Carlson LE, Goodey E, Angen M. A randomized, wait-list controlled clinical trial: the effect of a mindfulness meditation-based stress reduction program on mood and symptoms of stress in cancer outpatients. Psychosom Med 2000;62:613–22.

63. Carlson LE, Ursuliak Z, Goodey E, Angen M, Speca M. The effect of a mindfulness meditation-based stress reduction program on mood and symptoms of stress in cancer outpatients: 6-month follow-up. Support Care Cancer 2001;9:112–23.

64. Carlson LE, Speca M, Patel KD, Goodey E. Mindfulness-based stress reduction in relation to quality of life, mood symptoms of stress, and immune parameters in breast and prostate cancer outpatients. Psychosom Med 2003;65:571–81.

65. Canter PH. The therapeutic effects of meditation. BMJ 2003;326:1049–50.

66. Ott MJ. Complementary and alternative therapies in cancer symptom management. Cancer Pract 2002;10:162–6.

67. Mansky PJ, Wallerstedt DB. Complementary medicine in palliative care and cancer symptom management. Cancer J 2006;12:425–31.

68. Pan CX, Morrison RS, Ness J, Fugh-Berman A, Leipzig RM. Complementary and alternative medicine in the management of pain, dyspnea, and nausea and vomiting near the end of life: a systematic review. J Pain Symptom Manage 2000;20:374–87.

69. Rajasekaran M, Edmonds PM, Higginson IL. Systematic review of hypnotherapy for treating symptoms in terminally ill adult cancer patients. Palliat Med 2005;19:418–26.

70. Liossi C, White P, Hatira P. Randomized clinical trial of local anesthetic versus a combination of local anesthetic with self-hypnosis in the management of pediatric procedure-related pain. Health Psychol 2006;2:307–15.

71. Marcus J, Elkins G, Mott F. The integration of hypnosis into a model of palliative care. Integr Cancer Ther 2003;2:365–70.

72. Montgomery GH, Weltz CR, Seltz M, Bovbjerg DH. Brief presurgery hypnosis reduces distress and pain in excisional biopsy patients. Int J Clin Exp Hypn 2002;50:17–32.

73. Spiegel D, Bloom JR, Yalom I. Group support for patients with metastatic cancer: a randomized outcome study. Arch Gen Psychiatry 1981;38:527–33.

74. Oster I, Svensk AC, Magnusson E, Thyme KE, Sjodin M, Astrom S, et al. Art therapy improves coping resources: a randomized, controlled study among women with breast cancer. Palliat Support Care 2006;4:57–64.

75. Nainis N, Paice JA, Ratner J, Wirth JH, Lai J, Shott S. Relieving symptoms in cancer: innovative use of art therapy. J Pain Symptom Manage 2006;31:162–9.

76. Monti DA, Peterson C, Kunkel EJ, Hauck WW, Pequignot E, Rhodes L, et al. A randomized controlled trial of mindfulness-based art therapy (MBAT) for women with cancer. Psychooncology 2006;15:363–73.

77. Wardell DW, Weymouth KF. Review of studies of healing touch. J Nurs Scholarsh 2004;36:147–54.

78. Cook CA, Guerrerio JF, Slater VE. Healing touch and quality of life in women receiving radiation treatment for cancer: a randomized controlled trial. Altern Ther Health Med 2004;10:34–41.

79. Burden B, Herron-Marx S, Clifford C. The increasing use of reiki as a complementary therapy in specialist palliative care. Int J Palliat Nurs 2005;11:248–53.

80. Olson K, Hanson J, Michaud M. A phase II trial of Reiki for the management of pain in advanced cancer patients. J Pain Symptom Manage 2003;26:990–7.

81. Vickers AJ, Straus DJ, Fearon B, Cassileth BR. Acupuncture for postchemotherapy fatigue: a phase II study. J Clin Oncol 2004;22:1731–5.

82. Alimi D, Rubino C, Pichard-Leandri E, Fermand-Brule S, Dubreuil-Lemaire ML, Hill C. Analgesic effect of auricular acupuncture for cancer pain: a randomized, blinded, controlled trial. J Clin Oncol 2003;21:4120–6.

83. Filshie J, Bolton T, Browne D, Ashley S. Acupuncture and self acupuncture for long-term treatment of vasomotor symptoms in cancer patients—audit and treatment algorithm. Acupunct Med 2005;23:171–80.

84. Milazzo S, Russell N, Ernst E. Efficacy of homeopathic therapy in cancer treatment. Eur J Cancer 2006;42:282–9.

85. Thompson EA, Reilly D. The homeopathic approach to symptom control in cancer patient: a prospective observational study. Palliat Med 2002;16:227–33.

86. Ernst E. Complementary therapies in palliative cancer care. Cancer 2001;91:2181–5.

Index

Page numbers followed by letters *b*, *f*, and *t* refer to boxes, figures, and tables, respectively.

A

Acupuncture, 148–149
Adenocarcinoma
  clear cell, of the cervix and vagina, 49–50
  early-stage, in cervical cancer, 64–65
  with squamous differentiation, 77
  of the vulva, 37, 39, 44
Adenocarcinoma in situ, 60–61
Adenosarcoma, 84
Alcohol consumption
  as breast cancer risk factor, 23
  as cancer risk factor, 5
Alternative medicine, 139
American College of Obstetricians and Gynecologists
  on cervical cancer screening, 53
  on colorectal screening, 6
  on ovarian cancer referral guidelines, 92
Amsterdam criteria, 17, 18*t*
Amsterdam II criteria, 17, 18*t*
Anemia, 131, 135–136
Angiogenesis, 52
Anthracycline regimen, 32
Antidepressant use, 127*t*
Antidiarrheal agents, 134*t*
Antihormonal therapy, in breast cancer treatment, 29
Anxiety interventions, 144*t*
Anxiety manifestations, 128*t*
Anxiolytic use, 128*t*
Aromatase inhibitors, in breast cancer adjuvant therapy, 33–34
Aromatic amines, 111
Art therapy, 148
Ashkenazi Jewish population, 10–11, 23
Ataxia–telangiectasia, 12, 12*t*
Autonomy, 123
Avastin, 19
Axillary lymphadenectomy, 32
Ayurveda, 149

B

Bartholin gland carcinoma, 39, 44
Basal cell carcinoma of the vulva, 39, 44
Behavioral risk factors, 3–5
Beneficence, 123
Bethesda guidelines
  for cervical neoplasia, 51*b*–52*b*
  for hereditary nonpolyposis colorectal cancer (HNPCC), 18*b*

Bilateral salpingo–oophorectomy
  in breast cancer risk reduction, 21
  in endometrial cancer treatment, 78–79
Biologically based therapies, 141, 145–146
BI-RADS. *See* Breast Imaging Reporting and Data System
Bladder cancer, 110–111
Bladder-conserving surgery, 111
Blue dyes, 121
Body mass index, as cancer risk factor, 4–5
Botanicals, 141, 145–146
Bowel obstruction, 134
Brachytherapy catheters, 31
BRCA mutations
  in breast and ovarian cancer syndrome, 10
  breast cancer surveillance for carriers of, 34*t*
  in endometrial cancer, 8
  in fallopian tube cancer, 98
  features associated with, 13*b*
  lifetime risks associated with, 11
  prophylactic surgery and, 14–15
  risk assessment models for, 13
  screening and follow-up of high-risk patients, 13–14
  tamoxifen benefits in, 16
*BRCA*PRO, 13
Breast and ovarian cancer syndrome, 10
Breast biopsy
  fine-needle aspiration, 27, 121
  history of, 21
  image-guided percutaneous, 27
  surgical excision for, 27
Breast cancer. *See also* Hereditary breast and ovarian cancer
  biologic markers and prognostic factors in, 28–29
  body mass index as risk factor for, 5
  with *BRCA* mutations, 11
  BRCA mutation surveillance, 34*t*
  chemoprevention, 15–16
  diagnostic evaluation of, 27
  documentation of, 24
  ethnicity and diet as risk factors for, 23
  exogenous hormone use as risk factor for, 23
  family history and, 21
  hereditary syndromes, 11–12, 12*t*
  invasive, 28
  mammographic screening for, 24–26
  nutrition as survivorship factor in, 140

Breast cancer *(continued)*
  pathologic evaluation, 27–28
  in pregnancy, 120–121
  prophylactic surgery for, 14–15
  risk factors for, 5–6, 21–23, 22*b*
  screening guidelines, 4*t*, 6
  special issues, 34
  staging of, 29, 30*t*–31*t*
  treatment of
    adjuvant therapy, 33–34, 33*b*
    axillary lymphadenectomy, 32
    neoadjuvant chemotherapy, 33
    sentinel lymph node biopsy, 32
    surgical, 29, 31
    systemic, 32–33
Breast-conserving surgery, 29, 121
Breast-feeding, chemotherapy effect on, 122–123
Breast Imaging Reporting and Data System (BI-RADS), 24–25, 25*t*
Breast reconstruction, 34
Breast self-examination, *BRCA* mutations and, 14
Breast ultrasonography, 26–27

C

CA 125 levels, 89–92, 92*b*
Cachexia–anorexia syndrome, 136
Calcium intake, 5
Calmette-Guérin bacillus, 111
Cancer, modifiable risks of, 3–5
Carbohydrate intake, 140
Carboplatin, 96
Carcinosarcoma, 84
Cellulitis, 43
Cervical cancer
  human papillomavirus (HPV) vaccine for, 6
  invasive
    diagnosis and staging, 61–62, 62*t*
    early-stage adenocarcinoma, 64–65
    fertility-conserving surgery, 68–69
    stage IB2, 66–69
    stage IB1–IIA, 65–66, 65*t*
    stage IIB–IVA (locally advanced), 69
    stages IA1 and IA2, 62–64, 63*t*, 64*t*
  in pregnancy, 56, 58, 116–118, 118*t*
  preinvasive
    Bethesda system in diagnosis of, 51*b*–52*b*
    etiology of, 52
    human papillomavirus (HPV) in, 51
    incidence rate of, 53
    risk factors for, 51–52

153